DOCTORING THE SOUTH

∼ STUDIES IN SOCIAL MEDICINE ∼

Allan M. Brandt and Larry R. Churchill, editors

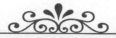

~ Steven M. Stowe ~

DOCTORING THE SOUTH

Southern Physicians and Everyday Medicine

in the Mid-Nineteenth Century

THE UNIVERSITY OF NORTH CAROLINA PRESS
CHAPEL HILL & LONDON

© 2004 The University of North Carolina Press
∽ All rights reserved ∽
Manufactured in the United States of America

Designed by Heidi Perov
Set in Monotype Garamond and Copperplate
by Keystone Typesetting, Inc.

The paper in this book meets the guidelines for permanence and
durability of the Committee on Production Guidelines for Book
Longevity of the Council on Library Resources.

Library of Congress Cataloging-in-Publication Data

Stowe, Steven M., 1946–
Doctoring the South : southern physicians and everyday
medicine in the mid-nineteenth century / Steven M. Stowe.
p. cm. — (Studies in social medicine)
Includes bibliographical references and index.
ISBN 0-8078-2885-8 (cloth: alk. paper)
1. Medicine—Southern States—History—19th century.
2. Physicians—Southern States—History—19th century. I. Title. II. Series.
R154.5.S68S76   2004
610'.975'09034—dc22
2004005103

08 07 06 05 04   5 4 3 2 1

≈ for my mother ≈

~ Contents ~

ACKNOWLEDGMENTS ix

INTRODUCTION: *Physicians, Everyday
Medicine, and the Country Orthodox Style* 1
Sickness and Health in a Southern Place 4
Physicians: A Mid-Nineteenth-Century Profile 7

PART ONE. CHOOSING MEDICINE

ONE. *Men, Schools, and Careers* 15
Family, Intellect, and the Manly Choice 16
Medical Schools and Reform: Stretching Orthodoxy 19
The Porous School: Apprenticeship 27
The Porous School: City Life and a Man's World 32

TWO. *The Science of All Life* 41
Lectures: Synthesis and Practice 42
Clinics: Foreign Bodies and Appended Charity 52
Anatomy: Opened Bodies and the Moral Urge 59
The Medical Thesis: Enlightenments 69

THREE. *Starting Out* 76
New Degree, Fresh Doubts 77
Calculation for Survival 80
The Community Chooses Its Own 84
First Patients, "Monster" Disease, and
"Inward Satisfaction" 90

PART TWO. DOING MEDICINE

FOUR. *Livelihood* 101
Logging Patients, Seeing Race 103
Self-Interest and Moral Judgment 108

Health Talk across the Racial Divide 114

Rounds 119

Livelihood, Subjectivity, and the Country Orthodox Style 127

FIVE. *Bedside* 131

Summoned to the Social Bedside 133

Seeing Bodies: The Physical and the Social 141

Changing Bodies: "Experience" and the Charm of Drugs 149

Borrowing, Experimenting, and Violence 156

The Shadow of Bedside Practice 162

PART THREE. MAKING MEDICINE

SIX. *The Lives of Others* 167

Co-attendance and Conflict 168

Writing Orthodoxy at the Bedside 175

John Knox: Effacing Pain 177

Charles Hentz: Making Case-time 182

Courtney Clark: Looking for Connections 192

SEVEN. *Landscape, Race, and Faith* 200

Landscapes of Knowledge 201

Slavery and Race 208

Faith: Knowing What "Passeth Understanding" 218

EIGHT. *Witnessing* 228

Case Narratives: Orthodoxy's Stories 229

Dr. Patteson: Technique and Transcendence 236

Dr. Dowler: Scientist and Community 239

Dr. Yandell: The Eclipse of the Personal 243

Dr. Bassett: The Eclipse of the Professional 249

EPILOGUE: *The Civil War and the Persistence
of the Country Orthodox Style* 259

NOTES 273

BIBLIOGRAPHY 327

INDEX 365

∼ Acknowledgments ∼

Many people have helped in the research and writing of this book, many more than I can hope to acknowledge here. I am grateful for funding received from the National Library of Medicine (#1R01LM05334-01), the Indiana University Center for the History of Medicine, and Research and the University Graduate School at Indiana University, Bloomington. Kate Torrey at the University of North Carolina Press kept me going with critical support from the inception of this project.

This study had its beginning some years ago when I found myself teaching history in the Department of Humanities at the Pennsylvania State University College of Medicine in Hershey, Pennsylvania, where I got my feet wet in the modern world of medicine with the help of colleagues Al Vastyan and K. Danner Clouser. At Hershey and in many other places since, I have benefited from the expertise and thoughtfulness of archivists and special collections librarians who knew something about the relationship between history, caregiving, and medicine that I hoped to discover. I have appreciated, too, conversations with graduate students at Indiana over the years, especially with Roark Atkinson, Hyejung Grace Kong, and Lynn Pohl. In this regard, I am particularly beholden to Scott M. Stephan not only for his intellectual contributions but also for his invaluable research assistance.

My colleagues in the Department of History at Indiana helped me in countless ways, and I especially wish to thank John Bodnar, Ann Carmichael, Ellen Dwyer, Michael Grossberg, Jim Madison, Joanne Meyerowitz, and David Ransel for their interest and good advice. Elsewhere, colleagues in the Southern Intellectual History Circle and participants in the workshops and conferences where I had the opportunity to present my research gave me many welcome insights. In particular, I wish to express my appreciation to Susan Donaldson, Ann Goodwyn Jones, John Harley Warner, Bert Wyatt-Brown, and to the anonymous readers for UNC Press. Charles E. Rosenberg offered an especially cogent and timely critique for which I am grateful.

David Thelen's ideas, provocations, and friendship have been a light of inspiration in my thinking about past and present—and about tomorrow, too. David Nord, a warm friend, has pushed me to see more clearly how to be a historian, teacher, and editor. Lisa Gershkoff's help shaped this book as a whole in many different ways. In southern studies, Michael O'Brien has been a thoughtful critic, a constant friend, and a source of many ideas about the South and history, and Drew Gilpin Faust has never failed to both affirm and challenge my efforts. Naoko Wake continues to show me that everything familiar is new.

DOCTORING THE SOUTH

PHYSICIANS, EVERYDAY MEDICINE, AND THE COUNTRY ORTHODOX STYLE

This is a study of physicians and medical practice in the southern United States during the mid-nineteenth century. It seeks to describe and interpret the work of ordinary practitioners who struggled to understand disease and care for the sick. For those readers who know little about medical care in this era, I hope to show why it was an important aspect of social and cultural life. For those acquainted with medical history, I hope to defamiliarize, and thus illuminate, features of ordinary practice in this time and place, which will deepen our understanding of what everyday doctoring signified in the medical past.

In one sense, sickness and health are impersonal processes. When an individual becomes sick, it may be seen as the result of the implacable objectivity of living in a complex biological world. Few people think of sickness in this way alone, however, because sickness and health are intensely subjective experiences, too, arising from people's understanding of their own bodies and personalities. Becoming sick and getting well thus are expressive of an inclusive sense of living in a world of danger, reprieve, and the possibility for solace. All of these are the subject of this book. They are explored by looking at the labors and perceptions of ordinary M.D.s in the South during the years from 1830 to 1880, a span of time just before their style of medicine began to make the shift toward what became accepted as "modern" healing, with its emphasis on biomedical science, institutions, and specialism.[1]

This transition was, of course, a fundamental turning point in the understanding of disease and the effective provision of care everywhere in the United

States. The three decades after 1880 are recognized as the formative years of what Paul Starr has called the "sovereign" authority that twentieth-century physicians possessed in defining disease and therapy. In view of this, not surprisingly, the decades before 1880 have been historically framed in terms of physicians' later success. Their brand of medicine, widely termed "orthodox," is seen as emerging from a welter of different approaches to healing, all vying for patients' trust and acceptance. M.D.s stood out in this mix, but it was not because they could more reliably cure. Rather, it was because they shared a certain notable approach to healing. They were unusually outspoken (arrogant, said their rivals). They embraced a tradition of book learning and an allegiance to an ideal of natural "science" with roots in antiquity. They favored close empirical observation of the body and the patient's environment, and they aggressively employed an array of potent drugs. Too, more consistently than other kinds of healers, physicians argued that their distinctive professional trappings—medical societies, formal schools, and, importantly, reliance on the written word—would serve a public interest by increasing medical knowledge generally. After a protracted economic and ideological struggle, rival doctors gave way by the end of the nineteenth century to physicians' superior organization and the promise, if not the realization, of clinical success.[2]

Whether admiring of physicians' increasing efficacy or critical of their dominance, this established view of physicians' rise tends to emphasize the ways in which M.D.s broke away from their commercial competitors and the domestic medicine wielded by patients. In what follows, I attempt to restore a complexity to this view of an ascendant, unitary modernity. I look at less-studied, ordinary physicians whose perceptions and decisions, and the underlying subjectivity that held these together, made them agents for a creative continuity in orthodox medical practice. Reading their words, I began to see the significance of what I call a country orthodox style. I use the term "country orthodoxy" to denote a style of practice rooted in physicians' sense that their orthodoxy grew from local sources, as well as from abstract traditions. As we will see, country orthodoxy tied a doctor's sense of his work to his imagination of self and place, and thus to a sense of continuity that both inspired and troubled him. Rather than seeing this style as a drag on "modern" medicine's twentieth-century incarnation, my approach is to see it as evidence that modernity itself is a recurring condition, conflicted and constantly redefined. Holding to the conviction that medicine was *essentially* shaped by a doctor's subjective grasp of the physical and moral identity of local places and people, mid-nineteenth-century physicians embraced a fully realized sense of work and meaning, whose continuity needs understanding on its own terms.

In particular, this study argues, the country orthodox style is important because it derived from, and produced, physicians' persistent allegiance to a distinctly personal vision of illness and health, fluid and alive, and deeply resonant of the South as a region. It was a style founded on a way of working that exalted the individual practitioner's search for the "experience" that gave substance to orthodox principles. Thus it was a medical style that made routine work with bodies and disease inseparable from physicians' moral imagination of what defined "good" medical care in various contexts: in their ideals of learnedness, in their relations with neighbors and patients, and in their attempts to find larger meaning in the realms of science and faith. As explored in these pages, then, we see a modernity implicated not only in the insights of physicians cutting against the grain of popular ways but also in their desire for collaboration and belonging.

This approach is fruitful because in each of the three contexts for medicine explored here—physicians' training, the bedside, and the wider meaning of their labors—M.D.s created a flood of written texts. Their medicine was inseparable from their need to pronounce it. These texts—ranging from rough notes to what I argue is physicians' prime literary achievement, the case narrative—captured not only the "facts" of daily labors but also the subjectivity at work interpreting them. In this sense, then, mine is a study of historical ethnography, understanding physicians' writing not only as mirrors of their satisfactions and discontents but also as productive of them. Specifically, I argue that physicians' daily work as an experienced reality, the heart of the country orthodox style, involved a tension between two desires. One was their deep attachment to orthodoxy as a special intellectual and professional realm that was (and deserved to be) a world apart from the everyday and domestic. The other was a need to belong to their communities, to inhabit the very essence of the "everyday," with its here-and-now focus on livelihood, neighbors, and practical care. Physicians' writings reveal how the uneasy balance of these two—a balance of critique and belonging, acting and witnessing—was a central dynamic of their troubled identities. This tension, I argue, went to the heart of a physician's subjective sense of his own worth, leading him to cherish his personal, hands-on "experience" as the essence of good medicine. This individual experience, reified and exalted, was read back through his texts to become the heart of orthodoxy itself.

Before sketching basic features of the southern setting for sickness and health and giving a brief profile of midcentury physicians, a word about how region and chronology shape this study is useful. Although there is no study comparable to mine outside of the South, I did not undertake a regional comparison. Rather, I decided to make a close cultural reading of practitioners who lived in the South, confronted diseases that flourished there, saw themselves as "southern," and thus gave what might be called a southern accent to nineteenth-century medical work. However, it would not be surprising if certain aspects of their daily practice in, say, rural Alabama, were similar to those of their counter-parts in rural Ohio. I hope, in fact, that my research will contribute to the study of country doctors in other regions. As for the period under study, most of the material here is from the antebellum years. But understanding the powerful continuity of southern practice in this century, as I seek to do, means under-standing that much of what physicians were perceiving and saying about their work in 1830 was echoed by their brethren in 1880. Despite certain changes in elite medicine, sketched below, many of the specific things local M.D.s did with bodies and medicines remained remarkably consistent over time. Thus, the Civil War, that hoary dividing line in southern history, and in U.S. history generally, does not loom so large with regard to the community practice that is the focus here; an epilogue explores the significance of country orthodoxy's persistence through the war.

SICKNESS AND HEALTH IN A SOUTHERN PLACE

This study of everyday medicine highlights two main ways in which a southern accent is audible. First, certain distinctive features of southern social and cul-tural life can be seen influencing physicians' daily work: the comparatively large number of African Americans (as patients and healers); the racial order of slavery and its legacy; the commitment to a sense of professional localism; the encounter with particular diseases and remedies typical of the region. Second, there is a southern accent in the way that most southerners *believed* the South to be distinctive. Sickness informs the image of a place much as it transforms a person's sense of her life. Just as becoming ill raises urgent questions about an individual's behavior and resources, so a region's sickness raises questions about why it flourishes *here*, in this place. Illness forces people to look around them and to wonder if its terrible transformations (how did this happen? when did it begin?) were latent in the happy mindlessness of being well. So, for southerners (and other Americans, too), the Sunny South was believed to have sickness im-plicated in its climate and diet, its social relations and cultural preoccupations—in what we might call its health ecology. Thus, important for southerners—and for us—in trying to understand their struggle against sickness is not only the region's biology and people's habits but also their ways of seeing and saying—of finding a language for illness.[3]

Fever sweeping across the southern land, like the weather that was thought to engender it, was the most visible—and for outsiders, the most exotic—feature of the southern ecology of sickness. In most instances of sickness, people saw themselves facing *disease*, not diseases. Disease was a unified thing, though dangerously capable of shifting its appearance and potency. We now see malaria as implicated in most of what southerners described when they talked about "fever"; both the malarial parasite and the requisite mosquito flourished in the South. Contemporary physicians and others, however, lived with many forms of "the fever" and were fascinated by their local origin, timing, and relationship: swamp fever, country fever, summer fever, bilious fever, broken bone fever; remittent, intermittent, recurring fever. By the nineteenth century, epidemic yellow fever, too, was seen by most Americans as a southern disease entirely. The turning of the southern seasons, the very lay of the southern land, were more than mere backdrop; they were part of fever's very identity. In this way, fever stood for all disease. It was a force described as descending upon communities yet also perceived as somehow always present, requiring only the right combination of local conditions to release its malign power.[4]

Along with fever, the biracial population was seen as an obviously distinctive feature of the region, as were aspects of social class and gender. From the eighteenth century on, southerners perceived certain racially determined differences in health, a few of which twentieth-century medicine in part confirmed: for example, that African Americans as a group were somewhat less susceptible than whites to malaria and yellow fever and were somewhat more vulnerable to respiratory disease. However, of equal importance to this study, southerners of both races also believed that sickness easily crossed racial lines, blurring, as well as bolstering, the divisions created by slavery. For instance, southerners in general believed that specific items of diet either fostered or thwarted sickness regardless of race; it was common sense for everyone, for example, to avoid eating too much fresh fruit during fever times. From our point of view, if not from theirs, the monotonous, limited diet of poorer southerners of both races made them vulnerable to certain regionally specific dietary deficiency diseases, as well as to intestinal worms and other parasites of impressive tenacity. Even wealthier southerners regularly consumed slightly spoiled meat, just-turned milk, and water alive with unseen creatures, bringing on widespread gastrointestinal havoc interpreted as arising from the vapors of a hot climate. Also at the mercy of climate and diet, childbearing women of all classes brushed against death with each pregnancy, and all children were looked upon as we might look upon the aged, as having one foot in the grave. Though not perceived as exclusively southern, of course, women's and children's vulnerability to disease nonetheless was considered to be exacerbated in the South by a "debilitating" climate and heated thickets of wet vegetation, the latter widely condemned by doctors and agricultural reformers as breeding grounds for deadly "emanations" invisible to the eye.[5]

Finally, there were certain other influences bearing on health that many southerners saw as having a regional cast. Whether they did or not, they clearly were widespread throughout the region. Heavy consumption of alcohol and tobacco among nineteenth-century southerners undercut health; sexual diseases were everywhere; occupational hazards were widespread (cotton gins seem especially treacherous), as was personal violence. Mental illness, uniquely difficult to see from a historical distance in all but its most dysfunctional instances, afflicted many more than can be counted.[6]

Broadly speaking, what could mid-nineteenth-century southerners do in the face of all this? For one thing, they could have strength of character. Most people, physicians included, saw a clear link between recklessness and sickness, and they were ready to assign blame to anyone careless or complacent. Prevention of disease called for commonsense caution regardless of class or race: bundle up at night; stay out of drafts; get enough sleep; be careful about getting wet; do not sneeze on your sister. Personal rituals of cleanliness and diet, charms worn on the body or spoken, and well-timed doses of potent mixtures to lift the spirits or clean out the bowels also were daily things one could do to avoid sickness. For most southerners, these measures were joined to a cosmology that accepted illness as part of life and, often, as a trial of faith. Over and through everything, a great many southerners believed, trust God and do not "murmur" at his mysterious ways whether it be toothache or smallpox.[7]

In between prevention and acceptance, though, southerners took steps to do battle with sickness in their homes and communities. The personal, intimate scale of routine caregiving was perhaps its most important feature and is a keystone of this study. It is easy to overlook, or to sentimentalize, this daunting reality. For everything from traditional lore to the latest popular drugs, sick southerners turned for help first—and often only—to family caregivers, especially to women. The contents of their medicine chests might be sparse, but, at the same time, there were no legal restrictions on what might be found there; opium was over-the-counter. In neither underplaying nor romanticizing self-care, it is crucial to keep in mind how dramatically different it was from our own. There were no vast, well-funded, technologically innovative institutions involved in tracking or defining disease; no "insurance"; no regulated pharmaceuticals or standard diagnostic instruments; no edifice of health law; no special *place* to go to be a special, sick person. Self, family, and, to an interesting extent, as will be seen, community shaped the culture of health and sickness—these, and the doctors. ·

PHYSICIANS: A MID-NINETEENTH-CENTURY PROFILE

Like their remedies, nineteenth-century healers were numerous, diverse, and unpredictable on first use. The comparatively wide open world of medicine with its unregulated array of legitimate caregivers (that is, those women and men who were not deliberately deceptive quacks) is another striking way to appreciate the difference between the mid-nineteenth-century medical world and our own. Democratic in one sense, entrepreneurial in another, it was a world of laissez-faire improvisation and caveat emptor results, with healers coming forward in every community with roots, pills, powders, and various mixtures in generous solutions of sugar or alcohol. Many healers were family, or the family of neighbors; others were strangers. Midwives were busy in every neighborhood; herbalists and local-lore healers abounded; slave healers visited the master's bedroom, and physicians visited the quarters. Effective or not, all were legal and all were pressed for help.[8]

The fierce, hard-fought economic and professional battles between physicians and alternative healers in this century have been well studied. And, as noted earlier, M.D.s are featured in the historiography because, by the end of the nineteenth century, they had won a largely ideological battle against their competitors—a victory that actually preceded their across-the-board therapeutic success. With new urgency by the late 1880s, elite, reformist physicians began to convince enough people (including a sufficient number of legislators and wealthy philanthropists) that orthodoxy's institution-based, biomedical model of medicine offered the most promise for future success. Building on this history, I seek to show in a southern context that beneath the surface of this professional change was a widespread country orthodox style of medical practice that continued to tie ordinary physicians closely to the knowledge and morality of their communities. As much or more than any other influence, the continuity of this style profoundly shaped physicians' definition of modernity and what counted as "good medicine." It is a style visible even today in the ideal of a unique doctor-patient relationship based on mutual understanding and trust, and in the popular image of the brilliant or quirky or compassionate individual physician at the heart of otherwise cold and impersonal institutions.[9]

A sketch of the basic approach and means of mid-nineteenth-century M.D.s—a kind of "ideal-typical" sketch—will help set the stage for the more in-depth story of everyday practice that follows. Generally speaking, orthodox M.D.s, as mentioned previously, were notable for favoring harsh, mineral-based drugs, for their surgical skills, and for aggressive procedures in general. The term "allopathic," often applied to orthodox medicine, referred to the use of measures that produced physiological effects radically different from the patient's symptoms in an effort to "reverse" disease. Allopathic M.D.s were partial to the language of warfare; they aimed to attack disease and throw it down. They placed a premium on "science," by which they meant a knowledge that was empirically based but that also required a theoretical synthesis linking specific measures to principles governing the natural world at large.[10]

By our standards, informed, skilled M.D.s in the mid-nineteenth century had achieved the ability to do certain things well. They could perform smallpox vaccinations and certain "exterior" surgical operations. They understood certain kinds of difficult childbirths, and they could reliably set broken bones. They possessed drugs that relieved some afflictions: certain kinds of pain, constipation, indigestion, and some kinds of poisoning. After 1846, general anesthesia proved an enormous advantage in surgery, and quinine against malarial fevers probably was southern doctors' most widely effective drug. By the 1870s, antiseptic procedures became more widely accepted as a sign of responsible practice, even though many ordinary physicians remained skeptical about the significance of "germs"; in fact, doctors were scarcely more effective in the face of infectious disease in 1880 than their counterparts had been in 1830. Instead, physicians' skill throughout these years was measured less by straight-out "cures" than by their ability to weave a complex pattern of palliation, persuasion, and sympathetic insight. The social and cultural context—and consequences—of this style of therapy make up a large part of the story to be told here.[11]

In terms of numbers of physicians in the South, the U.S. Census suggests that they increased at an unprecedented rate in the final decades before the Civil War, and then, not surprisingly, their numbers dropped off. Census figures throughout the 1850–80 period support contemporary physicians' dismay at the harsh, competitive market for practitioners. Indeed, the antebellum increase in the number of physicians in the South—especially in states with booming populations like Texas—was at a faster clip than elsewhere in the United States. The census for 1850 (the first to enumerate occupations) listed 40,546 individuals in the nation who identified themselves as physicians. One-third of these, 13,500 in round numbers, lived in the South, a region with 36 percent of the nation's population in 1850. This means that there was one physician for every 614 southerners, compared to a ratio of 1 to 550 in the rest of the nation. By 1860, however, the number of physicians in the South had grown more swiftly than the southern population at large, which had declined relative to the rest of the nation: the South now had only 33 percent of the U.S. population but 34 percent of all doctors, with 1 doctor for every 554 southerners in 1860 compared to a ratio of 1 to 596 outside the South. Moreover, considering the legal and clerical professions together with medicine, it is eye opening that physicians made up 49 percent of all southern professionals, compared to 42 percent in the free states. There were nearly two physicians for every lawyer in the South during the 1850s, and, strikingly, given the showy historical image of southern preachers, two physicians for every clergyman.[12]

Physicians in the aggregate may be further characterized in terms of race and gender. Orthodox practitioners in the mid-nineteenth-century South were by definition white males; the exclusions and pretensions of race and gender thus were inseparable from orthodoxy itself. Although there were African American practitioners among the free black populations in cities like Baltimore, Charleston, and New Orleans who doubtless included men with orthodox training or allegiances, almost nothing is known of them as individuals, and black medical schools were not founded until the 1870s. Vernacular African American healers, slave and free, were everywhere in the countryside, and although they appear only fleetingly in white sources, it is clear that physicians frequently worked with them and often respected them. White women occupied a differently liminal place with regard to the orthodox profession between 1830 and 1880. Women did not enter the orthodox fold anywhere in the United States until 1849, and then only in the North. Even after the Civil War, southern women were excluded from orthodoxy, even as women elsewhere were founding medical schools of their own. Although a handful of southern physicians gave serious consideration to having female colleagues specializing in "women's problems," most were skeptical not of women's caregiving skills but of their capacity for learning science and doing surgery.[13]

Despite the importance of race and gender, most midcentury male physicians, of course, spent little time thinking about what they considered to be the "natural" exclusions that followed from them. They were much more concerned with a final way in which we can profile the profession, namely the legal and financial contours of practice. The story of physicians' struggle to dominate medicine by having the state license or otherwise legally privilege M.D.s has been ably told. It was a struggle orthodox physicians seemed to be losing in the years looked at here. Legislators everywhere accepted the argument advanced by physicians' competitors that regulation protected no substantial public good by favoring a brand of medicine that was no more effective than any other. Although self-serving in its own way, this argument was much more democratic and carried the day, with state after state repealing even the minimal regulation that existed prior to the 1830s. The one notable southern exception to deregulation shows that the difficulties of excluding other doctors only added to physicians' woes. Louisiana established the *Registre du Comité Médical de la Nouvelle-Orléans* in 1816 to examine and license practitioners, requiring candidates to take an oral examination and to produce testimonials from physicians as evidence of their orthodox training. Although it is difficult to say exactly how this worked in practice, approval was not automatic. Records of the examiners indicate that during the 1820s, for example, about one-fifth of all applicants for licensure were rejected, often tersely, for such things as their "secret methods" or because they were "not deemed competent." Nevertheless, the procedure was in effect voluntary, and because the examiners could do nothing to enforce their decisions, many rejected applicants doubtless went on to practice anyway. Indeed, at least some orthodox physicians themselves opposed the examinations on these grounds, or because they were embarrassed by so many orthodox men failing the examination.[14]

If the struggle over regulation was a struggle over professional image and power, it also was a more immediate struggle for livelihood. Doctors making a living will be considered in what follows, but it is useful here to recall that just as mid-nineteenth-century medical practice was nowhere near the authoritative profession it would become, neither was it financially lucrative for the great majority of practitioners, many of whom practiced part time. Although this was a national reality, southern physicians frequently wrote about its southern accent, emphasizing the particular difficulties of living in a cash-poor, rural-isolated, staple-crop economy. Some practitioners supplemented their incomes by practicing veterinary medicine or selling drugs. Others picked up occasional employment as coroners' witnesses or by examining slaves for buyers in slave markets. But these latter opportunities were neither frequent nor widespread for the majority of rural doctors. As a very broad generalization, most ordinary physicians seem to have charged somewhere between $500 and $2,000 a year for their services during this era (a figure that inflated just after the Civil War), but they collected perhaps one-half or less of this in cash and barter. While the upper end of this range would put a man comfortably in the middle class, it was by no means wealth.[15]

~

These are the broad outlines of the physician's world explored in this book. It was a world, everyone agreed, saturated by local, dangerously protean sickness alive in the very grain of people's age, race, sex, and habits, as well as in the climate, topography, and history of the South. Physicians strove to make their medicine something unique amid the crowd of other doctors, an effort that has been seen mostly in terms of elite M.D.s' increasing professional power and intellectual authority. Complementing this picture, my approach is to look at the routines of everyday practice through which ordinary physicians shaped the "art" of their healing. Here they encountered the key tensions that marked their work: they wished to be seen as innovative men of science, but at the same time they embraced traditional, local ways of healing. They were inspired by the ideal of an overarching professional brotherhood of fellow M.D.s, and yet they found themselves deeply attached to their communities and dependent on their neighbors' esteem.

But if the everyday practice of medicine raised these tensions, it also suggested how to resolve them. The country orthodox style of practice implicated something more than the particulars of either craft or profession. It employed a moral energy rooted in physicians' identities. The work of doctoring thus became meaningful through the telling of each practitioner's personal story—hundreds of stories stretching across the South—which located the essence of orthodoxy in what each man cherished as his personal "experience." By so locating orthodoxy in the everyday rhythm of a man's work—his very identity—physicians' embrace of "experience" became a powerful source for continuity in medicine throughout this era. Although this was satisfying for many physicians, it made altering one's view of good medicine more complicated. Change was not defined by ideologies and interests alone; it involved far more troubling questions of self and imagination.

The three parts of this study look at three different contexts in which the bond between orthodoxy, identity, and everyday medicine took shape. Part I centers on men choosing medicine as a career and how, by the 1830s, increasing numbers of them chose to attend medical schools, by far the most visible place for orthodoxy's new cosmopolitan claims. Schools aimed to be a world apart from the ordinary, but in reality they were permeable in all sorts of ways to the surrounding social and intellectual world. Chapter 1 looks at men's personal context for choosing medicine as a career, stressing issues of gender and family. It then considers how schools struggled to organize medical knowledge as something apart from the "lay" world, even as they remained dependent on it. Chapter 2 takes up the culture of medical education, relying primarily on the words of students and teachers to trace a phenomenology of learning shaped by schooled standards but also inflected by the world beyond the school. Chapter 3 looks at what happened to the ideals and identities of young doctors as they left the school and began practice. Community expectations and relations of power sharply reminded graduates that orthodoxy grew from local health needs in local terms, a reminder that muted and redirected physicians' schooled commitment to universal values.

Part II shifts the focus from the school to the bedside. Here we see how—and with what significance—physicians realized that the essential skills and values of orthodoxy resided in their personal style of practice and in the southern setting for disease and illness. The bedside was the crucible where the doctor transformed random calls for help into the pattern of his cherished experience. He learned, case by case, body by body, that medicine was a moral work as he adhered to what he believed was good medicine, improvising with other people's suffering, his own compassion, and the contingency of bedside events. Beginning with a look at doctors' daybooks as key texts of actual practice, Chapter 4 focuses on physicians' livelihood and on the broad social setting for rural and small-town practice. These framed the stark difference between objective disease and subjective illness and revealed the power of patients to define both. The bedside itself as a social place shared by physicians and others is the focus of Chapter 5. In the sickroom, ways of healing clashed and combined as a physician forged his own personal style. Chapter 6 continues this theme by looking at physicians' confrontation with the daunting otherness of somebody else's illness. Physicians not only struggled to achieve—and sometimes to coerce—a practical co-attendance with others at the bedside but also plumbed the mysteries of body, spirit, and moral purpose.

Part III is a consideration of how physicians made the larger meaning of the country orthodox style when they stepped away from the bedside, re-imagining their work by seeing its continuity in the broad sweep of medicine's social promise. Chapter 7 explores the identities physicians shaped for themselves against the backdrops of southern landscapes, race, and Christian faith. Chapter 8 looks at the physician's case narrative as the most widespread, durable, and intellectually flexible way to configure the meaning of his experience. Shaping the materials of medicine to the varied, surprising realities of concrete lives—especially the doctor's own—such narratives emerge as much more than records of others' illnesses. They inscribe the physician's autobiographical bond with illness as his own prey and predator.

PART ONE

CHOOSING MEDICINE

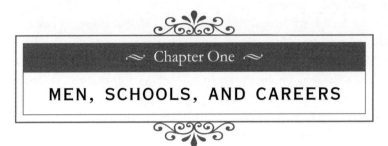

Becoming an M.D. in the mid-nineteenth-century United States was not an outlandish choice for a young man; it was not like running away to sea. But medicine, straddling the line between trade and profession, filled with economic and therapeutic uncertainties, was anything but the main chance. In the South, before and after the Civil War, the ideal of manly success was to master a flourishing plantation, the traditional seat of a man's economic power, political influence, and social esteem. Nonetheless, thousands of southern men made orthodox medicine their choice during the mid-nineteenth century, and increasing numbers of them (including some men already in practice) decided that formal medical schools were the best place to pursue it.[1]

This chapter focuses on southern men making this choice, viewing it as an encounter between their ambitions—framed by family, gender, and the local context of medicine—and an orthodox profession itself in the throes of change. Indeed, the fact that students were defining their personal goals at just the time physicians were rethinking education makes schools a particularly good place to analyze the tensions shaping medicine in this period. What follows builds on the well-known picture of medical innovators using schools as the means of reforming orthodoxy into a more intellectually unified and therapeutically sound medicine. The main focus here is on schools as the *local* institutions they were, sites for a distinct, ground-level orthodoxy in the making. Socially speaking, this means looking at schools as strikingly visible, urban institutions built on—and helping to define—a fraternity of physicians. From an intellectual point of view, it means understanding how the new medical education was caught in the friction between two goals that, as we will see, influenced physicians' view of their medicine throughout their careers. On the one hand, faculty and students imagined the school, and therefore orthodoxy, to be a cosmopolitan world apart from the surrounding vernacular culture of healing. On the other hand, they discovered that the outside world constantly impinged on the school in ways both useful and troubling.

Thus, even though most faculty and students after 1830 eagerly embraced the idea of an institutional world of their own, they were unable—and in many instances unwilling—to isolate themselves from a surrounding social matrix of ideas and influences on doctoring. In this respect, this chapter reexamines the fierce competition among schools during the nineteenth century as being about more than money, professional standards, and gatekeeping. On a deeper level, the struggle over schooling reveals that even the largest institutions, notwithstanding their genuine effort to make education more universal and abstract, actually privileged a local context for learning that encouraged physicians to focus on issues of self and locale. In particular, by fostering fraternal bonds among men, schools helped create a fluid, personal context for the very essence of medical knowledge.

This chapter considers, first, some of the moral and material realities that men—mostly young men—pondered as they made their decision to become doctors. This is followed by a look at the significance of medical schools' struggle to shape a unique world after 1830. A struggle over academic requirements, it also was a struggle over the question of physicians' identity: were they to be the harbingers of a cosmopolitan medical science or should they be content to be the repositories of familiar, local practice. Finally, this chapter considers how the issues raised by schools' academic tensions also were shaped by their continuing commitment to apprenticeships and to an urban setting. In all of these contexts, schools embraced elements of a vernacular world that they also wished to hold at bay.

FAMILY, INTELLECT, AND THE MANLY CHOICE

Family as the cradle of young men's prospects and character profoundly shaped how men imagined becoming physicians. Throughout the mid-nineteenth century, no clear professional career "path" in medicine existed to help men make their decision. Most men more or less backed into medicine. In the 1830s, for instance, J. Marion Sims thought that medicine was interesting mostly because it seemed more inclusive and less rigid than either law or the ministry. Another young South Carolinian, Lafayette Strait, after attempting "to go through the Citadel and fail[ing]," chose medicine in the 1850s for the simple reason that "I am very anxious to go at something." William Whetstone's older brother hoped that medicine would give William something to "put your mind upon" if only to "take it off the *women*." So, too, Hamilton Weedon was advised in 1851 that medical study might be a good alternative to "frolicking & Spanish segars, and extravagant clothes." Some men undertaking medical study did not foresee careers as physicians but rather hoped to acquire skills useful in planting, the ministry, or even business.[2]

Men framed their goals with the language of masculine willfulness and license—and with its obverse, the idiom of honor and sober morality. "Now is an import[ant] time in my life, and I must 'make hay while the sun shines,' lest the sun might refuse to shine for me," one young South Carolinian wrote in 1856 as he prepared for medical study. Another young man felt that his "*manhood* had been reached" with his decision to study medicine and that with it he had "started out on Life's voyage . . . to try to make something of myself." Making it while the sun shone; starting out on the voyage—the familiar images of manly effort gathered their power. Young men's families added their views, not always supportively. J. Marion Sims's father was appalled at Sims's decision to take up medicine. It was a mere trade, he told Marion: "There is no science in it. There is no honor to be achieved in it; no reputation to be made." Another South Carolinian faced family disapproval in 1856 for the quite different reason that medicine was deemed too difficult. His physician uncle "curled his nose in disgust" and said "that I would never succeed" because of a lack of self-discipline needed for a successful practice.[3]

Other families, though, supported their sons' desire to study medicine, defining an honorable career not by wealth or fame but by social usefulness or their son's intellectual bent. Lunsford Yandell, whose father practiced medicine, "cannot remember the time when I was not spoken of in the family as an embryo doctor." Charles Hentz's father, too, had studied medicine, and although Charles's mother insisted that the seventeen-year-old attend the University of Alabama for a year, she agreed with her husband that medicine suited Charles's interest in nature and his skill with his hands. Russell M. Cunningham recalled the "beautiful night" in Alabama when he told his parents, with some apprehension, "I am going to study medicine." But his mother told him, "Go it, my son; I rejoice in your ambition."[4]

To be sure, men worried along with their parents about the practical consequences of their decision. Charles Hentz had second thoughts in 1845 when he learned that "there are nearly a thousand young men turned out annually" from medical schools; he feared that there was too "little sickness to divide amongst so many." Hentz's mentor, Daniel Drake, himself recalled wondering whether his "home-body" self would be happy at a school so far away from home. Doubtful men turned to practicing physicians for reassurance. "Now you know me and . . . something of the physiognomy of mankind, [tell me] if you think it would do for me to undertake that kind of enterprise," a fellow Alabamian asked Dr. William Wylie in 1857. Dr. Charles Harrod reassured his friend in 1845 about her prospective medical student grandson, telling her that all would be well if the youth would "come down here [to New Orleans]—I will introduce him to several of the physicians." What Harrod's quite typical offer reveals is how much the midcentury medical profession was still little more than a hit-or-miss network of personal contacts, making a man's choice of medicine inseparable from the social and moral contexts of local, individual practice. Although, as we will see, the larger medical schools by the 1840s aimed to make admission to the profession something more, this personal scale of information and aspiration stayed largely intact.[5]

This should not suggest that the intellectual appeal of medical study did not count; for many men it mattered a great deal. Although medical students have been portrayed as a rowdy, unscholarly lot, many seem in fact to have been attracted to the intellectual challenges of medicine. Even so unfocused a young man as Lafayette Strait expected medicine to demand "the strongest mental exertion," which he welcomed as a test of his maturity. Similarly, Daniel Drake recalled that most of his fellow students took seriously the "learned, technical, and obscure" science they had chosen. "The physician, unlike the mathematician, is not the creator of his own science," one mentor observed. "Unlike the astronomer, he has no simple relations of matter to deal with; he cannot, like the chemist, make any two things which he examines or uses identical; the objects of his study [that is, his patients] are more variable than the winds and tides." Although doubtless understating the complexity of astronomy and chemistry, this view was common among physicians who saw medicine as uniquely difficult because its science would never be free from the vexing need to apply it.[6]

Even so, many intellectually curious students embraced medicine as the only field of study at midcentury that unified the natural sciences into a single realm of knowledge. For young Lunsford Yandell, reading through the lectures of Benjamin Rush in the 1820s, or for William Holcombe, working through French and English books on zoology and biology twenty-five years later, medicine was by definition "scientific" because it required an omnivorous reading that promised synthesis, as well as detail. The usual preparatory reading for medical students throughout the century included not only the natural sciences but also works in literature and moral philosophy, suggesting that nothing was intellectually beyond the physician's curiosity. The sense of medicine as the key to discovering a unifying "science of life" was sufficiently strong that many students would have agreed with Charles Hentz, who wrote in 1845 that his most compelling reason to become a medical doctor was his intellectual desire "to make the study of Nature one of my great occupations as well as pleasures."[7]

Men's interest in the intellectual domain of medicine is all the more significant in that it was not matched by an expressed desire to care for the sick and relieve suffering. In the correspondence among men, their families, and their advisers, there is scarcely a mention of helping sick people or of illness as a subjective experience. Although some advisers, rather abstractly, referred to the need for "constant attention at the bedside of the sick," it was not caregiving so much as an ethic of hard work they were recommending. It is tempting to think that the silence about caregiving implies that helping sick people was so axiomatic that it did not require words. But this view sells the significance of the silence too short. The silence may well suggest, once again, that many physicians conceived of medical learning as a world apart from its application to patients. To say "I wish to study the science of all life" was to be filled with a unique aspiration and sense of adventure; to say "I want to make people well" was far less ambitious, not least because it might not be possible.[8]

The subjectivity of illness, however, does make one brief but interesting appearance in the retrospective writing of certain physicians. In telling how they chose medicine, they include childhood memories in which someone (often themselves) is injured or suffers. Only glancingly seen and said, these allusions nonetheless suggest a personal tie between the desire to become a doctor and the realm of bodily infirmity, pain, and dependence at the heart of hands-on practice. Charles Hentz, for instance, recalling his earliest memories, remembered falling and injuring his head while chasing his sister around a tree as a child in the late 1820s. "Father sent for a doctor," Hentz remembered, "who trimmed my eyebrow & put on plasters, which filled me with a great sense of importance." Similarly, James Still remembered being vaccinated by a doctor, and throughout his career, "the sting of the lancet yet remains." Lunsford Yandell linked his decision to study medicine to the fact that he was frail as a boy, "called by the negroes 'splinter-shanks,'" and that his parents worried he might not be strong enough to work at anything. He proved everyone wrong by becoming a physician.[9]

MEDICAL SCHOOLS AND REFORM: STRETCHING ORTHODOXY

Before 1830, relatively few American men with an interest in medicine attended medical school. Apprenticeship, which is considered later in this chapter, was the traditional means of recruiting "practical" men into the orthodox profession. But after 1830, new institutions—larger and more intellectually ambitious than any that had preceded them on this side of the Atlantic Ocean—challenged and reconfigured what it meant to become a physician. Reformist physicians seized upon formal schooling as providing an education far richer than anything solo apprenticeship could offer: ideally schools provided a concentrated intellectual environment guided by experienced men and shared with a brotherhood of inquisitive fellows. To achieve this ideal, schools aimed to be an intellectual and social world apart from the larger society. But here a striking tension arose. Attempting to create a world apart was deeply problematic given a school's obvious dependence on local resources and goodwill. Thus, even as educational reformers pursued an idea of medicine as a realm of universal values and techniques, schools remained quite permeable to the surrounding world of local health practices and assumptions.[10]

For the most part, the history of these two linked worlds has been told as a story of how successful orthodox schools managed to break free from both competitors and the larger society alike. It is a story of linear change, the making of a twentieth-century institution. What follows here is a different kind of story. Mid-nineteenth-century medical schools are not seen as transitional institutions on the way to "modern" medicine. Rather, they are seen as an experienced *now*, a social and intellectual place in which orthodoxy was a fluid, protean body of knowledge stretched between two equally powerful visions of its potential. One imagined medicine as cosmopolitan and open-ended; the other focused on medicine's local roots and vernacular insights. The tension between these visions of orthodoxy gave rise to three interrelated debates over academic structure and form that profoundly shaped the expectations of nascent M.D.s. The first had to with the timing of a student's course of study, and the second with the expansion of the curriculum; here were questions about how complex (and therefore how remote from local society) the world of the school ought to be and how long a man needed to stay within it. The third debate concerned the relation between practical training (how to suture a wound; how to compound a medicine) and orthodoxy's traditional commitment to an ideal of a broad learnedness that went beyond such specifics; here were questions about schools' intellectual purpose and elitism. Understanding the importance of these debates is a way of understanding how physicians learned to straddle two worlds of healing and what they were choosing when they chose medicine as a career.

Before considering the debates, however, some context for midcentury orthodox schools is useful. The six orthodox schools in the United States in 1810 increased to twenty-two by 1830 and to sixty by 1870. During the 1830s, in the

United States as a whole, certain institutions achieved greater success amid the large number of small trade schools producing M.D.s. The ascendant schools flourished through a happy combination of ambitious faculty and an increasingly active market for prospective students and, most important, by attaching themselves to fast-growing cities and to universities. This latter move not only gave medical training an academic cast but also linked schools to urban elites interested in boosting their city's status. This in turn attracted physicians and students who joined their intellectual and career goals to a cosmopolitan vision of broad learning and to a city's ready supply of sick people. Six southern schools took this shape beginning in the 1830s. The earliest (and the first such institution west of the Appalachians) was the Transylvania Medical College in Lexington, Kentucky, founded in 1799 though not in operation until 1817. Next was Charleston's Medical College of the State of South Carolina (MCSSC), opening in 1824, followed by the Medical College of Georgia, in Augusta, which began granting degrees in 1832. Three years later, the Medical College of Louisiana, in New Orleans, and, in 1837, the Louisville Medical Institute, in Louisville, Kentucky, joined the now fully competitive southern scene. Between their founding and 1861, some 700 men per year sought degrees from these five schools. In 1851, these institutions were joined by a sixth, Tennessee's University of Nashville, which rose quickly to become the South's largest school just as the nation fell apart in war.[11]

For the most part, historians have not been kind to these schools in the South and elsewhere. "A century ago," writes the leading historian of twentieth-century medical education, "being a medical student in America was easy." While this may seem so with hindsight, a look at schools' efforts to define their purpose and strategies shows that shaping the intellectual contours of medicine was anything but easy and that students, as well as faculty, often became engrossed in the struggle to define good medicine. A good school, reformer Samuel Dickson said in 1826 at the Medical College of South Carolina, challenged a man intellectually by drawing him into a fraternal company where debate and the need for empirical proof were the essentials of a universal medical science. At the same time, Dickson acknowledged, schools were local places, teaching men that medical practice always was practice *somewhere*, alive to "the variable influences of habit and climate . . . [and] local rules for the management of the sick." Like Dickson and other reformers, Daniel Drake saw geographical region as crucial in this regard. Southern schools would become centers of a distinctly southern medical empire based on a "union of interests powerfully attracted into communion by a common channel of . . . intercourse in the south." On a personal level, too, the southern ideal of education seemed peculiarly fitting to students who, like one South Carolinian in 1856, saw the value of learning medicine in *his* South, "within a few miles of 'sweet home.'"[12]

All of this proved an inspiring vision of education for many, in both its emotional and intellectual intensity. And, as others have shown, the rise of such institutions was marked by fierce differences of opinion often aired in public. Schools battled each other for primacy. Alternative healers condemned orthodoxy's emphasis on formal schooling as yet another attempt to monopolize medicine. Many ordinary physicians thought schools went too far and were skeptical that classrooms imparted truly useful knowledge compared to the bedside. Some orthodox reformers themselves—most of whom either were or aspired to be faculty—criticized existing schools on the grounds that they did not go far enough. Beginning in the 1840s, they urged the more radical changes that ultimately resulted in the twentieth century's adoption of watershed reforms: academic admission requirements for students; a mandatory four-year course of study; a "graded" or progressive curriculum with courses in basic science preceding clinical work; rigorous examinations; hospital internships.[13]

But emphasizing the twentieth-century outcome underplays the significance of the debates that preceded it, to which we now return. At the heart of these debates over timing, curriculum, and learnedness was the question of how much schools should aim to be, or could afford to be, a world apart. Like the schools themselves, the debate faced in two directions, addressing the orthodox profession inside the school's walls, as well as the public outside. This is plainly seen in the descriptive circulars (also called "catalogues" and "announcements") published annually by schools. These circulars are a particularly revealing text because they aimed to recruit students even as they articulated demanding reforms that might drive students away. Circulars typically described the school and touted its material advantages; they announced fees and listed faculty and courses. However, in their relentless self-advertisement, circulars also traced the uncertain line between medicine's public mission to supply communities with reliable healers and the school's identity as a separate world marked by a distinctive intellectual quest.[14]

Indeed, changes in the basic form of these texts reveal how schools throughout the century increasingly, though cautiously, defined an ideal of themselves as a world apart. In the 1830s, for instance, circulars usually listed, to the exclusion of much else, the names of all current students and their apprenticeship supervisors. Featuring these linked names implied that a phalanx of students and supportive community practitioners was the school's most impressive attribute. Earlier circulars also emphasized how the school harmoniously fit into its urban community, enhancing it yet modestly beholden to its larger fortunes. Throughout the 1840s, however, these circulars became more inwardly focused, moving lists of students to the back pages or eliminating them altogether. Instead, circulars drew attention to distinguished faculty and such institutional attributes as the library and specimen cabinets. Highlighted, too, were descriptions of the curriculum, opportunities for rounds and special classes, and information about what a student could expect to actually *do* in medical school. As tellingly, circulars slowly detached the school from the city in which it was located, usually placing the school in the context of the medical profession at large (or its own institutional history) rather than its immediate urban context. These changes inscribed a shift toward an ideal of learning in which schools were institutionally freestanding and intellectually complex, suggesting not just a way station like apprenticeship but an entire world.[15]

First among the debates that followed from this shift, arising by the late 1830s, was the matter of the proper timing of the medical degree. Schools worried the question of timing in two ways: the length of the school term and the total length of time needed to complete an M.D. In part, the debate arose from the economic competition among schools for more students. Longer terms and more years would mean additional income for schools, of course, and yet a school that unilaterally lengthened the required time risked losing students who would seek out less demanding institutions. More deeply, however, the debate over timing arose from the conflicted image of schools as either inward-focused bastions of esoteric knowledge or as suppliers of doctors for communities. How long should it take for a man to become what most communities wanted—a solid, ordinary practitioner? For how long a time did the pursuit of learning justify withholding a doctor from the communities who needed him?

In the 1830s, at the beginning of southern schools' expansion, the standard term lasted four months. To earn his M.D., a student needed to successfully complete two of these terms (literally, he repeated the same run of classes) over no less than a two-year period. Because, with hindsight, this baseline requirement seems woefully inadequate, and because it was not permanently altered during the mid-nineteenth century, the importance of the debates surrounding timing has been underestimated. For one thing, schools were truly agitated over the four-month standard, with many faculty acknowledging that it was arbitrary. As early as 1830, the Medical College of Georgia, proclaiming that there was nothing sacred about four months, expanded its term to six. Although the school beat a hasty retreat shortly thereafter when other schools did not follow suit, the Georgia school's precedent was lauded by the fledgling American Medical Association (AMA) when it called for longer terms in 1848. This time, several schools expanded the length their terms, though they, too, soon retreated to the four-month standard. Thus, though inconclusive, the term length issue was a graphic instance of midcentury orthodoxy's struggle to achieve the desired balance between medicine as a learned ideal, determined within the school, and the equally pressing image of medicine as rightly grounded in the communities that supported and rewarded doctors.[16]

Much the same thing happened in the debate over how *many* terms were needed to achieve an M.D. This debate, too, was far more than a technical nit-picking, raising the troubling matter of whether a physician's dual allegiance to his community and his profession might prove fatally divisive. Although the existing standard (two terms required for an M.D.) remained unaltered during the midcentury decades, the debate stirred up revealing tensions—and compromises—in schools' desire to turn out a supply of doctors while not abandoning their ideal of a learned physician. Even as they stood by the two-term standard, schools established other requirements that resisted popular and market pressures, refusing, for example, to permit a student to rush through both terms in a single year. Although schools would have made more money by permitting this, the larger schools agreed that collapsing the two terms without time for reflection (or for the leavening effect the interterm apprenticeship was supposed to have) would result in inferior doctors. Too, schools debated the difficult matter of whether experience in bedside practice might in some way substitute for time spent in lectures. Allowing practice time to count toward a school's degree was an obvious way to attract working doctors to become students. At the same time, a simple equation of practice to schooling obviously undercut schools' claims to being unique bastions of medical learning. During the 1840s, the major institutions agreed to equate four years of "regular" practice to one term of lectures, an arrangement that did not close the door to established practitioners but did underscore the superiority of schooling.[17]

Equally indicative of schools' conflicted efforts to compete for students yet establish themselves as a world apart was their adherence to essentially the same required courses throughout the era even as they experimented with a growing array of other, unofficial courses. A core curriculum acted as a stabilizing force in education, of course, attesting to orthodox medicine as something certain and tamping down competition among schools. The core courses changed little over the midcentury years; botany was phased out by the 1840s; obstetrics was phased in. Other standbys included chemistry (inorganic), materia medica (pharmacology), anatomy, surgery, and a course involving bedside diagnosis and prescription, usually termed the "practice" or "institutes" of medicine. However, during the 1840s, the larger schools began to foster a substantial parallel or "shadow" curriculum around the edges of their required courses, offered as optional or "pre-term" courses. Although some faculty worried that the peripheral courses might detract from the regular term or exacerbate the competition for students, many others favored them because they could teach their personal interests, in the words of one student who had benefited, "without being tied down to . . . their publick lectures." Many faculty doubtless were aware that their extracurricular courses mirrored the trendsetting Paris clinics; others simply saw a local opportunity and took it. Regardless, students responded enthusiastically to classes where the faculty were engaged intellectually and taught, as one teacher put it, "*con amore*—from the love of science, or of fame."[18]

Arising from the combined interests of teachers and students, then, the shadow curriculum plotted whole new areas of endeavor three decades before schools usually are given credit for such depth. By 1850, for example, all of the major southern schools were offering an early (October) session of gross anatomy for students eager for experience with cadavers; other popular courses included ones on medical jurisprudence and on the diseases of children. In advertising these courses, schools stressed that they would not count as part of the stable core curriculum. And yet they used enticing language that suggested that students would lose out if they did not participate. The extra courses provided "ample opportunities" for hands-on experience (Medical College of Georgia); they would cover topics "which *will not be fully discussed in the regular Session*" (University of Nashville); students would "have the privilege of attending many surgical operations" (University of Louisville). Thus, even though they were on the margins, such courses inevitably called into question the established way of doing things. Teachers and students may be seen as working together to define a schooled orthodoxy with broader and deeper intellectual goals than a school's official curriculum permitted, and goals far superior to those found in the "outside" world of community practice.[19]

Equally telling as a sign of schools' cautious but determined effort to be a world apart was the value they placed on learnedness, evidenced by their esteem for academic experience and for writing. Despite charges of elitism by alternative healers and rival doctors, the larger orthodox schools supported modest but persistent efforts to promote a broad intellectual grounding that had no immediate practical application. By the 1850s, for instance, most of the major schools openly recommended some sort of preparatory "liberal" study and honored those students who had it, singling out "academic" students for special notice in circulars and giving awards for essay writing and other evidence of liberal attainments. The chancellor of the Nashville school was even bold enough in 1860 to say that his school would recruit men with at least some attendance at a university, arguing that such experience gave an individual "the literary and scientific grounding necessary to a perfect comprehension of the [medical] lectures."[20]

More strikingly, the career of the written M.D. thesis reveals how schools attempted to balance their claims for intellectual uniqueness with the need to fit into the larger society. At their founding, all of the major schools required a written thesis, even the Nashville school, which started up two decades after the others. In its form, the M.D. thesis was remarkably consistent throughout the century, a brief (ten to fifteen copybook pages) academic essay on some aspect of a student's work. The thesis was not meant to be an original piece of research, although a small number of them were, but instead was an openly derivative essay drawn from lectures and, sometimes, clinical experience. Schools highlighted the thesis as a mark of learnedness, as did the Louisville school, which observed in 1838 (somewhat optimistically) that students might write "in the English, French, or Latin tongue." In practice, it seems, most students disliked writing the thesis and many faculty thought it was an anachronistic exercise at best. Yet schools did not abandon it, holding to the conviction that, as a learned man, a physician should express himself in writing. Recognized at graduation, bound into volumes in the school's library, the thesis was a small but important first step in a man's attempt to speak from the physician's seat of authority.[21]

Through all of these curricular and academic tensions, then, schools' efforts to define themselves as distinct intellectual realms are best seen not for how well they approximated the "modern" but rather for how they expressed schools' conflicted relation to the larger social world outside their walls. At the heart of this relation was an ideal of a good doctor who could bridge the gap between the school and the community. He was a southern man steeped in a regional identity. He was intellectually curious and accepted the fact that medicine was a time-consuming effort combining practical skills with intellectual demands. He was unafraid of undertaking broad study, accepted the discipline of schools' courses and terms, and understood the need to speak and write, as well as to act, in the M.D.'s tradition. And, perhaps most strikingly, he was eager to join with his fellows in a special, fraternal setting that leavened competition with collective purpose.

This desire to be in but not of a wider social world was tested and further shaped by two other problematic features of schools' institutional life, both of which had particular significance, especially in terms of gender, for how schools framed orthodoxy. The first of these was the place that local apprenticeships continued to occupy in medical training, tying older men to younger in terms of work habits and social visibility. The second was the urban setting for most schools, tying medical learning to city life and highlighting both as a man's world.

Apprenticeships, an ancient tradition in medicine, were the most permeable point in the line between schooling and community, defining the creative tension between the two. Typically in mid-nineteenth-century apprenticeships, local physicians worked with young men with whom they were personally acquainted and whose families they knew, imparting to the relationship a commitment deeper than a mere labor contract. Usually the master (or "preceptor," as he was called by reformers who favored a more academic term) agreed to teach the apprentice a variety of surgical and medical techniques and to oversee a course of reading. The apprentice agreed to apply himself to such study, as well as to help his preceptor in routine tasks such as feeding his horse and cleaning the office. If the apprentice learned well, the preceptor had the authority to create a new M.D. simply by declaring in writing the apprentice's fitness to practice.[22]

The shortcomings of this way of learning are easy to see and are precisely what reformers thought schools should remedy: careless preceptors valued only the apprentice's labor and did little teaching; ignorant apprentices were turned loose on helpless patients; medical knowledge was chopped up into the peculiar habits of hundreds of individual mentors and taught as science. Even when these abuses were avoided, most solo practitioners, no matter how well-intentioned or skilled, had "no library, no apparatus, no provision for improvement in practical anatomy," as one critic put it. Moreover, doctors regularly apprenticed the sons of friends with little regard for screening the youths for "brains, purity, and force of character."[23]

Nonetheless, despite the quarreling, apprenticeship existed in a kind of creative tension with schools. While some reformers wished to do away with apprenticeship altogether, others advocated reinventing it as a source of grassroots professionalism that, among other things, would supply schools with motivated students. Even so thorough an antebellum critic of traditional standards as South Carolina's Samuel Dickson, who complained that loosely structured apprenticeships were the cause of "the comparative failure of so many good intellects [in medicine] & the elevation of so many inferior ones," acknowledged that a successful career in medicine was not only a matter "of thought, reading &c, but also of manner & conduct." Apprenticeship, Dickson admitted, was unmatched for putting these two realms together. Whatever its intellectual limitations, apprenticeship engaged the complexity of practice by pushing the novice into the midst of the values and relationships of both community and profession from which actual practice was made.[24]

Indeed, apprenticeships, as both supporters and detractors perceived, were an aggressively democratic means of training doctors. One preceptor's solo practice was the equal of any other's in turning out the next generation of M.D.s. That many preceptors took this responsibility seriously is suggested by the elevated, masculine language of the certifications they wrote. For example, Dr. George Logan said of his student in 1826, "*This certifies* that *Doctor Robert Lebby* of this city [Charleston] has been upwards of two years a student of medicine in my office during which period he has diligently applied himself in the acquirement of the knowledge of his profession." Invoking himself, and thus placing his own honor on the line, Logan concluded by saying that Lebby's manly "conduct and deportment" made him "entitled to my best wishes for his success in life, especially in . . . the practice of medicine, surgery, & midwifery." The power of preceptors to pronounce a man complete appears, more darkly, in two letters from Robert Montgomery to his former teacher, Dr. J. S. Copes, in 1841. Montgomery, it seems, had quit his apprenticeship and commenced practice sooner than Copes thought appropriate. Montgomery wrote Copes in an effort to jolly him along into a certification anyway. He would look forward to Copes's letter, he said, adding brazenly, and a little obscurely, "Be sure to commence my name in large letters with 'Dr' ha ha, so much for quackery." When Copes did not respond, Montgomery wrote again, this time showing the unmistakable edge of personal honor: "Now dear Doctor my character is at stake and their [*sic*] is only one thing which will enable me to sustain it: and that is a certificate from you showing that I am competent to practice." For good or ill, this bond between community preceptor and apprentice was loosened but not discarded when apprentices entered the world of the school. Indeed, because students were supposed to pursue apprenticeships both before and during their two terms of academic work, schools in a sense cooperated in diluting their own authority.[25]

The tension between school and apprenticeship can be seen, too, in students' reading, which was shaped by apprenticeship despite schools' efforts at control. For instance, it appears to have been common practice for a man to begin his apprenticeship by reading medical texts with little guidance. "I groped in darkness nearly all my way," wrote one physician of his first weeks' reading in anatomy in the 1820s. This seems to have been the point. He was meant to struggle against the sheer weight of the arcane words and shadowy acts that filled the pages of his mentor's books or else be crushed by them. Rising to the occasion, many apprentices took their reading seriously, recording when they began and finished a certain book, and taking notes. Most apprentices by the 1840s seem to have begun with basic science (anatomy mixed with some physiology), although some mentors, interestingly, had their students take a more social view of practice by having them read books of popular self-help medicine. This made sense, as one preceptor put it, because the young physician "would be expected by the people to know as much about the practice as the old women" who were well acquainted with such books. In any case, after groping for a while, the sharper students began to understand how to read. In 1854, for instance, after nearly a year's study, apprentice J. M. Richardson achieved a critical grasp on his reading that permitted him to say of John Eberle's *Practice*, "It is decidedly the best written work on medicine. His style is vigorous, poetical and fascinating. . . . He never says a foolish thing." In contrast, Richardson found William Dewees "rather too obscurely expressed" and "too litigious entirely." Some students read widely during their apprenticeships, working toward a general breadth of learning. "I read twenty pages in Bell [on anatomy], about thirty in Mrs. Cross [apparently on social etiquette]," young Richardson recorded in his diary, and then he read "Uncle Tom's Cabin till daylight."[26]

An apprentice's solo sessions of reading were offset by work in his mentor's office. Not merely drudge labor (though it included that), office work gave the apprentice a sense of the material world of everyday practice. Even the simple work of looking after the doctor's horse and keeping the instruments and medicines organized was an important first experience with the tools and physical space of doctoring that signified preparedness and professionalism. Apprentice William Whetstone, in Columbia, South Carolina, was satisfied to be apprenticing in 1853 "in quite a grand stile," tending the office and ordering about a young slave who the doctor "gives up to me" to help keep the office clean. Another apprentice liked the "many little things which come under my observation in the office," as he set up chemical experiments with his preceptor and macerated the bones of small animals, making skeletons that served to ornament the office and to instruct. Charles Hentz's memory of making gum opium in the afternoons when his mentor was out on rounds captures something of the tactile world of apprenticeship and the particular skills it required: "I took the Gum in its soft, rough state, and pulled it out into small pieces, & dried it in the sun, until it was as friable as I could get it, and then I pounded it faithfully in a mortar—into the finest powder I could make."[27]

When he had earned his mentor's confidence, the apprentice sometimes presided over the office alone. Thus playing the doctor, local youths were reintroduced to their community as nascent physicians. Some patients refused to allow an apprentice, whom they had known as a boy frolicking about town, to take hold of a sprained finger or a sore tooth. In Henry Clay Lewis's sketches of an apprentice's life in Louisiana in the 1840s, all of the patients who came under the care of the rowdy and competitive group of apprentices were either slaves, who had little or no choice, or Irish river boatmen and local ne'er-do-wells who either did not know or did not care who they were getting as a doctor. In fact, a large proportion of apprentices' first patients seem to have been slaves, which suggests that one way wealthier whites in the South tested an apprentice was to send a slave with something relatively minor and see what happened. In this way, many antebellum southern physicians began their careers by working on the bodies of people they called Uncle David, Judge Doty's Margaret, and Mr. Houseman's Sandy.[28]

Gradually, the successful apprentice moved outside the office and into his mentor's neighborhood rounds, learning that his social skills were indistinguishable from his therapeutic technique. In this way, the broadly "medical" things an apprentice learned were inextricable from the local context of practice. Exactly when a novice first laid hands on a seriously ill patient depended on some combination of confidence and curiosity on the part of preceptor, apprentice, and patient. One apprentice, deeply mortified after he passed out during a surgical operation in 1853, was reassured by his mentor that "it is quite natural" to do so, and the student resolved, "I will try and not fainte next time." Abraham Jobe, assisting his mentor with an amputation, was showered with a sudden spurt of blood ("I could taste it, hot and salty") and surprised himself when he realized that it "did not effect me in the least." Life and death happened up close in neighbors' homes. William Whetstone, his preceptor indisposed, was sent to a childbirth alone for the first time in the spring of 1855. It was an important call; she was "a respectable woman." Fortunately, the baby was delivered soon and well, "so I can brag on my maiden case." At the other end of the emotional spectrum, apprentice J. M. Richardson spent several days in 1853 attending, with his preceptor, a young slave girl named Lindy. She died even though Richardson "dressed her blisters and waited on her as much as I could." He was moved to tears at her death and "felt awfully" for days afterward.[29]

In such ways did an apprentice learn to engage somewhat with the subjectivity of illness, and engage, too, with medical practice's ragged terrain of boredom and emergency, failure and success. Attentive young men began to understand how important it was in daily practice to be aware of one's own skills, preferences, and character as a healer. It was this openness to the social world that makes apprenticeship seem more important than its detractors allowed. Consider young Thomas Wade's developing routine in the spring of 1852 in Louisiana. On May 21 he mixed his first medicine, a tincture, and four days later, his first ointment; "had a laugh at myself" for making it incorrectly. A day later, Wade's preceptor "was called off in the evening and left two patients, both women, for me to attend to." Wade wrote cautiously that he believed he had gained their confidence. The next day, with the doctor again out, "Mr. Pepper brought one of his negro men (Anthony) to town with a toothache." Wade had pulled one tooth and was struggling with a second when his preceptor returned and finished the job. On June 8, Wade was disappointed to miss "a very interesting case" because he did not have his horse, but a week later he was able to accompany the doctor to Mr. Oliver's, "and we 'doctored' him a while and he got better." Or consider one afternoon of Charles Hentz's Tuscaloosa, Alabama, apprenticeship in 1846. He manned the office alone, chatting with a neighbor or two who stopped by merely to talk. Then he "pulled one big tooth for Mr. Daley, prescribed & gave a large dose of pills to a negro man, *like to have pulled* a tooth for a negro woman, but she backed out—made & labeled a vial of colic drops for Mrs. Parson White—& made up as usual many vials of mixtures & lots of pills." Although Hentz had worried that an emergency might occur while he was alone, the day passed quickly, and when it ended he wrote with satisfaction, "I've been quite a doctor today."[30]

Such experience underscores how apprenticeship, as a mode of medical learning, was wholly configured by a mentor's personal style of practice and his willingness to delegate his work. What apprenticeship lacked in intellectual depth it supplied in social breadth, and thus it cut with a double edge into schools' efforts to establish a unique world. The same rootedness in a preceptor's (and a community's) ways of doing things that might blind the apprentice to the school's innovations also taught him how to pool local resources and gain public acceptance. If the world of the school attracted the novice doctor as a world of exclusive learnedness, apprenticeship impressed him with the importance of keeping himself within the life of his community. And if patients were exposed to his improvisation and error, an apprentice at least learned that he might choose to be open to people's preferences and demands, and thus confront his own emotional response to sickness. William Whetstone's mentor had him "trotting around Town pretty constantly" in the mid-1850s, activity that taught him that a practitioner of medicine "must not be above putting his hands to anything connected with it, no matter how nasty, and disgusting it sometimes is." This was the insight, too, of one young man who decided against a medical career in 1834. Doctoring, he learned, demanded "the 'art of pleasing' " people, which he detested, and, moreover, "you have no rest, and are liable to be disturbed at all hours of the night." Such were the gritty lessons of apprenticeship that many men learned early and learned well and that schools did little to alter or control.[31]

The world of the school was open in another way to outside influences that challenged and qualified the institutional goal of creating a special place for orthodoxy to flourish: the urban setting for the larger schools, too, cut with a double edge. The city fostered a sense of fraternity among students, and even among students and their teachers, which schools approved. But the urban scene also competed with the school, breaking men's discipline by highlighting the dullness—or the strangeness—of being a medical student. From the beginning of students' education, the city accented their sense of being in a man's world, and it shaped the way they fashioned themselves as nascent professionals.

Medical students were a discernible seasonal presence in most cities, noted in newspapers, welcomed by merchants, and recruited by churches. Students arrived each October or early November, purchasing lecture tickets at ten to fifteen dollars a subject and matching up with roommates at boardinghouses. Here they paid three to five dollars a week to live and eat with salesmen, working women, bachelor preachers, and others on their way to something better. One prominent teacher commented on the typical variety of students he had seen: the "bullies and desperadoes," the "gross and sensual," the "genius" youths driven by a love for science, the fugitives from school teaching, the boys good at fixing things, and the sprinkling of the "middle-aged . . . practical" men already in practice. Students settled in and sized up the "greenness" of their fellows— discovering who had studied elsewhere and already knew a thing or two, who were fellow Alabamians or Georgians or Louisianans. "I have found a fine, airy room . . . in a delightful part of town," Virginian Fayette Spragins wrote his brother from Lexington, Kentucky, in 1841. "I think I shall make great progress in the study of my profession." Another student depicted himself as a newborn infant, arriving on the scene "face first & head up" and looking forward to beginning his studies in Atlanta, which impressed him as "the grandest place to get a medical education in the world."[32]

From their rented rooms, the rural boys headed out into the streets. "New Orleans is decidedly a great place . . . for seeing a bit of the whole world in miniature," one student wrote to his brother in 1850. He was amazed to find attractions like "Mons. Adrien the magician; Shakespearian readings by two different celebrities, wonderful panoramas of all the curiosities on earth . . . harpists, and beer shoops, tamborine girls and grog shops, duck gardens and masquerade balls." Thomas Wade, also in New Orleans, first thought "the noise hustle and compression is disagreeable in the extreme." But an unusual snowfall brought him outside to throw snowballs with "the ladies," and as the days passed he loosened up, venturing into art galleries and finally the theater. Students explored the sheer variety of the city, from newspapers to eating establishments to churches—some attending, for the first time, Roman Catholic services. Groups of friends gathered for midnight serenades of young women, their professors, and each other. They went to libraries, picnics, and, by the 1840s, to the new ice-cream salons.[33]

There were dangerous pleasures, too, costing young men in money and morals, just as their parents feared. Students went on rounds to the grog shops—"frolicking" as it was called—and to women. Faculty at the Atlanta Medical College in 1874 granted a student petition for "two days to frolic in & to see our sweethearts, if we had any, or to make them if we hadn't." John Robinson's friend discovered that among "the young ladies . . . a medical student stands verry high among some of them. I have gave several of them a round." Thomas Wade, living in Mrs. Goodwin's New Orleans boardinghouse in 1852, met several young working women who also roomed there, and in the evenings they played cards, "blindfold," and "tinker's wedding." Wade discovered that the women "don't appear to care much about being kissed, stand and take it and sometimes kiss in return." In fact, he continued, "[I] believe I kissed every girl in the house except Mrs. Goodwin." If this was not enough, there was commercial sex. "Frigging will go on it seems," Marmaduke Kimbrough wrote to his friend at school in Philadelphia; he included the addresses of some "cock churches" and instructions on what to do to prevent venereal disease. Another student in Charleston in 1843 wrote that he had not "set my foot in a *white* whore house since last winter" but "there are some things which I cannot give up altogether until I get married." Parents urged discipline, and correspondence between students and fathers, especially, often was barbed with disagreements over money. Joseph Jones, who seems from his letters to have been the model of studiousness, nonetheless ran critically short of cash in 1855 and wrote home to suggest that his father sell a certain slave to raise some money. The elder Jones replied sternly about the need to economize, warning Joseph that he should "not anticipate the sale of your Boy by the purchase of Books & apparatus." J. S. Copes's older brother wrote reluctantly that he would send Copes more money but added that he was "affraid to send you cash" since students' letters from home were known to contain money and were easily tampered with.[34]

The school's daily work routine to some extent pulled students away from the city's temptations, tightening the fraternal bonds among them in another way. Most students seem to have worked at their studies, although it is difficult to say how many men dropped out; schools did not keep attendance records or give "grades" for classes. "I am digging away at my studies—have not missed a lecture lately," wrote one student; there is no reason to disbelieve him. Students quickly learned to share in the brotherhood of close quarters, novel scenes, and new knowledge in this man's world. At Louisville in the mid-1840s, as elsewhere, days were marked by camaraderie and competition. As Charles Hentz recalled, students attending surgical demonstrations (held on the top floor of the school so that daylight could be admitted from the ceiling) daily raced each other up three flights of stairs to get the best view. "In we burst, leaping downwards over the backs of the seats" in the pitched amphitheater "to a small area at the bottom, where the Professor stood" with a "revolving table before him, on which lay the corpse . . . or sometimes a living patient who underwent an operation before the class." Like other students, Hentz found great satisfaction in his studies, and when he landed the position of librarian and curator of the Louisville school's specimens, he exulted in having "the greatest possible advantages for learning." He told his diary, "I'm very much pleased with everything." Adopting the school's expectations in another way, student A. V. Carrigan, in Charleston, wrote to his brother in 1854 that he was excited about staying in the city over the Christmas holidays. A recent steamboat explosion had killed a half dozen people, "mostly negroes," which would give him "plenty of subjects for Christmas" dissections. At such times, the school's routine folded around students, sheltering them in a world apart. "Oh! the power to work and [to] love it," wrote Charles Johnson from Nashville, "is the most munificent boon ever granted by kind providence to man. . . . Sweet labour! how I love it."[35]

So students went from lecture hall to boardinghouse and back again; they sparked the ladies and then returned to make tinctures and Cook's pills and memorize the number of bones in the human hand. Students were apart from the city yet surrounded by it, taking the measure of their peers and future competitors in a way that highlighted the young man's prerogatives of free movement, loud talk, and insupportable dreams. But their routine fostered misgivings, too, which arose from the fact that the outside world of getting and spending—also a masculine realm—never fit comfortably with their studies. Sometimes the grind of classes seemed merely a way of estranging themselves from the active world. Even as he looked forward to disemboweling the steamboat victims, Mr. Carrigan thought that "things are as dull and monotonous here as walking around a tree." Mr. Johnson woke up another day and saw himself "plodding along my weary way like an old plough horse." Bored students watched their teacher prescribe the same harsh drug to yet another round of patients, and they livened things up by placing bets on which of the sick would not survive the treatment. At such times, school seemed an uncertain path to the manly world students felt entitled to. Henry Ivy felt "Damnably blue" in 1878 because his first weeks at school had confirmed his fears that no fortune was to be won in medicine; he saw his future sunk in "the wretched nightmare Poverty . . . I can't throw it off. Am I doomed for life?" And even this might not be the worst of it. The same school that enfolded a man inside blessed work, tilted at just a slightly different angle, might be seen as keeping him apart from "the world," that crucial masculine mirror that confirmed reputation and held out fame. In 1860, Charles Johnson heard the world saying, " 'But who cares for the Medical Student? We have no interest in him. Let him plod away over his books, his disgusting dissections, his nauseating drugs . . . we have nothing to do with him.' " Lunsford Yandell thought that medical school focused too much on scholarship and thus encouraged a life perhaps too quiet for a man. "We read our books in solitude," he wrote to his father in 1824, half appreciative, half complaining. "[I]n the great tide of human affairs we have no part; we play no part in the grand theatre of public business."[36]

On top of students' fear that the male world of the school contained spots of ripe unmanliness was a more specific anxiety that they themselves might fall victim to disease or debility. Significantly, this fear, too, prompted a gendered language, casting studiousness in a pale, feminine light. Under the heading "The Student," Joseph Eve Allen wrote in his notebook, "See the youth bending with anxious look over yon huge volume of forgotten lore, the pale midnight lamp sheds a pale radiance upon his sickly features." After weeks of study, he takes to his bed, "a sigh breaks from his lips a peacefull radiance o're spreads his face and he is gone. Consumption has done its work." Published obituaries of medical students played upon the same theme. With the death of a student ("of disease") at the Medical College of Georgia in 1849, a medical journal pointed out that hard study and healthy manhood were at odds: "Forgetful of the claims of Nature," the journal wrote of the deceased, "the morning star often found him absorbed in his studies . . . until disease supervened, and he fell an early victim to its violent ravages, a melancholy, but instructive lesson to the living." Lunsford Yandell remembered "becoming a confirmed dyspeptic" while in school, and Louisiana student Jeptha McKinney wrote to his wife that he was "almost ready to break down . . . endeavoring to keep myself Posted up with the Lectures. . . . All nature Decays so am I but a small part of its decaying matter."[37]

Although the image of the student pondering weak and weary was an image belonging to students of letters or law, too, the frightening twist added by a medical student's routine was that his work led him literally into the midst of sickness and death. Indeed, students wrote more about their personal exposure to disease than they did about a desire to help the sick. "Did not go to the Hospital, had rather not come in contact with cholera," Thomas Wade noted in his diary, hoping that his teachers would not disapprove. In fact, schools seem to have had no single response to the risk faced by students. Jeptha McKinney's teachers advised their charges not to go to New Orleans' Charity Hospital after typhoid and typhus spread through the wards in early 1852. But I. H. Blair, in school when smallpox broke out among Charleston's hospital patients, wrote that his professor called students who stayed away "d——d cowards."[38]

In this and other ways, a school's teachers were a crucial factor in the permeability of the school to the world outside. The faculty gave a focus to learning by personifying it, giving it a flair and a voice. What emerges from student writing is the way in which teachers and students came together in a striking mix of fraternity and professional hierarchy to give schooling a deeply personal cast. Schools fostered no uniform "corporate style" to smooth out the wrinkles of teachers' individual personalities. Quite the opposite, personal style was at the heart of mentoring and thus became inseparable from the heart of orthodoxy itself.

Within a flexible, often dramatic, style of learning, schools used their prominent faculty as major drawing cards. When Daniel Drake came to the Louisville Medical Institute in 1839, for instance, the school devoted an entire page of its circular to noting his "long experience," "great popularity as a teacher," and "the high estimate" made by the profession of his talents. A few men such as Drake, a prickly character, took part in founding several schools. Other faculty became prominent throughout the South by staying put for decades; Louis D. Ford spent fifty years on the faculty of the Medical College of Georgia, and J. Ford Prioleau was at MCSSC for nearly as long. Competition for positions at the larger schools quickly became intense as schools grew in the 1830s, and although some schools included well-known non-M.D.s on their early faculties— Horace Holley at Transylvania, Milton Antony at Georgia, and Stephen Elliott at MCSSC—by the end of the decade only M.D.s were deemed suitable for highly visible faculty positions.[39]

At first, students wrote about their teachers cautiously, sometimes a little reductively, but in ways that show how they quickly learned to think about their schooling in terms of faculty personalities and style. "I think I am tolerable well pleased with [the] college faculty," Medical College of Georgia student J. E. Walthall wrote to his hometown mentor in 1842. His teachers were "familiar affable polite . . . but they must be amply remunerated." Similarly, another student felt he "was graciously received" by the faculty in 1842, but he figured that might be because he came "with the money in hand." With a blend of skepticism and curiosity, students sharply inscribed the personal display that was inseparable from the influence of an established physician: an aged Charles

Caldwell, "twirling his walking cane often like a boy," was both a "splendid figure" and a man "shocking" for his "total want of anything like religion." When Daniel Drake entered the lecture hall in the 1840s, students quacked appreciatively, or mockingly, or both. Drake often appears in letters and memories as the image of professional manliness, a practitioner-scientist with "an alert and masculine mind," in the view of one former student; a man "justly distinguished for his powers of mind and useful attainments," according to a colleague and frequent antagonist. Another well-traveled professor, surgeon Samuel D. Gross, "might well be styled 'le beau Docteur,'" student Courtney Clark thought in 1841. "He is tall, handsomely made . . . has a smile stereotyped on his countenance." Gross is an example of a teacher who seems to have been almost universally popular with students; he was the only faculty member Henry Clay Lewis did not caricature, finding Gross "a man of too much good sense to wheedle or fool with." Such men clearly relished the masculine world of the school through their long careers. "Gross is a little humorous sometimes for an old man," another student wrote thirty years later of the surgeon's off-color jokes. "It seems a little strange that he would be so full of it."[40]

Student portraits of faculty deepened over time, revealing how orthodox learnedness was bound tightly to a paternalistic style that flourished in the school's world. "It is the business of the medical professor to lighten the labours of the student," one teacher explained, "to suggest materials for reflection—trains of thought." Walter Porcher appreciated how his mentor asked questions so difficult that "my heels would go where my head ought to be, and he would then proceed to rake me fore and aft." Joseph Jones learned from his teachers how to "refresh the memory, & promote habits of accuracy, attention and careful investigation. . . . Every one must feel a pride and ambition to appear to the best advantage before his professors." Faculty seem generally to have been willing to review and correct student notes, share their private collections of books and "preparations," and take students along with them on neighborhood rounds on weekends. More than a few professors entertained students by taking them into their homes for parties and dinners, thereby further mingling the personal with the professional. Some of this seems to have been calculated to please. "Dr. [Benjamin] Dudley gave a party to the students last night," wrote a young colleague. "This will attach them, still more warmly to him, & consequently to the school." But spontaneous celebrations occurred, too, and students saw their teachers in less official or even unguarded moments. Students reciprocated formally by publishing resolutions of appreciation for individual faculty at term's end and informally by giving gifts to favorite teachers. Charles Hentz presented his anatomy demonstrator, who had an interest in comparative anatomy, with "the snake I had preserved in the act of swallowing a wood-pecker—he . . . thanked me warmly—It gratified me very much." Like other students, Hentz learned what it meant to be a physician by learning to admire a particular mentor's combination of personal and intellectual qualities. Indeed, there was no clear distinction between the personal and the intellectual, between a mentor's style and the substance of the orthodoxy he encouraged his students to master.[41]

By the same token, then, their self-indulgence or aloofness opened some teachers to student criticism. Although he later apologized, Charles Caldwell once disappointed a group of student musicians honoring him with an early morning serenade by snapping, "Come, get done with that song, will you!" Caldwell was a teacher who seems to have inspired both intense admiration and dislike, doubtless because he was dogmatic, competitive, and, by the end of his career, loudly defensive of outdated preoccupations like phrenology. Young Lunsford Yandell, arriving at Transylvania in 1824, was in awe of Caldwell and flattered by the older man's attentions, praising "the vigor of his intellect, & the profundity of his learning & science." Much later, however, seeing how formative his attachment to one man had been, Yandell ruefully reflected that "if I had chanced to take the fancy of [Benjamin] Dudley or [Daniel] Drake . . . I should have left the University much better qualified." Teachers sometimes failed to show up for lectures or delivered ones on unexpected or odd topics. There were times when entire faculties seemed inept. "Dr. Ford did not attend at his regular hour," wrote Georgia student John Knox in disgust. "But afterwards at Dr. Means' hour which was to have been occupied by Dr. Dugas, he [Ford] gave us a lecture on Metaphysics." His professor of obstetrics, Thomas Wade noted tersely, "did not lecture[;] expect he is unwell or drinking." Opportunities for socializing with teachers sometimes proved a burden as well. Of one faculty member's upcoming party, a Louisville student wrote in his diary, "Wonder if he'll invite Bob & myself—hope not indeed."[42]

In the main, however, school was a place where student self-fashioning eagerly adopted the personal style of faculty as its template. It was at its core a moral, as well as a practical, pattern. Many teachers truly encouraged students to think about the moral values underpinning a healer's role as a socially prominent figure in rural communities. Because excessive drinking of alcohol was a social problem encountered by physicians inside the school and out, for example, student-faculty temperance societies existed in all major schools. Meetings combined testimonies against alcoholic drink with lectures and discussion on the physiological consequences of alcohol and the management of delirium tremens. Students and faculty together created philomathic societies or "honors" study groups, and many schools sponsored occasional religious meetings and opportunities to teach Sunday school, which kept at least some students attached to the expansive evangelical culture in which so many of them lived. John Robinson, recently graduated, heard from a friend still in school that students "are going to have a sermon preached for our especial benefit from the 11th Chap Ecclesiastes, 9 verse," and another student told of hearing a "very practical sermon" on self-control—a good idea, he thought, as "there is no class of young men who exercise it in a less degree than medical students." Milford Woodruff assured his absent friend Charles Hentz that "the prayer meetings you used to attend every Sunday night" continued to flourish and that "our beloved Philomathic Society . . . is everything you could wish." Through the entire range of student-faculty relations, then, the authority conferred by medical learning assumed an immediate, personal shape in students' experience. Students knew their teachers in a way that mixed their esteem for formidable men of science with times of rough equality when everyone belonged to the same great enterprise.[43]

~

Despite an unevenness apparent in hindsight, the new commitment to formal schooling after 1830 was a striking achievement of orthodox medicine, an investment in a special institution founded on the belief that collective, systematic study was the route to a better medicine. It was a striking achievement not least because schools housed tensions of aspiration and identity that would mark a physician's work long after his schooling. With his choice to become a physician, a student joined orthodoxy's efforts to map a distinct medical terrain from within the walls of the school. And yet here he discovered that schools straddled the very line they drew between their standards and the supposedly inferior means of everyone else. He was encouraged to immerse himself in an institution that represented M.D.s as standing apart and above, intellectually and socially. At the same time, however, orthodox schools remained necessarily open to the local knowledge and support flowing into them from apprenticeships and from the surrounding social world of the city.

In particular, through their structural and curricular reforms, schools struggled to realize physicians' faith that, ultimately, their knowledge was sufficiently stable and unified to win out over competitors. Simultaneously, though, schools placed great emphasis on the fluid personal relationships that configured a professional fraternity, trusting that these relationships themselves would give essential shape to a knowledge useful outside the school's walls. How this dynamic of learning general truths through intensely personal relationships shaped the particulars of students' daily routine is explored in the following chapter. It considers how students and teachers in school together created what counted as universal medical knowledge through a particular, personal way of imagining a doctor's work. As they did so, they also created an underlying subjectivity that defined and justified the ways of local practice as the heart of orthodoxy.

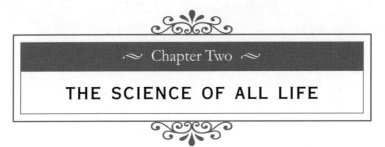

~ Chapter Two ~

THE SCIENCE OF ALL LIFE

Just as medical institutions created but also crossed a line between their world and the larger society, so the culture of learning inside schools made orthodoxy less of a realm apart than many students and teachers supposed. Histories of medical education have focused largely on broad institutional and professional changes and have had surprisingly little to say about the everyday modes of teaching and learning. This chapter looks at midcentury medical education in this immediate sense, seeing it as a matrix of ideals and practices created by teachers and students together, one shaped by happenstance, as well as by design. This means looking at how the intellectual substance of orthodoxy was shaped by its fraternal setting, which flooded medical learning with a moral light as men learned that judging others' character was essential to the work of doctoring. And it means understanding how teachers and students, even as they reached for broad principles and general skills, turned again and again to individual practice as the touchstone of learning.[1]

Specifically, what follows is a look at four contexts of learning that students and teachers themselves emphasized in their writing: lectures, hospital wards, anatomical dissection, and the written medical thesis. Each context was a way for men to master information and fulfill "requirements." But, more important, each was a way for them to imagine what good medicine should be in its southern setting. As men's writing reveals, these four contexts, despite undergoing some change during this period, helped create a remarkable continuity in the physician's identity. Essential to this continuity was the profoundly subjective cast imparted to learning by physicians' reliance on their individual experience in community practice. Although breadth of knowledge remained a powerful goal for orthodoxy, it is crucial to understand how frequently teachers discovered in their own work the most compelling way to articulate what was truly orthodox. By this means, often inadvertently, vernacular ways of interpreting sickness and therapy flowed into schools, inflecting traditional learning with elements of a country orthodox style.

LECTURES: SYNTHESIS AND PRACTICE

Bound for medical school, men often said they were "going to the lectures," making lectures a synecdoche for the entire experience of schooling. Classroom lectures were the badge of physicians' claim to a unique learnedness, and, indeed, among all midcentury healers, M.D.s were the ones most committed to the formal lecture as a way of both conceptualizing and performing the intellectual attainments of a good doctor. Historians since have tended to overlook this dual feature of lectures, for the most part concluding that nineteenth-century schools overemphasized them at the expense of more active forms of learning. And yet, as a flexible, focused means of instruction, lectures were an important means of bringing students and teachers together, moments alive with subjectivity and the performance of an intellectual style. As such, lectures are difficult to recapture; they were oratorical moments, now gone. Still, notes and other writings from both teachers and students together form a rough, composite record of the intellectual work of lectures, inscriptions of a medical mentality as it was being made.

What follows, then, is a look at the rhetorical form of lectures that cut across specific subject matters, giving all of them a distinctive shape. First, lectures typically combined an attempt at grand synthesis with an admonition to be closely empirical. As we will see, these awkwardly joined imperatives were especially important in the mid-nineteenth-century's long-running debate over whether physicians should modify their traditionally aggressive approach to therapy. Second, lectures usually included an injunction to be skeptical, especially charging students to question vernacular wisdom. This charge often was couched in moral language and framed in terms of anecdotes drawn from teachers' practice that took on a unique explanatory power. Finally, lectures peripherally included certain topics, notably race and sexuality, which found no intellectual home of their own in the curriculum (unlike, say, surgery or materia medica) but rather floated free in a way that reveals lectures' conceptual limits and their southern context.

Because lectures were performances, students frequently commented on the teacher's rhetoric and staging, thus helping to integrate a man's personal expressive style into the very substance of medical knowledge. Lectures were not about information only; they demonstrated how to explain and persuade. Louisiana's Dr. Thomas Hunt, as one student noted, became so carried away by physiology that his "oratorical flights [were] hard to follow." Hunt calmed down when it came to pathology, however, because "diseased lungs, livers, and ulcerated bowels did not furnish inspiration to flights of fancy." Teacher John Esten Cooke at Louisville was so soft-spoken and shaky in 1841 that student Courtney Clark wondered how Cooke was able to persuade patients of anything. By contrast, in another student's view, Daniel Drake was a physician in his persuasive prime, exemplified by his ability easily to project his voice to the far reaches of the lecture hall and to command complex explanations "extempore." Similarly, a Transylvania student admired Benjamin Dudley's gift for intellectual organization and was especially moved by Dudley's breaking down in tears as he was narrating a desperate case history.[2]

As student Joseph Jones observed in 1860, an able lecturer demonstrated that the medical mind was capable of synthesizing nothing less than the "phenomena and laws of the universe." Orthodox medicine opened a vision this inclusive, this vast; it was, teachers said repeatedly, the science of all life. And the aim of this synthesis was to understand that Nature was complex but complete, always supplying an "antidote . . . to the poison of the viper." Nature's synthetic patterns lay beneath the fearsome riot of disease and beneath every aspect of medicine from the bloody challenges of surgery to the "dry technicalities" of chemistry. But how, exactly, was this insight concerning Nature to be acted upon? Increasingly after 1830, physicians thought the key was a subtle sense of timing; medicine meant taking action, but it also required a measured patience. Timing was at the center of what was probably the most significant conceptual debate in orthodoxy before the 1880s, the debate over the proposition that many diseases were by nature "self-limiting" and that an aggressive doctor did more harm than good when he immediately assaulted the patient with full-bore therapy. Sometimes called the "nature-trusting heresy" by its opponents, this point of view put forward the "heretical" suggestion that good medicine did not necessarily require immediate therapeutic intervention but rather the deployment of the body's natural recuperative powers. As others have shown, the debate betrayed M.D.s' growing fear that they were perhaps abusing the well-known toxicity of their traditional medicines, as their opponents had been saying for years. Physicians inclined to trust Nature spoke approvingly of what they called "expectant" medicine, that is, a medicine poised to intervene but also alert to the body's cues.[3]

In this way, knowing *when* to act, not simply which procedure or drug to adopt, was the mastery physicians aspired to. And in this sense, "expectant" medicine was a term that nicely captured their ambivalence about where they stood with Nature. On the one hand, to be "expectant" suggested hopefulness and self-confidence. On the other, doctors worried that "expectancy" might turn out to be a fancy term for failing to do something, or doing it too late. Here the battle was joined. Physicians favoring expectancy charged that aggressive, preemptive treatments created a haze of misleading symptoms, interfering with the body's natural efforts to throw off disease. Rejecting this view, critics of expectancy saw little or no distinction between disease and its symptoms. "To treat symptoms," as one exasperated critic said in 1859, "is the motto of every sensible, discerning physician" because there was no other way to relieve patients' suffering. Nature perceived as a feminine force was a crucial aspect of the debate, for feminine powers were known to be both formidable and in need of rational direction. The gendered language underscored the high stakes of getting the timing right. Where advocates of expectancy depicted themselves as engaged in the masculine tasks of active observation and seizing the moment, opponents depicted expectancy as merely waiting, a passive, feminine role.[4]

Joined to lecturers' attention to synthesis and "expectant" timing was a second imperative, that of empirical observation and the mastery of typologies. Thus most lectures included exhaustive lists—of body parts, physical functions, drugs, fever types, chemical reactions. The implication was that a physician was someone who should seek to be neck-deep in small, relentless facts. Indeed, some lecturers, after invoking the marvelous expanse of Nature, spent much more time arranging it into typologies. Charles Short loved Nature's fecundity and its beauty but nonetheless lectured on botany by fixing his eyes on a point at the back of the room and dispassionately ticking off typologies of plants. In his materia medica course at Randolph-Macon Medical College in Virginia in the 1840s, one student carefully listed twenty-one types of therapeutic agents, including emetics, cathartics, diaphoretics, expectorants, astringents, tonics, excitants, sedatives, refrigerants, revellents, entrophics, disinfectants, diluents, and more, each classification further broken down in terms of its "direct" and "indirect" action in the body. Thomas Keller's 1848 notebook suggests how the drumbeat of empirical lists itself became a kind of authority: "Plethora is accumulation of blood. . . . Enemia is deficiency of blood in any part. Hyperenemia is congestion or oversupply of blood in minute vessels. . . . Tone is firm organization [of any body part]. Excitement is healthy action in the organ." The effect was to elevate orthodoxy as the supremely empirical intellectual discipline, and thus to possess Nature not only by sensing her vast rhythms but also by way of inventory.[5]

Thus, the distinct rhetorical power of lectures consisted of a tide of grand, synthetic claims about Nature and the importance of timing, which flowed into streams of particular diseases, symptoms, and medicines and then circulated back into the vast ocean of knowledge. Although physicians shared an empirical impulse with other kinds of healers, the systematic movement from lists to synthesis and back again was distinctive to orthodox medicine. Indeed, M.D.s underscored the importance of this dynamic by braiding moral instruction into their lectures, suggesting that, through his unique intellectual grasp on knowledge, a physician might lead his patients and even his community to systematic thinking and right behavior. Teacher Francis Porcher's lecture notes, for instance, show that he laced his teaching of materia medica with impassioned reminders to students that medical practice was a moral endeavor, highly visible within the community and best employed carefully. A doctor's knowledge of medicines could not be separated from a "delicacy, tact, sagacity" in using them.[6]

In all, the message was an interestingly mixed one. Though treating popular knowledge with some care, most lecturers also voiced an intense skepticism of it. They especially emphasized the moral necessity of confronting popular ignorance of the sensory and perceptual complexity of the human body. The physician thus appears as a kind of intellectual gadfly, stinging credulous medical students first. Edward Geddings at the Medical College of Georgia, for instance, was at pains to tell his students (in a lecture on the eye) that stars do not twinkle, despite what lovers say and what students' mothers had told them; the twinkling star is a deception wrought by imperfect vision. And despite what they might have read, table-tapping and levitation are not caused by spirits, or even by con artists, but by "a fatigue of the sensitive nerves of the fingers." There is a relentless physical reductionism in this skeptical approach; like Geddings, many teachers relentlessly implied that medical knowledge cut against the grain of a profound popular reluctance to think about the sheer physicality of life. For some teachers, this meant probing the borders of students' religious faith by using religious imagery and stories to drive a point home in a challenging way. Samuel Gross provoked one student in 1873 by arguing that the symptoms of Job and King David suggested that "they were affected with some loathsome disorder. . . . you know what affection I mean—." The student wrote to his friend wondering if such a shocking assertion might be true.[7]

Most lecturers modeled the good doctor's obligation to set his neighbors straight by telling brief, personal stories drawn from practice. The narrative simplicity of these practice anecdotes, their seeming offhandedness, should not disguise the explanatory power invested in them. As we will see in following chapters, lecture anecdotes were related to daybook entries, case notes, and case narratives as the conceptual bedrock of physicians' identity. Teachers often told a personal story at just the point in the lecture where the clinching argument had to be made, and so anecdotes became far more than illustration; they became the point of the afternoon's talk. Anecdotes sharply cautioned students that everything they were learning about disease, the body, and medicines was brought into focus *only* by seeing it applied in a particular setting and with individual patients. Examples of failure served as well as examples of success. One teacher, lecturing on pleurisy, drove home his point by saying of his wrongly placed trust in a certain medicine, "I have killed some by this kind of treatment."[8]

By way of anecdotes, then, a teacher introduced into lectures something about himself, as well as about practice. A lecture on the treatment of children with diphtheria, probably by Warren Stone at Georgia in 1866, gives a sense of how such glimpses of the sickroom—scattered liberally throughout lectures— drew on the warmth of a teacher's bedside work. As a practitioner, Stone appears both authoritative and conflicted. In treating children with diphtheria, he said,

> You are justified in blowing alum or tannin down the larynx and even strong solution of N. Silver. I have seen so many bad effects that I am discouraged in its use. . . . Children sometimes get up from playing with toys and die. You should warn parents of the fatal tendency to the larynx for sudden symptoms of suffocation. . . . Tracheotomy has failed so often here in this climate. . . . If you treat a child for diptheria [*sic*] and it gets better don't let it go out of the house nor out of the room for the disease is apt to return when the child is exposed to visicitudes [*sic*] of temperature. I touched the patch [that is, the characteristic membrane in the throat] with nitro muriatic acid and the child got well but its foolish mother took it to the circus and it relapsed.[9]

Here are realities of practice captured midflight. By couching his therapeutic information in a confidential, almost confessional tone, and by drawing upon a domestic world familiar to students (children at play, the circus), Stone invites their acceptance and agreement. And yet because key elements of the story do not sit easily together, a seemingly simple recitation of detail yields a glimpse of the difficulties of practice. For instance, although Stone articulates a physician's moral duty to warn parents, he speaks with contempt for "foolish" ones who do not take his advice. With equal ambivalence, he details a particular therapeutic mode—the alum, tannin, and silver nitrate—about which he also admits being "discouraged." And again, his observation that tracheotomy often fails in the South (an allusion to the well-known link between warm climate and the risk of "fever") does not lead him to positively disallow it. In these ways, Stone's narrative portrays the complex reality of practice more forcefully than if he had simply pronounced it: recommendation and risk go hand in hand; general rules have particular exceptions; families cannot be wholly trusted as caregivers.

The larger intellectual implication of such anecdotes was that the many truths flowing from orthodox synthesis and empiricism might be—in practice *must* be—compressed into essential, authoritative maxims or rules of thumb. For instance, student John Knox heard Louis Dugas, at Georgia, conclude an 1843 lecture on intestinal worms with this single maxim: "[worms] never cause disease until you are called to treat for some [other] disease." Similarly, another teacher summed up his encyclopedic remarks on liver and skin disease with his personal rule: "the liver has no more sympathy with the skin than with *the boots* a man wears." Period. By transcribing anecdotes and maxims in their notes, students made these small certainties a satisfying end to their journey through a forest of names and principles. At the same time, for teachers, maxims elevated what they had seen on their rounds to the status of general knowledge.[10]

Although one anecdote might be countered by another, and several of them could together open up more questions than they answered, neither teachers nor students seem to have criticized this way of knowing or to have questioned its limits. As a consequence, students and teachers invoked the world of practice in lectures without having to analyze very far the social relations that went into creating and maintaining that world. Anecdotes gestured, in a lifelike and enticing way, toward an entire world of doctor and patient, bedside and community, without letting students see very far into the complex assumptions and persuasions necessary to inhabit it.

This was true regardless of whether the lecture concerned materia medica, obstetrics, or some other formal subject matter. And it was the case for certain subjects that never quite became lecture topics at all. These latter are especially interesting because they suggest how physicians, using anecdotes to shape knowledge, in effect dispersed certain subjects throughout the curriculum rather than giving them their own intellectual home. Sexuality is a particularly striking example of how an area of human experience with obvious implications for health had no clear place in the curriculum. Teachers of obstetrics, not surprisingly, most often approached the subject of sex, but only in the most halting, oblique way. Even into the 1870s, empirical evidence of human sexuality was almost nonexistent and synthesis tentative, and, just as important, bedside anecdotes were especially awkward. Although able to describe in great detail labor and delivery in childbirth, midcentury teachers of obstetrics remained puzzled by the physiology of sex, debating the function of menstruation and unsure about how the sexual act resulted in conception. Only women—not men—were puzzled about at any length. M.D. theses on obstetrical topics, a fair measure of what lecturers talked about, show a sharply dichotomized view of women as sexual beings. One kind of lecture abstracted women as "woman" and "the feminine," while the other focused on close, anatomical descriptions of childbirth. In both approaches there is almost complete silence about sexuality.[11]

Sex occasionally appeared in physiology lectures as a nearly irresistible force with a disturbing potential for both harm and rescue. An MCSSC student learned in 1854 that engaging in sex before marriage, which his teacher called "premature concubinage"—a wonderful blend of scientific and moral language—was "very injurious and [he] says nothing exhausts, and enervates the body more, or hurries old age faster." Masturbation was the Scylla to the Charybdis of "concubinage." Harmful physiologically in obscure ways, masturbation clearly was adverse in its social consequences, as the guilty man avoided good company. In a weirdly circular way, sexual intercourse now became a therapy. For a man far gone in "onanism," a Louisiana teacher told his class in the early 1830s, "the only rational advice you can give is one that will not fail to cure. It is to tell him to have intercourse with females." He understood the irony here but told his students that sex was replete with moral and physical difficulties and that while "an angel from heaven could give better advice," this was his best.[12]

Although such frankness could be refreshing, it also raised the troublesome extent to which the world of the medical school was—or should be—a realm apart from vernacular knowledge. Faculty themselves walked the permeable boundary between the vernacular and the orthodox. Student J. E. Allen transcribed at length the remarks of MCG physiology professor Edward Geddings in 1874 as Geddings (and Allen) danced around the topic of sexual intercourse. Geddings began by noting that sex was a subject of art and literature, putting his spin on a familiar and never inappropriate text, the Bible: "so Adam begot Abel & so they begat each other to the end of the chap[ter]." From here, Geddings offered brief observations on the variety of sexual behavior with reference to Mark Twain's sexually willing Sandwich Island girls and included learned references to Jupiter and Io and to the Old Masters' explicit sexual scenes (which he assumed his students would know). Finally, he arrived at his own status as "an old bachelor," although, he added, he was not entirely without information. Once he witnessed "a fellow student sup the celestial nectar." What struck him was "the beastly visage of the male while the female was as if asleep all composure." All told, Geddings concluded, the whole matter of sex was still pretty much a mystery, for "the sexual act is one done in private in the cover of darkness & between sheets, & no one has hardly ever seen it performed, the reason is no doubt because as the Frenchman said that although 'the feeling was nice the position was dam ritacule.' "[13]

Geddings's remarks are a colloquial tour de force, self-deprecating, with a bit of pandering mixed into what seems genuine embarrassment. Strikingly, he does not claim to be saying anything uniquely orthodox; in his tale there is little to separate school from society. And so teachers relegated sexuality, about which they knew little as physicians, to the broad cultural realm of gender, about which as men they knew much more. This approach did not remove sex as a medical topic but left it vague and at large within the walls of the school.

Perhaps most striking of all, because it had none of sexuality's personal awkwardness, and because it was a uniquely "southern" concern by the 1840s, the matter of race similarly was dispersed throughout the curriculum. Thus, as with the subject of sex, orthodox views mingled with popular ideas about the nature of African American health. Of course, lecturers' oblique view of race does not imply the absence of racial theory in scientific thinking at large. Such theory serving white dominance became more sophisticated and extreme during the century. What is significant in terms of medical lectures, though, is that broad racial theory did not find its own clear place in the curriculum. Schools did not even offer separate courses in the diseases and health care of slaves, let alone racial theory, despite advancing the argument that a southern-trained M.D.'s familiarity with slaves was an excellent reason for slave owners to choose him over others. What little teachers had to say about African Americans aimed to illustrate orthodoxy's unique breadth, and here as elsewhere lecturers invested individual practice with sweeping powers of explanation. As a result, physicians' views did not stray very far from the those of most slave owners, especially in the way they uncritically mingled notions of race and servitude.[14]

The broad picture of black health and sickness that emerges piecemeal from lectures was that there were very few diseases unique to African Americans, although the "African race" had certain distinct "predispositions" to becoming sick. This meant that blacks as individuals could be treated with the same drugs and techniques as whites, although doctors were expected to be aware of certain broad, racial tendencies, always defined by a white "norm." African Americans were seen as more vulnerable to lung ailments, for instance, and to "congestion" generally, and thus to dropsy and to ailments associated with cold temperatures. Teachers considered a black patient more resistant to disease at first, but, as one student expressed it, "when his system does . . . succumb, it is completely overpowered." Blacks responded similarly to harsh drugs, and thus a good doctor used his medicines with special attention to blacks' lesser tolerance for them. These working assumptions were only briefly noted for the most part, mostly as asides in lectures on other topics. The clear implication was that whatever was the nature of "race," it was more important for a practitioner to have a few rules of thumb to take to the slave patient's bedside.[15]

Moreover, when teachers did hazard generalizations about black health they ambiguously combined a largely implicit racist physiology with a much closer attention to the environment created by slavery. Teachers sometimes spoke of "Negro" characteristics as if they were typical of Africans everywhere; other times, however, the implication was that the only conditions that mattered were the immediate ones of housing, diet, and general care under southern slavery. One affliction deemed largely (but not exclusively) a "Negro disease," cachexia africana, or "dirt-eating," received such attention. The disease, signaled by a victim's languor, his "depraved" behavior (dirt-eating, as well as lying about it), and his ultimate death, was almost always presented as deserving of more attention in school than it received. Indeed, authors of M.D. theses on cachexia africana included a disproportionate number of already experienced practitioners, who seem to have been gently rebuking schools for neglecting an important topic. In any case, even though students speculated that something in African blood, some "impurities of a specifically poisonous character," might support the affliction, the clear consensus was that poor diet, poor living conditions, and, interestingly, slave-master conflict were most important in explaining dirt-eating in slaves.[16]

Judging from the larger number of M.D. theses on "plantation health" than on "Negro diseases," at least some lecturers considered slavery's impact on health more broadly, though typically doing so in the midst of lectures on "regular" topics such as materia medica. And, again, the relation between race and environment was wholly ambiguous. In F. Perry Pope's 1837 thesis on the "management" of slaves, for instance, is fascinating ethnographic detail about the diet, clothing, work experience, and even the recreation of slaves. Pope, like other students, was able to see slaves as individuals and observed human variety in their social life. Yet now and again he hints at underlying assumptions about race that confound his picture of slavery as a social environment. At times, "race" has the sense of ethnicity, as when he writes that "our Negroes are a thoughtless Race of uneducated people, so their amusements are of the simplest nature." But at other times he implies that a biological aspect of race is somehow important, as when he notes that "from Color, Habit, and Diet, they are much more liable to chronic forms of disease." Here "color" clearly implies a biological dimension to African American "predispositions" to sickness.[17]

Among other things, by smoothing over the distinction between what they considered to be "natural" to blacks and what was imposed upon them by slavery, doctors avoided a conflict between what they thought was medically advisable and what masters considered the prerogatives of ownership. Thus, a South Carolina student took note of poor slave diet and "filthy huts" in the up-country of his state. But he tempered the implied criticism of masters by observing that, overall, blacks "enjoy as good health as any [whites]" living in "our most healthy sandhills." Students wrote, too, of slaves' long hours of hard field labor in bad weather but diluted the force of such observations by noting that slaves as a group foolishly ignored masters' sound advice, or feigned illness. Medical learning therefore tamped down what might have been expansive issues in public health into the confines of a common sense serving the institution of slavery: feed slaves good food, keep their houses in repair, do not overwork them. Other common threats to slaves' health that might easily have been highlighted in theses—how best to treat the wounds worked by the lash, for example, or the medical problems of rape or abuse—went unmentioned in obvious deference to slave owners.[18]

Thus, teachers and students together did not pursue very far the question of precisely how or whether "race" mattered in sickness. Racial assumptions had no clear context in the curriculum and were given no empirical scrutiny. This allowed some students to avoid, others to canonize, whatever half-formed racial theory filled their minds. Although this lack of analysis may have forestalled the more formal, oppressive theories of black inferiority that arose at the very end of the century, the immediate effect of lecturers' approach to race was to naturalize it as a passive setting for health rather than seeing it as an active set of assumptions and practices defining it.

As a result, slavery and race, along with sexuality, floated obscurely throughout the curriculum. They came into focus only as individual teachers allowed them to, revealing an area of orthodox thought built upon a disturbingly unstable line between medical school and the larger community young doctors would join. As teachers did not give either sex or race the solid-seeming reality of surgery or materia medica, there were fewer terms to memorize, fewer cases to study, and less "science" to be articulated. At the same time, not able to ignore them, physicians and their students approached these subjects obliquely, configuring them in a way that allowed them to remain in the popular domain. In this way, physicians learned not to innovate in matters of race or gender.

Instead, they sought to balance what they learned of blood and bone and other "purely" medical topics against vast areas of knowledge that remained at large in the community. In a medical school world seeking to be apart from the surrounding society, gender and race were, strictly speaking, nowhere in particular. But in another sense, they were everywhere and uniquely impervious to change.

Not only did this mean that popular, conventional wisdom continually gained new life inside schools; it also implied that an alert physician might discover genuine medical science in his own local practice. In the embrace of synthesis and empiricism, in the reliance on practice anecdotes, and in the careful handling of the sexual and racial values dearly axiomatic to most members of the free, white community is clear evidence of orthodox education's roots in popular values and its dependence on the vernacular world of practice. To be sure, some physicians were aware of this ironic contour to medical learning, and it spurred them to continue to define medical school as a world apart. But even for these men, there was no escaping the fact that lectures were shot through with evidence that professional exclusivity was neither as seamless nor as steady as they wished.

CLINICS: FOREIGN BODIES AND APPENDED CHARITY

As a counterpoint to lectures, work with sick people in clinics or hospital wards was eagerly awaited by most students. Kentucky student Lunsford Yandell spoke for many when he declared in 1826 that "a *bedside view* of diseases will be more profitable, than the hearing of lectures." Older histories of medicine suggested that students had virtually no hospital experience until the 1870s, and although recent histories have revised this view, emphasis still is on how episodic it was compared to the modern system of internships and residencies. The view here is that by the 1840s clinical work with sick people, while uneven and not living up to elite reforms of the 1880s, was nonetheless widespread and taken seriously. Students were drawn to the clinic's or hospital ward's world-apart strangeness compared to lectures or even apprenticeship. The clinic measurably added to students' sense of having a unique identity, becoming an important site for what it meant to be a doctor.[19]

This was so, especially, because the hospital opened up a world little known to most students, the world of the urban, immigrant poor. These were the people on whose bodies students put their hands and in whose lives students tested ways of exercising whatever authority they possessed. What needs exploring, then, is how the mid-nineteenth-century ward was a place not simply for learning skills but for imagining the social and moral implications of hands-on medicine. It was a place apart from familiar rural life and its configurations of class, gender, and race. And it was a place in which a subjective sense of caregiving as a form of charity became for many students the moral resolution of the ward's often brutal events.

Hospitals were a barometer of nineteenth-century urban social need. Thousands of sick poor people passed through the doors of institutions such as Charleston's Roper Hospital, Louisville's Marine Hospital, and the huge Charity Hospital in New Orleans, which had 1,000 beds by 1860. Working poor, transients, the homeless; inmates of almshouses and seamen's hospitals—these were the people described enthusiastically by schools as the "large, floating, and dependent population" offered up only by large cities for the betterment of medical training. In 1850 alone, more than 18,000 patients were admitted (and re-admitted) to Charity. Most suffered from acute problems—injuries resulting from accidents; a sudden, alarming illness. Most checked themselves in, and many, fearful or fed up or feeling better, discharged themselves, sometimes against doctors' advice ("absconded" was the term used in Charity's ward records). Indeed, aside from a small number of chronic cases who sometimes stayed two or three years, patients seem to have come and gone pretty much as they chose, a few paying but most not, and wards emerge as chaotic and largely anonymous in even the most favorable accounts.[20]

Arriving on the wards, students wrote about the riveting, ad hoc jumble of suffering, transience, teaching, and caregiving. The sheer strangeness of the hospital excited the young men and moved them to words that parsed medical learning into sets of novel skills. Few students commented directly on how what they were seeing comported with the lecture's demand for synthesis and empiricism. Rather, particular techniques commanded students' note-taking. Traill Green, for example, recorded the important observation that, contrary to his intuition, it was best "not [to] make a long stump" in amputations of the leg, for a long stump would prove a greater inconvenience once the patient recovered and began moving about. A Transylvania student was satisfied to learn a clever way to hold a convulsive patient's arm during a venesection so as to "not bespatter anything around." Similarly, Charleston student William Whetstone carefully observed a time-saving procedure for tying off arteries in surgery. Many students witnessed complicated events, such as childbirth, previously only read about, and they quickly became aware of new therapeutic discoveries, such as the advent of general anesthesia in 1846–47. Indeed, many students realized on the ward just what teachers hoped they would: a sense of the stark physicality of disease complementing the relatively abstract lessons of the lecture.[21]

Most students did not pause in their desire to "get rite down among the patients," as one said. Wading into the concentration of bodies, the open suffering, and the pressure to make decisions—however cushioned by mentors—students reached out to fellow students, tempering their fraternal bonds in the new heat of firsthand work. Thus many students understood for the first time how the actual treatment of patients realized orthodoxy's insistence that caregiving had moral, as well as intellectual substance. Student T. L. Laws grasped a key lesson when he realized that hospital work posed so many difficult choices that lofty principles often proved too rigid; there were no moral ends in this work, only moral means. The doctor therefore had an ethical responsibility to think of the greater good, rather than doing things by rote or enhancing his reputation; the good doctor would "*elevate* the *Medical Profession* and not be *elevated by it*." And yet students' words reveal them caught up as well in male bravado and callousness. "We are cutting and slashing away, tearing everything up by the roots," wrote Louisiana student William Bonner excitedly about the many surgical cases he was seeing several times a week on the wards. "Those we do not kill we cure &c.," he added, discovering the reality behind this cliché of allopathic aggressiveness. Killing and curing were side by side on the wards; what else would one expect? The hospital was a world of risk and bodies, and a man's job was to make his mark assertively in the spirit of such a place. Students sometimes apologized for their blunt descriptions, but they sent the letters home anyway. Francis Jones wrote to his wife, Cleopatra, "I have saw several people butchered since I got here," assuring her that this was necessary; to see such things firsthand "can't help but make [me] a good *Doctor*."[22]

It is not easy to separate nervous boasting from nervous brutality in this kind of writing; either way, the language was quintessentially masculine. Students knew that what they were seeing or doing had the potential to shock ordinary sensibilities back home. Even in quieter moments, students were struck by the dissimilarity between patients on the wards and patients in most rural, southern communities. For one thing, the wards housed very few African Americans, a fact that stood in stark contradiction to southern schools' claims that local practitioners' familiarity with treating blacks was "so important in the South" and a reason to patronize local schools. In large hospitals such as Charity and Roper before the war, for example, there were only small numbers of African Americans, despite the fact that slaves were a large proportion of the surrounding population. Slaves were scarce in hospitals because most masters preferred to have them treated at home, not only because it was more convenient, but also because slave owners feared disease-ridden hospitals and, perhaps, clumsy students. This situation could not have bolstered students' confidence in the axiom that southern doctors should be trained in a southern context. And it may have served to heighten students' uneasiness in diagnosing and treating black patients when they did see them.[23]

Indeed, antebellum students' infrequent work with blacks in clinics seems to have muffled, even more than in lectures, any systematic thinking about race. Even though they appeared in small numbers, slaves and slave bodies were not singled out as either exotic or alien. In fact, some schools pointedly reminded students that slaves were fully inside the social order, a "class of the community," in the words of the Medical College of the State of South Carolina. That is, slaves' place in the social hierarchy—not the mysteries that might be bound up in race—defined the slave as a patient. It was axiomatic that the surgical techniques learned on slaves' bodies were transferable to the bodies of whites, race notwithstanding. Similarly, when schools used female slaves as subjects for "practical instruction in Obstetrics," it appears that most of what students learned was assumed to be equally useful in white women's cases. Not her race but her availability and the calculation of her value as property is what chiefly differentiated the slave patient on the wards.[24]

In this regard, it was the treatment of the hospital's far more numerous white poor that opened up the full complexity of clinics as places for pedagogy, dependence, and morality. Objectifying the poor en masse as an "opportunity" for instruction, schools tried to recruit them, one school inviting "friends" to "send . . . persons in indigent circumstances," as if the hospital were simply a benign place to pass the time. Students commented on the strangeness of the immigrant poor, who had no "masters" responsible for them and who often spoke strangely and embraced suspect religions; they were alien in a way that African Americans were not. Many students easily mixed condescension with contempt, particularly with regard to immigrant women, who did not easily fit into the masculine bifurcation of females into either sexual objects or moral exemplars. That students saw poor women as not feminine like the women back home was made worse by the fact that many women on the wards were seen in childbirth, a prime setting for student anxiety. Southern student Marmaduke Kimbrough in a Philadelphia lying-in ward in 1859 wrote that "it feels just like sticking your hand in a soap gourd when you put it into these old Irish women" and commented on what to him was the dubious distinction of having "conducted two little Irish babies into America." Another student encountered a poor woman "from the wilds of Indiana" who underwent an ovariotomy in front of the entire class—an "awful array" of people but "not enough to daunt [her]." The woman's courage under the knife in so public a place both elevated and lowered her in the student's view. He saw in her something essential, something connected to the very "'bone & sinew' of our country." And yet he believed that her poverty had thoroughly dulled her feminine sensibilities, allowing her to withstand the surgery "as a pig does spaying," without full awareness of the event and with perhaps less pain.[25]

It is important that this view of the hospital's white poor was more demeaning than anything else students wrote about any other group of patients. Social class, as well as gender, thus became a key aspect of how students combined power and morality on the wards, learning ways to manipulate patients' compliance, as well as their bodies. Henry Clay Lewis's ward students, for example, are forever tricking poor patients instead of persuading them. Similarly, Nathaniel Siewers, disgusted by one "excessively dirty" hospital patient, discovered that he could get the man to bathe with "the strongest turpentine soap" if he first gave him what the man considered real medicine—a dose from a doctor's bottle. So Siewers gave him a flavored water to drink, and the man agreed to take the bath. Sometimes students witnessed the use of force so memorable that the words of poor patients enter into student notes. One afternoon in 1847, for instance, Charles Hentz accompanied his surgery teacher, Samuel Gross, to witness an operation under the new general anesthesia. Hentz soon realized that the patient, an "old man," had not been told that he would be given the new drug. Gross and the students tied the man down, which was normal procedure in surgery, but when they clapped the ether-imbued cloth over his face, the man panicked. Gross tried to "pacify" him, Hentz recorded, but the man would not be stilled: "Why doctor, I'd fight the devil," he told Gross. Even as he was slipping under the anesthesia, still resisting, he cried, "Dr., you put me in bodily fear."[26]

Clearly, however, caring about what poor patients thought or feared was not high on students' list of things to learn. Rather, as teachers and schools surely knew, how to assert one's power as a physician was the overarching lesson on the wards, linking visit to visit, procedure to procedure. Students' self-interested learning became inscribed in the most self-centered fashion. Nathaniel Siewers wrote that he would be "very sorry to lose" his first obstetrical patient if she died, but he was just as concerned that she "give me no trouble" should she live. And so another student, having dosed, bled, and blistered a man with ophthalmia, decided that while he would not "flatter" the patient with a cheerful prognosis, neither would he tell him the truth: the man was going to lose his eyesight. Most students seem to have welcomed the power to manipulate the information patients received; they took satisfaction, as Thomas McIntosh wrote to his sister in 1876, in discovering how to make hospital patients "think that anything that I tell them is law." Much more rare are students who wrote of suffering patients, "poor things, I pitied them"; or, who, like Solomon Mordecai, told of finding "pleasure in being instrumental in giving relief." Suffering was everywhere on the wards, but it became something familiar very quickly, an atmosphere in which to shape a repertoire of practice skills and paternalism. "[P]aradoxical as it may seem," one perceptive young doctor wrote, the hospital offered the poor "the kindest yet the grossest treatment imaginable."[27]

Thus, braided into images of blood, power, and Irish patients is a sense of how ward rounds closed certain moral avenues for students. Learning objective skills was essential; searching out the ways of sympathy was not. For the most part, the disparity in power between doctor and patient simply was accepted as a reality, clearing the way for novice doctors to act aggressively in the name of science and their own skills. Time and again, students were pulled toward this or that individual case only to move away, with what seems like relief, back into the flow along the rows of beds, along the pathway from admission, to diagnosis, to treatment and discharge, or, "if the disease proves fatal, . . . to the *dead-house*, with scalpel in hand."[28]

Throughout the midcentury decades, students grappled with the novelty of the ward and its inmates, using them to shape their identity as physicians. Most came away with a strengthened sense of joining a brotherhood that knew a special world of sensation and morality. They were impressed by what their mentors knew and did to make the ward into an orthodox domain, even as many were disturbed by the larger world of the urban poor that flowed into the hospital. Impressive, too, was what orthodoxy did not know. In a sense, an insider's knowledge of orthodoxy's limits—and their moral implications—became part of the exclusive knowledge M.D.s attained on the wards. After weeks in the hospital in 1873, student E. L. McGehee accepted, with as much relief as disappointment, that "the truth is, I thought till late there was more virtue in the drugs—that our noble vocation could do more with disease." William Cozart similarly emerged from his South Carolina clinical work in 1856 with a sense of limits, too, shrewdly understanding that medicine fundamentally was defined by what teachers knew from their own bedside practice. "In fact," he said, grasping an essential reality of country orthodoxy, "their practice is their teaching." The wards taught that knowledge was grounded not so much in lofty principles as in a practitioner's personal judgment and, ultimately, in his moral character. The hospital, wrote Albert Bachelor to his sweetheart, taught a mature student that the "wretched specimens of depraved & suffering humanity" were not only "fertile fields for inquiry . . . into the sad varieties of human pain & weakness" but also gave the doctor "a wide scope & exercise for the intellect." These realities, taken together, "tend to elevate the thoughts" and reveal the moral lining of orthodoxy's scientific claims.[29]

There is little doubt that this mix of personal experience and moral focus, bound up in the fraternal closeness of mentors and students, imparted a strong continuity to what students experienced in clinical settings throughout mid-century. It was a continuity resistant to change because it was so successful in permitting students to navigate at will the peculiar channels of class, race, and physical dependence found in hospitals. At the same time, however, hospital training did little to resolve the problematic relation of this world to the communities where students would practice. If anything, schools' claim that students would see on the wards "every species of human affliction, and specimens of nearly every variety of the human race," seems critically misleading. Compared to hospital patients, patients in rural communities occupied a far broader range of ages, classes, and afflictions, and they possessed a much greater independence from a physician's raw power. Moreover, except in major cities at the very end of the century, hospital practice did not remain part of ordinary practitioners' careers and did not shape the character of their brotherhood once schooling had ended. Strikingly, then, the novelty and intensity of the hospital during medical school obscured its idiosyncrasy, shaping students in ways not altogether suited for their practice to come.[30]

In this light, the problematic place of compassion in caregiving emerges as perhaps the most important reality of community practice that ward experience left essentially unaddressed. Apart from references to a collective "wretchedness," students' sense of suffering and sympathy is almost never put into words. This suggests that it was left up to each individual to decide the relation of medical authority to moral sensibility. It is not that hospital patients were treated as inhuman objects; it was unusual, in fact, as it would not be a century later, to hear students collapse individuals into their disease (calling a patient "the fibroid tumor on ward two," for instance). Even so, the closest approach most students seem to have made to fellow feeling with patients was not in terms of sympathy but in terms of charity—a very different calculus of caregiving. By adopting charity as a posture toward the sick, students gave a distinct texture to the tangled matter of class, emotion, and caregiving that they were learning along with techniques in amputations and childbirths. Thinking of oneself as acting charitably in the patient's best interests was a cleanly functional and self-protective image of doctoring. It acknowledged—indeed, expanded—the distance between doctor and patient, allowing the former to disengage emotionally while also giving him a welcome opportunity to smooth out disturbing issues of power, work, and his authority. Although this may have worked passably well on the poor wards, it remained to be seen whether it would suffice among neighbors at home. Hospital training obscured this difficulty from students' view and from their teachers' lists of things to be learned while walking through the wards.

ANATOMY: OPENED BODIES AND THE MORAL URGE

In different ways, lectures and clinics each bolstered orthodox medicine's allegiance to broad learning and its fascination with empirical discovery, thus defining how schools departed from the larger society's more utilitarian sense that what mattered in medicine was healing. At the same time, each context prefigured for students (and preserved for teachers) elements of a country orthodox style that privileged a practitioner's personal experience, inescapably local and moral, as basic to all medical knowledge. The resulting tension between these two modes of learning became strikingly apparent in the study of anatomy, a subject that uniquely stirred medical students to write in considerable detail. Anatomy was esteemed as the essence of current science throughout the mid-nineteenth century, combining well-defined practical goals, a learned tradition, and the newest instrumental and diagnostic techniques. Equally impressive to students was that anatomy required handling the bodies of dead people, something that challenged conventional morality in troubling but exciting ways. For these reasons, looking at how students and teachers together constructed anatomy as an academic subject—indeed, an academic *practice*—furthers our understanding of how orthodoxy was made on the border between school and society. And it sharpens our sense of how medical learning not only consisted of certain assumptions and techniques surrounding the body and disease but also was shaped by a volatile moral sense of medicine's realm.

By the 1830s, there was little disagreement among physicians nationally that advances in the understanding of human anatomy, from the eighteenth century forward, best exemplified the flowering of orthodox medical science. Anatomy brought physicians' commitment to empiricism and synthesis (looking at particular bodies, generalizing about all bodies) into a clearly "practical" context through the dissection of cadavers. By mastering the knife, saw, and trocar in disassembling a human body, students' immediate aim was to learn its skeletal structure, the placement and relation of the internal organs, and such things as how bones fit together, how muscles were attached to them, and how veins and arteries could be located. Such knowledge had obvious application in surgery and obstetrics. In a larger sense, anatomy mapped reformers' logic of why basic science deserved a featured place in medical school. The causes and transmissions of disease might be mysterious, but disease always was embodied; and bodies were to be understood, first of all, as structures (or in many teachers' religious idiom, as "temples"). Anatomy's province, the study of the body at rest, thus had a logical priority over therapeutics, and also over physiology (the study of the body seething with healthy growth and decay) and pathology (the body in the grip of disease).[31]

The privileging of anatomy was so intense that competition between medical schools in the South, as elsewhere in the United States, was framed largely in terms of who possessed the best resources for anatomical study. The language of school circulars is eager and superlative in this regard. At the University of Louisiana in 1838, for instance, the facilities for dissection were "nowhere equaled in this country." At every dissection table at Louisville in 1842, "there is a light fully equal to twelve candles" and the ventilation of the room was superior. And, of course, there was the supply of bodies. As the Nashville school noted of its cadavers in 1852 (with unusual frankness), never mind "how they were obtained, where they came from or to whom they belonged. . . . The whole secret consists in the proper combination of five magic letters—M-O-N-E-Y." Most schools were not so blunt, but they nonetheless found it necessary to assure students that they would never go wanting for "material" and noted, accurately, that there were fewer restrictive laws governing anatomy in the South than elsewhere. Another southern advantage was the large number of slaves. The South Carolina school's antebellum circulars, for example, assured students that "subjects for dissection are obtained in ample number, chiefly from the black population."[32]

At the same time, schools spoke of studying anatomy in coded, almost mysterious terms. Students were told that in the "dissecting room . . . the medical student must make himself *really* a physician." But what did this mean? Almost coyly, schools promised students an unspecified "practical acquaintance" with a kind of knowledge "beyond that which may be derived from books." In part, of course, such disembodied language was self-protective; schools wished to avoid roiling up unpopular images of a body on a table—*somebody's* body, after all. But such language also doubtless aimed to counter students' own revulsion or timidity. It served to frame the subject as remote from emotions of any kind, except for an avid empiricism. Even at its most precise, schools' language suggested something fine-grained and delicate, something almost alluringly hidden: students of anatomy would come to know the "intimate structure" of the body, the "morbid specimens" and "primary tissues" uncovered in "private dissections" that yielded "minute knowledge" of form and structure.[33]

Schools added to anatomy's exotic image by devising certain rules and behaviors delineating it as a realm apart, even within the school itself. At Louisville, for example, dissections took place in the large surgical room at the top of the building. The lighting was better there; also it was less likely that casual visitors would wander unsuspecting into the carnage. There was special dress, too. Students wore "black cambric aprons over their clothes, fitting with close buttons at the wrist & neck, & a band tied round the waist—, & a black cap." Groups of students began working together on a single body as a team, later dividing it up into parts for individual work. To attend J. Edwards Holbrook's anatomy class at MCSSC in the 1850s was to see the body—the solid-seeming body—disassembled into seven distinct systems of organs. Seemingly reduced, Holbrook implied, the body was in fact enhanced by the number of its remarkable functions, of locomotion, digestion, absorption, circulation, respiration and voice, urine and reproduction, and enervation, intellect, and the senses. Each of these functions in turn opened up to reveal further layers; for instance, the intellect seen as an organ system invited scrutiny of the "several parts composing the nervous system, as the brain and its coverings; the spinal marrow; and the individual nerves are next described; together with the senses—the eye, nose, ear, skin and tongue" and so on, deeper into the particulars of the body's interior. When exhausted, the cadaver was taken to the "dead room," in the basement, where the remains were dropped into a deep well. After each session, students washed their hands and arms thoroughly, although sometimes they could, "in spite of hard washing, smell the stench on our fingers even at the [dinner] table."[34]

So revealed, the body attracted the student not through its vital wholeness but through its being reduced to a "system" of related parts and tolerances. The work of the anatomist was powerful for its controlled exploration of both breadth and particularity, reaching beneath the surface with privileged instruments and nomenclature. Some students discovered a surprising personal significance in this work. Every discovery, and just as important, "every term" that he mastered in his work with the "decay" of cadavers, student W. H. Timmerman realized in 1854, "is expressive of some portion of [my] own frame . . . which is then perhaps vibrating, contracting, and pulsating" even as he worked with the anonymous and stilled body of another. In effect, the immobile, opened body became orthodoxy's most telling motif. For dedicated students, the study of anatomy demonstrated the superficiality of most other ways of understanding mankind. Knowledge of the body, student Joseph Jones wrote to his parents in 1854, made all other kinds of knowledge "only mere accomplishments." In short, by plumbing the stilled body, by demanding that all "anticipations [be] confirmed" by carnal reality, the student fashioned himself into the preeminent man of science. Without anatomical knowledge, in the view of a South Carolina student in 1845, "medicine is an humble art, and [a] degrading occupation. It reduces the physician to the level of the cook." But with anatomical knowledge, wrote Nashville student William Broyles in 1857, "science opens out to us the wide field of the fixed principles of the practice of medicine. It leads us gently to the bedside of the sick."[35]

Or so doctors wished. But the wisdom conferred by anatomical study proved more subjective and more problematic than this. Despite anatomy's general appeal, some students were deeply disquieted by it. In the opened body, disease was present in ways far more daunting than could be simply imagined—horrible in the "grey granulation in the lungs," in the "inflamed stomach and guts." Moreover, the huge gap between cadaver and the living patient troubled some students. In spite of Mr. Broyles's hopes, practical anatomy did not lead students so gently from the corpse to bedside care. Teachers understood this; consider the French, they warned. While French physicians were to be admired for having advanced the understanding of anatomy, they were regarded as notorious for being indifferent caregivers who could scarcely wait for the patient to die so they could get on with their postmortems. A student was wise to be wary lest his interest in anatomy fly too high, leaving therapeutic concerns far below. Becoming glassy-eyed with "diagnosticating between the thousand and one cutaneous eruptions" whose different names had no known bearing on healing made anatomical study just another form of "idle, useless theory," Nashville student William Miller reasoned in 1854. Static anatomical knowledge was of limited help at the volatile sickbed, Miller realized, where what a doctor needed to know was why "one thing sometimes follows another." In fact, anatomy had taught him the uncomfortable truth that the M.D. was, after all, "related to an empiric"—by which he meant an unorthodox tinkerer with the body—"a character which he has always taught himself to despise."[36]

The fear that actual practice thus opened up a huge gulf between the promise of orthodox science and the much deeper mysteries of sickness was joined in students' writing to something even more unsettling. This was the sense that the dissection of human bodies was odd in any event, having a strangeness that extended into dark regions of moral doubt. Students deflected some of their uneasiness through dissection room camaraderie, jokes, and initiation rites. Henry Ivy was relieved one grisly afternoon in 1878 when dissection finally "made me sick for the first time"; it meant that he was normal after all. His fellow students made fun of him, he drank the glass of sugar water prescribed by his teacher, and he got on with the cutting. There was memorization, quizzing, bravado; anything but silence over the bodies. A student placed "a chunk of meat" in the coat pocket of another student, who discovered it later when he reached for his handkerchief. Cigars appeared in the mouths of male corpses and roses on the bodies of women. Cadavers were reduced to parts and parts upgraded to "subjects." "Today, I did my first dissecting," Thomas Wade wrote in his diary in 1851. "My subject was the arm of a woman." For many students, nonetheless, just behind the jokes and the science was a raw fear of handling death. Joseph LeConte, who used his medical degree to prime a life in science, vividly recalled dissection as "strangely fascinating—the very horror of the thing adding greatly to the fascination." The journey from the well-lit, top-floor dissection table to the dead room below mapped the vast distance covered by medical learning compared to the ordinary run of life. Words chosen to describe the experience to the folks back home did so only awkwardly, dressed up with qualifiers that made the experience seem blandly remote or cautiously imprecise. Benjamin Lucas managed to say only that dissection was, all in all, "a 'spectacle,'" and when Solomon Mordecai wrote to his sister that she would be "*astonished* to see with what apparent nonchalance I apply the dissecting knife," the word "apparent" catches the eye.[37]

Indeed, part of the fascination was that the act of opening up the body to view eluded a single grammar of descriptions and tropes, even those of science. The body changed during the act, and the act changed the student's sense of the body, and informing everything was the mystery of life and death. Sometimes the horror of death was transformed into the liveliness of art, the "beauty of a masterly dissection." Dissection was inscribed as a journey into the "mysteries and intricacies of the human organism," and the body was beheld as "a great city" or temple, exemplar of all things "fearfully and wonderfully made" by God. For others, quite differently, the stilled body fascinated because it nonetheless remained sexual. Henry Clay Lewis, after "stealing a kiss from the pulpy mouth of my ladylove," found himself wondering if "even in death, electricity by some peculiar adaptation might not be able to continue [the mouth's] bewitching suction." The struggle was for intellectual footing against horror, and for some students the struggle became obsessive. Lewis portrayed himself as "becoming clean daft on the *subject*," scrutinizing every new social acquaintance as more or less suitable for the knife. Another student caused his friends great concern in 1844 by becoming "almost crazy about the human bones" that he had recovered and scraped clean. Too many different meanings opened to view.

"All the superstitions of ancestors way back in the ages focused in my mind," one doctor recalled about his nights spent dissecting alone, "and to my over-wrought imagination, the sheets covering bodies . . . seemed to be rising."[38]

Stranger still than these transformations were those that blurred the line between student and corpse, and in one way or another led the student to embrace death. Students wrote no more than a line or two in this vein, and the density of their feeling is difficult to gauge. Still, there were at least some students for whom the study of practical anatomy strayed into territory that bordered on the weird or the blasphemous. One student, home on a break from his lectures, took his friend to the family vault and there "admired the skeletons of my *sweet sisters*" and handled the scattered bones of his uncle Walter. Students like William Whetstone seemed bent on raising their family's moral doubts, and perhaps their own, with an enthusiasm for anatomical work that put everything else in service to it. "I like dissecting very much," Whetstone wrote to his mother from Columbia, South Carolina, in 1854. "Only here of late, people do not die fast enough for me." It was such sentiment, revealing a cold, atavistic underside to scientific acumen, that drove another South Carolina medical student, Dandridge Bibb, to reject medicine as a career. After completing his course work in 1846, Bibb wrote a dissertation explaining how the study of anatomy had driven him away from medicine. A youth such as himself, he explained, was "accustomed to reverence the Dead"; however, once in school, "familiarity with corpses hurries him into the opposite extreme." The "heart of the young student becomes tainted and his lips also polluted with impious jests; untill he looks upon the face of the dying, . . . or steps across a grave without a thought, or with only reckless or unholy ones."[39]

Not surprisingly, these fears were shared by parents who worried that their sons would emerge from the strange world of the school deeply immoral. Protestant Christianity animated much of the conversation between students and their parents on the consequences of studying anatomy. Joseph Jones, who after taking his degree at the University of Pennsylvania in 1855 would go on to become a medical teacher and author, responded to his pious parents, who worried that his medical study would diminish his moral, Christian character. Jones's father, the Reverend Charles Colcock Jones, a prominent Presbyterian clergyman, acknowledged that physicians needed to be "grounded in anatomy" but wondered whether it was "necessary to spend *two hours and a half in the dissection room every night*." He reminded Joseph that "in your uses of *the dead*, never forget that '*the Body is the Lord's*'" and that "disrespect & levity & coarseness [*sic*] & vulgarity are all brutish & highly derogatory & criminal." Replying,

Joseph met his father on his own ground, the fall of man. Yes, medical studies might "harden and corrupt the heart," Joseph admitted. But this was not the fault of science. "Does this [dissecting] render the sensibilities callous, brutalize the feelings and obliterate the fear of death?" Joseph asked his father. Surely the answer was no. Man's sinful nature, not anatomical study, was the source of this failing. If anything, the enlightenment of science worked to draw man away from sin.[40]

Joseph's mother, Mary Sharpe Jones, pressed him as well, not so much on the strength of his Christian principles as on her fear that the world of the school was replacing home in his affections. Her picture of him at school, "amidst all the allurements of science & the acquisitions of knowledge," suggested disregard for the moral values of his community. She urged Joseph to permit "the love of Christ to constrain you" and to be mindful that medical learning was not for knowledge alone but so that he might become "the instrument of incalculable blessings to your fellow beings." Mary Jones also wove scenes of home into her letters, tugging at her son with memories of the community—the Christian community—she hoped he would rejoin. She assured him that everyone was pleased with his accomplishments, including the mother of the young slave L'Fayette, "your *assistant demonstrator*" who had helped Joseph dissect "Rabits & squirrels & frogs" on the plantation; L'Fayette would receive "his full share of fame" through Joseph's studies at school.[41]

As Mary Jones's worries make clear, a moral risk of studying anatomy lay in running afoul of the community. Most obviously, medical students walked the boundaries of the law in every southern state that proscribed grave-robbing for any reason. As was typical of other students, Nathaniel Siewers reassured his parents in 1866 back home in North Carolina that "the students of course have nothing to do with procuring [cadavers]." But this was disingenuous, as Siewers knew. One of the common nicknames for a medical student was "grave rat" or, a little more flattering, "resurrectionist." And a familiar genre of popular literature and medical memoirs was the body-snatching tale, a story of student legerdemain and public opposition. Charles Hentz, for example, recalled working with his school's anatomy demonstrator George Bayless to procure corpses in Louisville, Kentucky, in the mid-1840s. Stealth and night were essential to this work, along with the cooperation of a church sexton named Gardner ("a traitor to his post") who supplied opportunities for snatching bodies at eight dollars apiece. The doctors themselves worked the shovels, masked against the smell (and against being recognized), cracking off the top of the casket, fastening a looped rope under the arms of the corpse (usually a German or Irish immigrant), and hauling it out onto a sheet of canvas and from there into a wagon or propped on a horse in front of the rider. Mishaps occurred, which Hentz related as a kind of Gothic farce. Bodies proved too heavy to lift; they "leaked"; ropes broke; horses bolted. Families watched over their graves to make sure none of this happened. Once, having stolen the body of "a colored woman," Hentz and his cohorts were forced to replace it the next night, after it was discovered that white "friends of the woman" and her family were threatening to take action.[42]

Body-snatching stories, however entertaining, thus played on the deep moral anomalies wrapped up in anatomical study and, by implication, all of medical training: the irony of would-be professionals sneaking about in the night breaking the law; the gap between lofty professional ideals and the desecration of graves; the clash between fundamental scientific values and the larger community's sense of right and wrong. All of this went far beyond midnight-in-the-graveyard melodrama. Serious students with an eye to future practice thought hard about the strategies, limits, and explanations they would adopt in their communities for something merely routine within the school's walls.

Indeed, notwithstanding schools' anxiety over popular disapproval of dissections, faculty themselves sometimes triggered public outrages. The dean of the Medical College of Georgia found it necessary in 1860 to remind the faculty that "no fragment of coffin nor of shroud nor any material calculated to give offense to [visitors] shall be allowed to remain on the premises." James Riddell, in a dispute with his faculty colleagues at the University of Louisiana in 1852, dealt them a heavy blow by reporting to city officials that anatomy classes were so out of hand that every day "guts had been strewn from the passage to the sink in the yard." Alarmed at possible reprisals, his colleagues censured Riddell for sensationalism and for arousing a public hatred of doctors. And in a stunning instance of bad judgment, a faculty member at the Kentucky School of Medicine in the early 1880s decided to play a joke on an anatomy student who had dissected the body of an infant "of good family" instead of burying it as he had promised the parents. His professor arranged a complicated hoax so that the student would think his misdeed was about to be made public. Before the hoax ran its course, however, word of the dissection did in fact find its way into a newspaper; the student was frightened and mortified, the family outraged, and the school hastily held an inquest to stanch the spread of public disapproval. The faculty instigator, however, in the messy aftermath, pronounced his amazement that such "a Hurricane [resulted] from such a little breeze," an attitude more incomprehensible than the hoax itself.[43]

Or maybe not. What this bad joke suggests is how easy it was, even for experienced teachers, to become inured to a medical school world at odds with the ordinary, a world where people were transformed into "material," a world that prized the close study of alarming things. Physicians became used to this world, but family and neighbors did not. And so, looking up from their work, students blinked in the harsh light of their community's judgment. Most fell back on concealment and irony, like Kentucky physician John Knox, who, even in his private diary, clothed his trips to the graveyard in a wry but respectful euphemism as a "stroll to the sacred depository of the dead." But whatever rationalizations students adopted, they discovered them without formal guidance from their schools. Perhaps with a mentor or two showing the way, students were left to untie the moral knots themselves.[44]

This suggests with particular sharpness how in the matter of dissections, as elsewhere in orthodox schooling, standards for morality and science came to be rooted in each physician's personal way of doing things, his "experience." His identity as a good doctor and a good man thus rested in large measure on his own subjectivity as a practitioner and in his determination to see his personal mode of doctoring as the heart of orthodoxy. In turn, this profoundly personal scale for professional values suggests why many practitioners retained an ambivalence about the tie between their medicine and local morality. A story told by one experienced physician suggests that even after long practice, with many corpses seen and dissected, the moral texture of anatomical study might remain troubling. It suggests, too, how a man's personal morality, not codified rules, served to negotiate the complicated encounter between the special knowledge of medical men and their communities. In his autobiography, Charles Hentz recalled being called out as a novice practitioner one night in 1850, some forty years earlier, by the employer of a young, unmarried, immigrant German woman. This young woman—"artless; not long in the country"— had become pregnant, and now, her employer revealed, "affairs had culminated in the birth of a big fat Dutch baby boy that lay dead in the next room, rolled up in a flannel petticoat." As Hentz recalled it, the employer and his wife, sympathetic to the young woman's plight, were unsure what to do with the infant's body until they

> thought that maybe the young doctor might be pleased to dissect it—
> which he was—I was real glad to get the nice specimen—and although it
> was really not the right thing to do, to hush up a matter that strictly
> speaking ought to have undergone a legal investigation, we all thought
> that it was erring on the side of mercy—that the poor girl would probably

not do so again—; so, I took charge of the little dead Dutchman, and, taking the diminutive trunk under my arm, walked down Broadway with it, to my office—where, at my leisure, I made some very nice dissections and preparations with it—; I had a coal closet in my office, very convenient · for secreting the little body, and the sink was very handy for disposing of the refuse—I have the skull of that baby yet with me—in good state of preservation—; had the baby lived he would now be a German burgher forty one years old.[45]

Although it concerns dead bodies and nighttime secrecy, Hentz's matter-of-fact way of relating this story is quite different from the way he had written of his student grave-robbing exploits. These he embalmed in the gothic prose of body-snatching tales, "rather a fanciful style," as he himself admitted, complete with a "glowing little stove . . . sending forth a cheerful murmur" and the corpse, "a ghostly thing . . . with fallen jaw, and glassy eye." In contrast, the story of the immigrant woman's dead infant, free from sentimental varnish, has a more complex mixture of motives and emotions. Even after all the intervening years, the doctor's pleasure at this windfall chance to do some "very nice" science was something to be savored. Moreover, Hentz's story reveals how a conscientious physician might construe the moral issues. The young physician plainly understood, both on that night in 1850 and many years later as he penned his account, that infanticide was a likely explanation for the newborn's death. Accepting the body, he confesses, was "really not the right thing to do" in the eyes of the law. But weighed against the law was not just science but "mercy." Here was the moral fulcrum of the story, and support from the unfortunate woman's employer and his wife was crucial in what the young doctor did. "We all thought" that turning the mother over to a murder investigation, a "poor girl" who would "probably" would not repeat her mistake, would be heartless. So, in this instance, the doctor and his co-conspirators defined their charity—and local morality—in a way that also served science. And yet even this decision did not sum up everything that Hentz told. His closing remark suggests that this long-ago incident was not quite dead and buried. It is not the fact that Hentz had kept the baby's skull that gives pause; doctors found such skulls useful as guides to how an infant's flexible cranial bones might be manipulated in a difficult birth. What is arresting is that Hentz imagines, even briefly, the long-dead infant grown up, a "German burgher." The image is an unexpected ghost at the end of a memory, a flickering sign, maybe, that for the doctor neither anatomical knowledge nor the greater good of mercy answered all of the mysteries of using the bodies of the dead.

As we have seen, students inscribed their responses to lectures, clinics, and anatomy in a range of notes, diaries, and letters home, although there was little in the way of formal writing to capture the experience of schooling. The exception to this was the M.D. thesis, the only required piece of writing in a student's career. Recall that nineteenth-century theses were not intended to be deeply researched or to contain "new" knowledge. And yet despite their rote qualities—in fact, because of them—they incorporated much of what students were able to make of their months of study and fraternity. In writing their theses—popular topics included particular diseases and medicines, surgical procedures, and women's ailments—students bolstered in two ways the continuity of medical schooling over the century. In one sense, the thesis was a retrospective act, testimony that a student's acquirements were within orthodox traditions. At the same time, the thesis officially was termed an "inaugural thesis," suggesting a man's debut on the professional stage. Thus, the thesis writer simultaneously inscribed orthodox medicine in terms of what he had accomplished and what was appropriate.[46]

Mentors' voices can be heard just beneath the surface of theses, of course, and that is one reason theses are so valuable as historical sources. And although many theses are technical and closely focused, something of the expressive style of mid-nineteenth-century American intellectual life resided in them, too: Romantic apostrophes to Nature; warnings about (or paeans to) the bustling, modernizing world; scenes from the medical past; an empirical toting up of objects seen and categorized. The composite nature of these texts—student and teacher, medical school world and the world beyond—is especially notable in the small but important number of theses devoted to characterizing the profession of medicine itself. These "art of medicine" theses, which will be the focus here, changed from the 1830s in ways that paralleled the rise of medical schools. They increasingly located medicine's art in the hoped-for fraternity of local M.D.s and in the moral challenges of community practice that awaited the graduate. That is, elements of a country orthodoxy gradually reconfigured the "art of medicine" thesis, drawing students' attention to a local, southern place.

Before turning to these particular theses, however, it is helpful to size up theses in general, regardless of topic, for what students said about the act of writing and how they tried out their new identities as physicians. Not all students, of course, took up the thesis with equal seriousness. Lafayette Strait began work on his in 1857 by writing to ask his sisters to send him anything they happened to read on medicine because "it will help to fill [it] up." Still, many students seem to have made a genuine effort. Even Strait confessed that he planned to devote "exclusively" two weeks to writing, and like many other students, his anxiety grew as graduation neared. A thesis's style was at once conventional and personal. In this way, theses illustrate precisely how the expression of orthodoxy was tied firmly to each man's personal engagement with it. Within a single essay, the prose might float along on passages of "airy" inspirational rhetoric and then suddenly descend into closely packed technical terms. Images became facts, and facts images. Many students openly characterized their writing as an important professional act, giving the reader directions on how it should be read. William C. Wright informed his readers in 1848 that he had taken two months to write his thesis, pointing out that it was "no small task" to study "Physical Sympathy" because so little had been written about it. He was proud that he had thus put himself at the boundary of knowledge, undertaking work on a subject "that will, I think, pretty generally engage the medical attention in the course of a few years." Other students were struck by the discovery of their own ignorance. "Having no practical knowledge of my own, but being a mere student," Jeptha McKinney realized upon choosing pneumonia as his topic, "of course I must be guided, entirely, by a knowledge from what I have read." Such modest disclaimers were a hedge against faculty criticism, of course; but they also gave voice to genuine fears of being unprepared for practice.[47]

Writing the thesis thus bared certain truths and anxieties about how the student would be judged by his peers in the world beyond the school. Nashville student M. A. Shackleford observed forthrightly in 1857, "What I shall have to say will be said from experience." But he immediately backed away: "And as my experience has been somewhat limited I hope as much leniency will be shown me as possible." Students also feared falling into the thick of medical controversies. While Albert Smith hoped that his 1837 Transylvania thesis would be more than just "the singing of an old song," he was worried that in choosing any topic a mere student was "at a loss . . . if he wishes to steer clear of conflicting elements" in orthodox medical thought. Indeed, Fayette Ewing thought that the thesis should be postponed until a man had gained some experience through practice, mostly because of the "pugilistic mysteries" of medical debate into which the student might blunder. His vision of the political purpose of theses was a shrewd one: it was "a sort of *confession of faith* by which the candidate was ascertained to be orthodox," and if he should later deviate from orthodoxy, the thesis was proof that "no blame could be attached to the professors."[48]

Thus, at the end of his schooling, the thesis writer condensed the intellectual and professional challenges it had raised into a brief textual moment in which he was free to be both learned and ignorant, professional and novice. Some of this talk curried favor with mentors, no doubt, polishing the writer's image as a serious, eager fellow. But in a larger sense, students were borrowing from and experimenting with a professional voice with which to speak to the world as good physicians. Theses in this sense were students' testimony, part demonstration and part elegy, to the time they had spent preparing for a world of practice they now realized they had only begun to imagine.

As a genre both personal and professional, then, the thesis opened easily to this wider narrative purpose, configuring what medicine might be by imagining one's place in it. It was not unusual even in the midst of a dissertation on, say, the nature of blood, for a student to include a few sentences on the historical progress of medicine or on the meaning of a medical man's good moral character. A few students, however, used their theses solely for the purpose of commenting on the profession they were joining, thereby advancing a complex vision of their own futures. And here the shift in the late 1830s to a new rhetoric in these "art of medicine" theses reveals a new focus on the local, southern challenges and continuities of practice as the heart of orthodoxy.

The image of the physician that underwent this change began as an image of a healer framed by vast historical backdrops against which the meaning of the student's novice work appeared certain. One of these backdrops was the ideal of natural science as medicine's ultimate goal, often portrayed as a beacon or a temple on a distant hill toward which the student journeyed. Another setting was a personified Nature, a female figure familiar from school lectures. Never mind that Robert Lebby was emerging from a world of dissections, bottled specimens, and hefty textbooks, his vision was of fields and forests ripe with Nature's power. He was inspired by Nature to learn and to hope. "Who knows," he wrote in 1826, "but that at the foot of the Allegheny mountain there blooms many a flower that is an infallible cure for Epilepsy?" Occasionally, the image was a harsh one, with talk of Nature's mysteries including talk of force; a student "interrogated" Nature, and she had been "compelled to yield up her secrets." But regardless of the tenor of the relationship, the physician stood backlit by the natural world, certain in his knowledge.[49]

Similarly, in many theses written before the 1840s, the influences that explained the physician's relation to science and nature tended to be grandly historical. Recommending their profession's strengths, students retold the history of orthodox medicine on the largest possible scale as a story of the heroism of great doctors who had kept alive the spirit of science against all odds. Typically, students wrote of medical knowledge as a flame, igniting in ancient Egypt, brightening under the Greeks, glowing (though not so fiercely) in the Rome of the Caesars, then finding refuge in "Arabia" during the dark night of medieval

Europe. In this epic tale, the flame or spirit of medicine/science, hounded by frauds of all descriptions, and by the dogma of the Catholic Church in particular, nevertheless lived on in a line of great men: Hippocrates, Paracelsus, Georgio Baglivi, Galileo, Bacon, Thomas Sydenham, William Cullen, and then in a leap across the Atlantic, in Benjamin Rush, Phillip Syng Physick, Phillip Hosack. Mythological figures mingle freely with students' other intellectual ancestors: the god Aesculapius works hand in hand with Galen, and one student observed in 1833 how "Chiron, the centaur, son of Saturne," was responsible for moving the spirit of healing from Egypt to Greece. All of these giants work toward orthodoxy's apotheosis: its arrival in eighteenth-century Philadelphia, a fortunate home free from ancient spell and amulet.[50]

This story was satisfying, it seems, because it placed new physicians into a history of difficult challenges but transcendent outcomes; it was classical in its proportions but Romantic in import. Retelling it, a student could feel pride— and relief—that a plan much larger than his own future lay beneath his wishes and fears. At the same time, however, the social vision of this narrative is from a perspective so remote that the student-author could be anywhere; certainly he is not in the wards or in lectures. He is not even in the South in any identifiable way. Questions about student's immediate future were thus swept aside by a tale that included all of recorded time in each physician's story and excluded others by placing M.D.s alone at the head of a single, ancient genealogy of truth-seekers.

When sick people and communities began slowly to enter into student theses, doing so dependably by the early 1840s, the shift suggests how students—and schools—began to struggle to reconceptualize a physician's most important purposes in terms of his relation to the world beyond schooling. Although pedigreed science and the great chain of immortal doctors never completely disappear from theses, a new narrative took shape that replaced the rise of Western medicine with stories that illustrate the duties and responsibilities of a local, southern physician. Most strikingly, it was not "civilization," or even science, so much as the practitioner's good moral character that was the key to orthodoxy's worth. Students' language, and doubtless their teachers', became more intimate and idiomatic; they strained less for literary effect and were more likely to look at their immediate surroundings. Historical change in medicine was like "the course of the Great Mississippi," one South Carolina student wrote in 1852, his southern image in sharp contrast to earlier theses in which Cos or Athens stood at the center of things. Throughout these later theses, in fact, students' tropes spring almost entirely from the nearby world: the fundamentals of medical knowledge are likened to the "traces, gauntlets, kinds of harness" that every country boy would know. The sick body appears in theses, and the sound of a diseased chest is compared to the "friction of two cornstalks," human tissue to cloth or leather, and the blood's nourishment to pabulum. Moreover, there were images of patients and fellow M.D.s. To be sure, mostly everyone is one-dimensional; patients, especially, are types rather than figures arising from a fully seen context of practice. But even these relatively featureless people are dramatic evidence of how the student's search to express what he had learned shifted to rely on local knowledge and expression.[51]

By 1850, the huge, heroic world of medicine and civilization portrayed in earlier theses cracked open to reveal a world built to an entirely different scale, one drawing upon an ideal clearly forged by students and teachers in the crucible of the school. It was a scale that evoked the importance of southern locale and a sense of the challenges of medical practice as primarily centered in community life. The torch of science once burning in a hilltop temple now burned most brightly in the hearth, and heroism was found at home. The images of the moral practitioner often were archetypes of manhood, but ones rooted more often in the romance of domesticity rather than the epic of civilization. The physician, a Transylvania student wrote, "alone can infuse hope into the bosom of the mother, who, with a tottering frame and a tortured soul watches at the side of her suffering child. He alone can raise up the strong man who has been bowed down by disease and restore him to the field of useful honorable exertion." Sacrifice, too, assumed a homely scale. Physicians appear as men deprived of the ordinary pleasures of life by their responsibilities. At night, "when all around is hushed to rest," as one student wrote, "and the busy cares and perplexities of life are forgotten . . . it is then the physician is called from the bosom of his family to go and mingle again with disease and wretchedness."[52]

Beneath the surface of these images of sacrifice and heroism, where the challenge to a man's character was all the more serious for being phrased in terms of cathartic sentiment, there was another vision of life after school, a darker one. It was a story in which a man's good character unraveled not because he failed to respond to peoples' needs but because he responded and failed. It was melodrama in a sense, but it may also be read as a remarkable confession of inadequacy and fear. Typically, the story features a young doctor opening up shop, and when his first patient appears, he "sets to work with bleeding, blistering, cupping, puking, purging, etc." But despite his honest work, something goes wrong, some detail is overlooked, and the patient dies. Embarrassed, full of remorse and second guesses, the young doctor withdraws from his community. He avoids his neighbors, slips in and out of church or, worse, stops attending services altogether. In some versions of this story, instead of withdrawing, the doctor caters to people's whims and relaxes his intellectual grasp on his work, finding the "halls of public entertainment more inviting than . . . silent study." Like wolves, rival healers circle around. The young man is gossiped about, and in frustration he breaks a confidence and "instantly the report flies that he is a traitor to private friendships; he has violated his honour." He now is shunned and "forced to wend his way to some remote region" in a vain attempt to regain his character and begin his practice anew.[53]

A great intellectual distance lies between these stories of moral failure and personal loss and the earlier ones, where physicians, as reifications of enlightenment, fly across nations and centuries. Here the significance of M.D. theses as texts woven of two voices—teacher and student—is brought home. From the success of the new schools in the 1830s, it seems clear, came a new if uneasy emphasis on orthodoxy's location not only in schools but also in the social world of ordinary community practice. A country orthodoxy now was central, evoked by images of individual success and loss, of morality and culpability, in a way that made *experience*, not pedigree, the text for a young doctor. By thus condensing the scale of a doctor's mission, and at the same time making it immeasurably more textured, thesis writers imagined the deeply personal, moral meaning of the practice that awaited them. A life of doctoring, the thesis writer told himself, was no saga of spirits and gods; it will happen to me.

∾

Overall, the words of students and teachers reveal a powerful and creative continuity tying together the various everyday modes of teaching and learning orthodox medicine throughout the mid-nineteenth century. This continuity lay beneath the more well known institutional shift toward greater organization and curricular reform in schools between 1830 and 1880. It was a continuity built not from abstract arguments for orthodoxy's superiority but from the personal relations of teachers and students as they confronted the kaleidoscope of places where "real" medicine was to be found: in the intellectuality of lectures, in the social confusion of hospital clinic, in the disturbing practices of anatomy, and in the first words they spoke as worthy professionals. Linking all of these together was an emphasis on the personal scale of medical learning and thus on the subjectivity of the individual practitioner. It was a subjectivity that infused the school's ideal of an exclusive scientific knowledge with a moral, as well as an intellectual, authority. It was a subjectivity that featured the school's fraternal bonds as the chief mark of professionalism. And, perhaps most important, it was a subjectivity rooted in individual practice as the clearest guide to what was orthodox. School provided the frame for what there was to know and how to know it, but it was a man's personal experience in practice to which everyone turned with the deepest regard.

At the same time, this way of learning placed new physicians into a keen predicament as they contemplated making a living. For all of the uniqueness of the school's intellectual and tactile world—its camaraderie and tensions, its lived-in air of ordinary men becoming something special—the school was at every point permeable to the surrounding culture. Indeed, the very breadth of orthodox medicine's ambitions that inspired M.D.s to seek an expansive social role through their schools left orthodoxy open to revisions flowing back into the school from local communities. Schooled orthodoxy thus bore the imprint of the social world it sought to rise above. And although physicians resisted the idea, we must see this world—a world of communities, families, competitors, the well, and the sick—as importantly *creating* orthodoxy. Not warring worlds, but aspects of the same world, accounted for the tensions new physicians faced as they started out in practice.

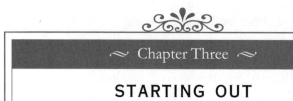

Chapter Three

STARTING OUT

"I am now in very fact a Doctor and feel fully repaid for all the sacrifices made and privations suffered," Samuel Van Wyck wrote to his wife in Anderson Court House, South Carolina, after receiving his medical degree in the spring of 1860. Two years earlier, he had quit the tannery business to plumb the mysteries of medicine. "So far I have done as well as my best friends could wish," he wrote, referring to his teachers and fellow students. "I now long to be a candidate for public favor and once more in the way of making a living." His letter may be read as a kind of graduation address, a farewell and a commencement. Many new physicians wrote similarly, announcing their new status to their families and in their diaries; older physicians, too, recalled this time as a major turning point in their lives. Taking this cue from doctors' writing, this chapter looks at physicians starting out in practice as a time when their sense of who they were was revealingly elastic—stretched between schooled ideals and the now pressing need to make a living and to come to personal terms with sickness. As a result, orthodoxy, too, took on a troubling but inventive elasticity. Men spoke with conviction about cleaving to orthodox ideals. But many a graduate, like Samuel Van Wyck, realized that as a "candidate for public favor" he would have to embrace an orthodoxy flexible enough to survive in a harsh, competitive world.[1]

Thus, stepping into the gap between school and acceptance into a rural community, graduates discovered that the world of the school quickly receded and the broader fraternal professionalism that it promised was in some ways a stark fiction. The professionalization of medicine in this era usually is written as a story of elite physicians mastering the values and organization that underwrote modernity. Here it is explored as a predicament of the novice practitioner on the ground, in many ways on his own. Men managed this rough transition by construing their first weeks in practice as a personal and largely moral challenge to their good character. They saw that the "experience" they would need to acquire was a difficult aggregate of medical skill, worldly calculation, and moral soundness. This realization marked the important shift toward a country style of orthodoxy in which schooled expectations were transformed by local realities of personal achievement and the encounter with illness. Though exaggerated in some ways, the resulting tensions nonetheless prefigured the medicine physicians ended up practicing as orthodox men.

NEW DEGREE, FRESH DOUBTS

Amid the inspirational oratory on graduation day, most new M.D.s pledged to be more than just another kind of doctor. There was music, and young women tossed "flowers from the hot house." Ministers refreshed the day with prayer, journalists with irony. A Louisville newspaper in 1848 congratulated the city's ninety-four new physicians, but with a wink it pointed out that all of them were now to be "turned loose on the community." Professors gave their farewell lectures, gifts were exchanged between faculty and students, landlords were paid, and leave taken of friends, all of which "reminds us of the final conclusion of all things," as one participant remarked. Parents pronounced their words, too, highlighting the occasion with the language of worthy manhood. "We congratulate you and now write to be the first among your relations and friends to address you by your title, *Doctor*," one father wrote to his son in 1856. An older brother in 1832 admired his sibling's new sheepskin; it was proof "that you are what you are cracked up to be." Wilson Yandell transcribed and sent to his son the letter of a professor who had written, "Your son will not disappoint your hopes. His mind is well furnished, and his ambition is manly & honourable. With him I am pleased—fully pleased." The moment was so heavy with words of approbation that the young men receiving them seem comparatively speechless. Some students who had worked hard admitted to feeling as exhausted as they were fulfilled. Walter Porcher recalled realizing "how severely I had applied myself" to his studies at South Carolina only when his father took him to see "an exceedingly emotional play" and he "found it impossible to let myself down." Oliver Stout worked hard for his degree at Transylvania, he wrote to a friend in 1823, but admitted "whether I deserved it, or not, time alone must determine."[2]

For most of the students, graduation worked a kind and bestowing magic, opening up a view of the world beyond school time and boyhood, proclaiming them finished doctors and men. But no ritual is seamless, and around the edges of graduation were outsiders of various kinds. For some students who had run "hastily over the . . . meagre list of text books and manuals; listen[ed] drowsily, carelessly and irregularly," there would be no diploma. One such student wrote angrily to his parents of the "trap" he felt the faculty had set for him by raising his expectations and then humiliating him at exam time. Among several students failed by the faculty over the years at the Medical College of Georgia was one man in 1835 who had submitted as his thesis "an almost literal transcript from the works of Thomas Cooper." There also was a Mr. Thompson who was examined twice in 1842 with such mixed results that he was given his degree only after he pledged in writing that "he would not practice medicine but devote himself to the [further] study of the Profession for 12 months." Other students on the margins of the day included those slave-owning men who intended to practice only on their own plantations, and those who, like Joseph LeConte in the 1840s, had discovered that medical science, not practice, was what interested them. Practice was a kind of hubris, he decided. It was about nothing less than "life and death," and even graduates of good schools were "utterly unfitted . . . to assume the terrible responsibilities of medical practice."[3]

South Carolina student Dandridge Bibb shared these worries. Indeed, his 1846 M.D. thesis was a discussion of reasons *not* to practice (he was awarded his degree nonetheless) and voiced doubts about medicine's moral compass, doubts that were far from uncommon. With its tight relationships among men and its edgy pride in knowing and doing things most people avoided, medical school had created its own moral atmosphere that Bibb now considered dangerously thin. He was confident in his skills and his science, he wrote, but worried that he had drifted away from the moral sensibility of southern communities and, worse, from his own religious convictions. His schooling had ignored "the little daily influences of [a physician's] life" necessary for acceptance in close-knit rural neighborhoods. Worse, it had tainted his religious faith with the "impieties" of anatomical dissection and had introduced disturbing class prejudices. Recalling his hospital rounds, Bibb was appalled by the "different effect produced upon the mind by witnessing the death of one belonging to the lower class of society, from that experienced by the deathbed of the wealthy and educated." Though no advocate for the poor, Bibb nonetheless rejected medical school's implicit message that "our perception of spiritual things should be . . . blunted and perverted by externals" such as a patient's relative wealth. Overall, his "imagination had been degraded instead of softened" by his schooling, so much so that he now lacked the moral peace of mind that would allow his "ideas [to] flow into the right channel" at the bedside of the sick.[4]

Certainly most students did not anticipate feeling as alien in their communities as Dandridge Bibb feared he would. Nonetheless, his sense that the medical school world cut against the grain of southern social relations in the rural, small-town areas where most men would seek employment is a theme easily found in young men's graduation talk. Actual practice was not only a matter of bodies, judgment, and medicines, Transylvania graduate Willard Taft reflected upon his graduation in 1848, as if only just realizing it; it was far more open-ended and unpredictable. For one thing, in community practice a physician did not have the luxury of deliberating only with other M.D.s. Instead, he must be "prepared to learn something, even by the wayside, and from the *illiterate*." Similarly, a Nashville student in 1854 suspected that in practice he would need what he called a "sensitivity" not taught in either clinic or lecture. Indeed, it was not a school-bred scientist but a worthy man—a good father— who now seemed to him the best model for a practitioner. "There is no occupation, nay no relation save perhaps, that of a parent, to which greater responsibility attaches itself" than medicine, he realized. Making a similar point, though ironically, Charleston graduate J. W. Keitt in 1844 understood that a shrewd practitioner must please people neither too little nor too much; the secret was to "draw a nice distinction between the pedant and the clown, and traverse the pleasant grounds between the two." More seriously, he saw that in a relatively isolated, rural setting, a physician had to command a wide range of natural, social, and "rational" knowledge. The difficult thing would be to make his work "enhance his utility and . . . support his dignity" both. In the mysterious balance of these two qualities lay the secret of being a good doctor.[5]

To be sure, mentors' advice echoes in these words. But the experimental tone of voice, the mixture of curiosity and anxiety, belongs to the neophyte M.D. At the close of schooling, novice doctors realized that the character of a new doctor, heretofore tested only by his mentors, now was to be tested by his neighbors in ways that did not privilege the school's version of orthodoxy. Lunsford Yandell's doctor father touched on the tenuous relation between being a good man and a good practitioner when he told his son that, once in practice, a doctor had to rely on his "faith"—by which he meant his moral, as well as religious, bearings—to unite all of the particular things school had taught him. A young doctor, the senior Yandell cautioned, would have many opportunities to choose between morality and expediency; either a man's "practice must be regulated by his faith, or his faith must conform to his practice." Much of the intellectual impetus of schooling rewarded the latter, but communities were seeking the former kind of man.[6]

Henry Clay Lewis's alter ego, Madison Tensas, looked at the gulf between schooling and practice in a different, though related, way at graduation; not faith but common sense would help a new practitioner attach himself to a community. In Tensas's story, his teacher of surgery surprises him during his final examination by asking him how he would make chicken soup. At first, Tensas thinks he is being toyed with and is prepared to be insulted. But the teacher says, no, he really wants to know about the soup; so Tensas gives him a recipe. The teacher listens, then points out that nowhere did Tensas say that he would kill the chicken first. This was the difference between schooling and practice: "Tensas, I knew you were well-prepared [for the exam], but I thought I would teach you that nothing that may be conducive to the recovery of our patient is too trivial to be remembered by the physician—also to try your temper. You have too much of the latter. The sickbed is a fine moderator, however. Go, my dear fellow, study hard, and in ten years I will hear from you."[7] School was over; now the hard lessons began. The memorized details, the principles and explanations, the clever fixes in the clinic or in apprenticeships, the interiors of dead bodies—all fell away with alarming suddenness. School had taught a man how to discriminate among the things he observed, asked, and did, so that courses of action were either ruled in or ruled out. But in practice, in the community of men and women, "nothing . . . is too trivial" to be of some import. The problem was not a tactical one of choosing this or that course of action but a moral one of framing the choices.

CALCULATION FOR SURVIVAL

The counterpoint to a man's moral intentions were his material ones. "For two weeks I have been engaged in resting mind and body—and now feel like work again," graduate Robert Battey wrote to his aunt in 1857. "I shall settle down and engage in practice as soon as I can." He made it sound easy, but just as new graduates worried over the fraying seam between professional means and popular morality, so they discovered the practical limits of professional authority beyond the school. Indeed, in considering where to work, a new doctor encountered a profession so dispersed across the South, and so rooted in the judgments (not to say whims) of individual senior men, that it appeared scarcely to exist at all. Some men had fantasies of places far away and adventure. Young Samuel Dickson wanted to be a ship's physician and travel to outposts of commerce and empire, "to Canton and Calcutta." Other men dreamed of Paris, or Italy, or, especially, of the American West. Interestingly, while a few men thought in terms of cities, most did not; the pedagogic attractions of the urban medical school did not carry over into a place to settle down. In fact, some advisers seem to have warned young men away from the city for some of the same reasons that it was prized as a place for education. In the city, even a southern city, Joseph Jones's teacher advised him in the 1850s, "the practice of medicine is much more difficult on account of the diversity of [patients'] temperaments, than in the country." Joseph Copes was given similar advice two decades earlier: "the young practitioner in the city seems to meet with little encouragement" from either fellow physicians or the marketplace.[8]

What emerged as the sensible choice of most southern neophytes and their advisers alike, then, was the rural life, imagined in terms of southern people and the southern countryside. Chief among men's wishes, even after the Civil War, was to establish the classic "plantation practice." As Alfred T. Hamilton of Franklin County, Tennessee, imagined it in 1858, this was a practice where "the country is good, planters wealthy, and society respectable." As a vision of success, it combined professional privilege with the manly challenge of working in the mainstream southern economy. In conjuring this ideal, young doctors in the antebellum years tied their imagined careers without much question to whatever allowed slavery to prosper. A location with a sizable population of slaves (so they imagined) meant planters willing to make contracts with physicians for a period of months or even years. Young Frederick Egan wrote excitedly to his mother of his extraordinary good fortune in having secured from a local planter "the promise of the practice on two plantations." Slaves were a captive patient population, of course, which meant a stable income; but as important in this vision was being ushered into local society by elite patrons. While still in medical school, Charles Hentz spoke with a wealthy planter in the mid-1840s about a position in which the latter would use his influence to "insure me an overwhelming practice among the neighboring farmers."[9]

At the same time, with good reason, new physicians were warned by senior men of the elusiveness of such a practice. Even when physicians did secure contracts, they were not the multiyear arrangements most novices anticipated. Before and after the war, plantation districts throughout the South were a market frequently glutted with healers, and planters had little reason to tie themselves down to one man. "The Country is so full of Doctors now that I'm afraid it will be a bad chance anywhere to succeed," William Whetstone wrote to his mother about the South Carolina piedmont in 1854. The shifting patterns of sickness were as impossible to control as the supply of doctors who hoped to take advantage of them. Although populated by flourishing plantations, "this country is too healthy to support one quack," a Louisiana doctor wrote to his brother-in-law in disgust. Abraham Jobe had a difficult time starting out in

Yancey County, North Carolina, for similar reasons, but then "sickness began to increase . . . and my calls came thick and fast until I had all the practice I could attend to."[10]

As Jobe cheerfully suggests—and as others pointed out with darker irony—a physician's prospects often depended on nothing so much as a community's bad fortune. Moreover, the individual locus of material success, like the emphasis given to individual moral character, pushed the school's image of an orthodox brotherhood further into the background. Apprenticeship may have given some young physicians a hint of the realities of competitive solo practice, but there was nothing like being faced with it as a matter of economic survival. Indeed, the "profession" at this crucial stage of a man's career stood revealed as not much more than a fiction when it came to offering any kind of support to a beginner. Throughout the century, men learned about prospective practices almost entirely from a loose, personal network of mentors and acquaintances, and from on-the-road hearsay. Alfred Hamilton was typical of most new physicians in following up on a suggestion from his mentor and traveling to Carroll County, Mississippi, in 1858. Here he was excited to find a community where a previous physician, or so Hamilton was told, had "only stayed five months and booked $3000," an eye-popping sum. Relying on this hearsay alone, Hamilton decided to try it. Samuel Dickson believed he had made a good deal by agreeing to pay a senior Charleston physician for the opportunity to treat some of the older man's patients for a period of three years, an arrangement that Dickson hoped would permit him to become known in the city. Thousands of similar individual deals were consummated—or fell through—as men launched their careers in this eclectic fashion.[11]

In all of this, a novice soon realized that his diploma was far from his chief advantage in the marketplace. Strikingly, both before and after the Civil War, even mentors continued to recommend students not as men with diplomas but as personal acquaintances within a network of respected individual practitioners. Letters of recommendation typically employed a language of manhood and honor independent of academic particulars, even by midcentury, when more senior men at least mentioned schooling. In praising graduate Edward Barton in 1820, for example, Richard Davidson wrote to his colleague, "You must pay him the same attentions you would pay to me my friend." Davidson also thought it important to mention that Barton "is the particular friend & distant connexion of our friend Mr. Chew." Similarly, in 1860, a mentor recommended Samuel Van Wyck in terms of his *own* character, noting that Van Wyck's parents "are among my most influential & fast friends." The implication is that it was the good man who made a good doctor, and mentors touted their students in terms of a broadly shared morality, for their "character & integrity . . . great industry & perseverance." In relying so heavily on personal ties, senior physicians in effect affirmed a reality that men in rural communities would soon learn firsthand: a graduate's excellence was recognized principally by the praise experienced practitioners heaped upon him. And, because established physicians used the language of personal honor and trust, the implication was that communities of like-minded citizens had much weight when it came to deciding who qualified as a doctor.[12]

Even so, advice from experienced men varied greatly on how to impress a community. The variety was a sign both of the orthodox profession's lack of dominance and of individual practitioners' ability to improvise: charge low fees at first, and patients will follow; do not charge low fees, because fellow practitioners will be annoyed and refuse to help you. Seek to know a few influential people at first, for through them others will come to you; seek to know anyone and everyone, and you will get a reputation as fair and open. Learn about rival doctors by associating with them as much as possible; learn about rival doctors by discreetly asking patients about them. Wholly subjective, often passionate in their formulae for success, a graduate's advisers created a climate of calculation and wish that privileged idiosyncratic, personal reasons for making what were anything but empirically researched choices about starting out. Once again, a man's own moral character emerged as decisive; his scientific attainments seemed oddly irrelevant in this wide world beyond the school, and the beneficial professional connections markedly absent.

Consider the mixture of personal judgment, hearsay, and worldly calculation that the young physician Joseph S. Copes received from his two older brothers in 1833, one of whom, James, had practiced as a doctor. Copes was thinking about setting up practice near St. Louis, Missouri, and both of his brothers agreed that the area was socially rough and already swamped with doctors. But while brother James thought Joseph would be wrong to settle there, indeed "lowered" in his moral character, Thomas argued that such circumstances were exactly right for a quick rise to the top. The area was booming, Thomas wrote, "one of the most thriving places in the western country." Some neighborhoods had no physician at all, and those that had several were marked by "much jealousy" among doctors, which, in Thomas's view, created openings for an aggressive, skilled younger man.[13]

Not so, wrote brother James. He himself had only recently relocated from one of the communities in question, St. Charles, and the status of the four physicians there was proof that professional competition made for the worst of worlds. All of the physicians were "dilapidated" from struggling over the slim pickings of St. Charles's French-speaking community. The doctor with the most patients kept them not because he was a better healer but because he spoke French; even then, he had to practice carpentry to make ends meet. A second physician was "supported in part by a small farm," acquired through some swindle involving shooting guns at a target "which no honest man can ever hit." Another doctor survived entirely by exchanging his services for credit on the tabs of various merchants, while the fourth physician "gets nothing at all to do and has gone to storekeeping." Thomas countered by arguing that Joseph should see all of this as an opportunity to display his school-polished manners and fresh skills. Joseph's real competition in St. Charles numbered only two, his brother insisted. One man, moderately skilled at surgery, remained a "notorious drunkard" who had arrived in town only to get last year's "cholera business" and would likely disappear soon. The other seemed to possess more skills but was "a petulant fop, and also a moist soul" and thus not well liked. And do not worry about speaking French, Thomas went on. "You would in 2 mos. learn more french than all of them together." Jump into the fray, was his advice; throw everything into impressing the locals: "bring all the best medical books you can with you and the trunk full of letters [of recommendation]—they cost nothing but a little time in collecting them and this world is such a place that even names carry much weight without substance."[14]

THE COMMUNITY CHOOSES ITS OWN

Whether communities were easily swayed by a physician's credentials, as Thomas Copes believed, or whether, as seems more often the case, people were not much impressed with paperwork, most doctors starting out were struck by their utter dependence on the preferences of local communities. And even though these communities were insular in many ways, they were not socially homogeneous. Every neighborhood had its locally prominent citizens, as well as its poor and its ne'er-do-wells. And in the South, of course, most communities had not only a class hierarchy but a racial order, before and after slavery—both saturated by Protestant Christianity and yeoman republicanism that imparted distinct character to social relations generally. Little about this social order was strange to most new physicians, of course, who had come from, and had apprenticed in, similar settings. However, starting out solo impressed them anew with the power of the community to define "good" medicine on its own terms, which sometimes coincided with schooled orthodoxy, sometimes not. Historians have generalized perhaps too easily about the "democratic" quality of the era's skepticism of orthodoxy, as if popular skepticism were simply a matter of majority rule. In fact, the particulars of how a doctor made his place in a community were far more complex and never more exposed to view than when a man began his career. Some of these particulars, as we will see, doubtless were common to rural communities outside the South, while others had a distinctly southern accent. Looming largest, in any case, were men's anxieties concerning social class, rural isolation, and confrontations with rivals, all of which shaped not only their first encounters with patients but also their sense of orthodoxy itself.

Graduate William Whetstone was pleased with his visit in 1855 to a South Carolina community where he was brought to church to meet people. He answered their polite questions about his training and his family and found that "they are all very anxious for me to practice for them." After hosting a similar meeting for Dr. William Reedy, J. R. Manning, of Manning's Roads, South Carolina, wrote warmly to Reedy, "We are still in need of a Dr. as much as ever. We still insist on your coming." Sometimes negotiations were surprisingly specific. In 1873, Dr. John Robinson responded to a newspaper advertisement placed by community leaders in Osyka, Mississippi, who were seeking a Baptist physician. Robinson, a Baptist, did not name the fees he hoped to receive but rather asked about the fees people were accustomed to paying. He also wanted to know how many Baptist churches the community was able to support. Among his reasons for leaving Due West, South Carolina, he said candidly, were the low fees, the laws favoring debtors, and the fact that a Presbyterian doctor got most of the business. W. E. Tynes responded to Robinson's letter by giving him the community's standard for fees (Robinson could expect $5 per visit—the going rate in much of the South in the war-inflated 1870s). But Tynes took the opportunity to spell out again his community's requirements: the new doctor must "be a good obstetrician. One who will make himself useful as a leading Citizen in every good enterprise. . . . A *Sound* and *Active* Baptist—and strictly a *Temperance man*, with personal skill and experience to succeed."[15]

In framing terms in this way, communities negotiating with physicians throughout the midcentury years reinforced the view that the ideal doctor was first of all a moral man who would fit in. Although this expectation was not necessarily at odds with physicians' own sense of the morality that underlay practice, the fact that community leaders took the initiative could prove unsettling. The self-image a physician had learned to cherish in school was now exposed as less a personal achievement than a matter of power—and of social class. When young James A. S. Milligan wrote to his father in 1846 that he was thinking of leaving his first practice in Harmony Grove, Georgia, his father (himself a physician) cautioned him that the views of one community leader, a Mr. Butler, would be crucial in any move. "Be careful that you do not displease him," wrote the senior Milligan, "for if *he* should array himself against you, you will find it a very difficult matter" to collect the money owed by patients and leave with good reputation intact. A South Carolina doctor was annoyed in 1856 by the thought of submitting to the "unpleasant interrogations" of community leaders concerning his style of medicine. It made him feel, he said revealingly, as if he were "acting almost the part of an ungrateful ser'vt" in having to argue for his orthodoxy. Even M.D.s returning to their own communities to practice wrote about feeling manipulated, subservient; in a way, it was worse than beginning somewhere completely fresh. As one graduate wrote in 1859, a new M.D. "returns to the home of his infancy and boyhood" only to find "many of his best friends slow of heart to believe that the stripling who lived amongst them . . . has attained a maturity" required of a doctor.[16]

While these experiences doubtless were true of rural doctoring elsewhere, some physicians starting out wrote of a distinctly southern rural insularity, contrasting it to the stimulating life fostered by the school. Tiny Mt. Meigs, Alabama, in 1835 seemed in some respects "a fine start for a Physician," young J. Marion Sims wrote tentatively to his fiancée, Theresa Jones, since the vicinity was "very rich, densely populated . . . & withal sickly." But, in part to prepare her, Sims worried aloud that most white people seemed quite poor and the slave-owning elite difficult to approach. He confessed to having strong doubts overall about "society" in Mt. Meigs, which struck him as rough and "dissipated." "At this very moment," he wrote Theresa, "there are about a dozen or twenty men of the most profane cast drunk & fighting in the street below my window, with a negro playing a banjo (I believe it is called) in their midst." That Sims was not sure what to call a banjo says something about his readiness for life in a place like Mt. Meigs. He was not alone. Fears of being marooned in small, socially and intellectually isolated communities, even the ones that welcomed them, sprouted like weeds in new doctors' diaries and letters home. "I pray that my isolation may be beneficial to me—God guiding me, I know that it will," young Florida physician Charles Hentz wrote in his journal during his first days in practice. Youthful anxiety over how much they really knew was made worse by their sense of exchanging the vibrant world of the school for the dreary prospect of tending the victims of street fights or teaching basic hygiene. Samuel Leland, for one, locating at Mill Creek, South Carolina, in 1849, was appalled to see that "people, all wash (both hands and feet) from the same basin, and have one comb, and towel in common."[17]

Dislike for hardscrabble communities, then, was not only fear for one's livelihood and a class-inflected distaste for certain aspects of southern rural life but also a fear that one's orthodox medicine would become hopelessly embattled by a popular ignorance greatly underestimated in medical school. It seemed to many physicians starting out that people had to be taught the most basic things about how professional physicians practiced. One man fresh from school came to a community where, he was amazed to discover, "the majority of the citizens . . . had never had occasion to employ doctors" before his arrival. They appreciated neither his need to "expectantly" observe before acting nor the importance of following his directions to the letter. Worse, in the view of many novices, people did not see the need to truly study medicine. Doctors observed that rural folks took more interest in the details of local politics and gossip than they did in the fundamentals of health, and yet people's ignorance of the body and drugs did not stop them from having strong opinions about them.[18]

Physicians' initial depictions of rural people may be read as sketches in ethnography. But even more powerfully, they are evidence of physicians' wavering self-image as they realized that they might well occupy only a marginal place on the vernacular landscape of healing. It was as if many of these young men clinging to schooled ideas were seeing rural communities for the first time, which in a sense they were. Interestingly, more than a few responded to the troubled transition to practice with an elevated rhetoric by which they attempted to infuse their predicament with a sense of moral mission. It was a rhetoric that depicted the M.D. as fair and philanthropic in the most lofty terms. As such, it was a class-inflected rhetoric that recalled mentors' homilies and the ideal of charity developed on hospital wards. And yet, strikingly, the imagery did not engage with the southern, rural circumstances at hand. A physician's services are equally open to all, wrote one graduate in this vein, "whether they are required in the gorgeous mansion of luxury & ease, or in the humble cabin of the beggar, upon his bed of straw." The good physician, wrote another, does not abandon "the humble cot of poverty and wretchedness for the pomp and glitter of the abodes of opulence." Such language raised the doctor's sense of his calling by way of sentimental tropes that were widespread throughout popular literary culture: opulence and wretchedness, pomp and poverty. It is a rhetoric that yearned for a community with clear, static class lines and a generally accepted paternalism. And although such words imply emotional engagement with suffering, they remove the whole disturbing matter of poverty to a realm remote from the southern community at hand: beggars, beds of straw, humble cots, and the rest of it bore only generic resemblance to the particulars of southern poverty, particularly in terms of slavery and its convoluted racial dimensions. Yet the language, much used, clearly served to express—in its power to sentimentalize and thus to control—a sense that the new physician would start out by testing his moral resolve.[19]

Many of the anxieties about class, rural isolation, and the proper response of a moral man came to a focus when new physicians confronted the hostility of senior M.D.s in the community. In fact, writing about such rivalry—a theme that runs throughout memoirs of this period, as well as letters and diaries—was even more compelling than writing about conflict with the citizenry or with alternative healers. The hostile older M.D. was a signal reality upending the mentor-student ideal, and a powerful way for young men to inscribe their fears of going it alone in a skeptical town without the fraternal bonds of the school. Stories of rivalry with senior men also witnessed the larger insight that the medical profession, as a corporate body, had little substance in rural practice beyond the ability of individual practitioners to come to personal terms with each other. And, as with the rhetoric of class and charity, this sense of rivalry marked a new practitioner's attempt to come to terms with communities' power without directly attacking people at large.

"A junior member of the medical profession is almost always in the power of older physicians who have . . . gained the confidence of the neighborhood," one young practitioner learned to his disappointment in 1853. Fresh from the world of the school, he had hoped to find a senior man who would be pleased to take him, "as it were, by the hand" and lead him into practice. But the reality was dangerously different. Thus, young J. Marion Sims was being realistic when he not only anticipated the opposition of a certain older practitioner but also used it as a yardstick for his own success, calculating that "if with such opposition as Dr. Lucas I can support myself & pay my debts next year," he could feel optimistic about his future. Some young men, like J. E. Clark in 1883, were flat-out combative, confident that their youth and energy would soon give them "quite a reputation . . . *over* these old cusses!!" Fogies, cookbook doctors, scandal mongers: many younger men characterized their elders as not only out of date but also selfish. Some older men responded exactly as younger men feared, publicly ridiculing a "young'un" as a mere "grave rat" (knowing cadavers but not patients) or a "dead shot" with his medicines (making only the most lethal mistakes). A novice's efforts had but one effect in the community: "to enlarge the grave yards." The kind of older man especially dangerous to a doctor just starting out, Abraham Jobe recalled, was a man in practice for twenty years in the same place, popular and outgoing, who attended several churches and was an "exceedingly plausible . . . fluent talker" who could make people "believe a lie quicker than I could the truth." In the writings of younger doctors—and in the memoirs of older ones—these competitive, complacent men are everywhere.[20]

Indeed, for Jobe, the memory of how older physicians had tried to obstruct his early practice still was fresh many years later, and still relevant. He wrote to warn younger men but admitted that he himself had not heeded a similar warning. His recollection expresses precisely how rivalry and local professional relationships reconfigured the school's vision of M.D.s' fraternity into a struggle over livelihood and reputation, setting aside orthodoxy's scientific energy and therapeutic claims. Locating in Elizabethton, Tennessee, in 1850, young Jobe decided to approach the community's established physician, Dr. Joe Powell, forthrightly: "I said 'Doctor, I have located here, hoping to gradually grow up into an honorable practice. I expect you to get the leading practice, of course, as you are established here, but there will be times when you can't take all the calls and demands made upon you, and in this way, I may supply a want in the community. I would always be glad to call you in consultations and would feel proud if we always get on in our respective practices on the best of terms.' "[21]

With a nice mixture of deference and determination, Jobe put his concern for honor first, thereby placing both therapeutic and business concerns into a moral register. No honorable man would make an exclusive claim to an entire neighborhood. Though portraying himself as an equal in this sense, Jobe gave the older man a chance to be his mentor and, finally, invoked the needs of the community as something larger than both men, thus underscoring the right of people to choose who they wanted to attend, touch, and medicate them.[22]

In response, however, the older man attempted to reduce mutual honor and professional cooperation to the hard knocks of "business": "Dr. Jobe, [he said], you have driven your pigs to a bad market. Dr. Rogan, my Uncle Gaston Powell and myself will form a copartnership, and we can do all the business the people can pay for; of course, you would get the kind of calls we would not want, and it would be doing us a favor, but it would starve you out."[23] Deciding to make a stand, Jobe replied as many young doctors doubtless did, telling Dr. Powell that he would stay no matter what and "try lives with you" to see who came out best. As Jobe told it, his story had a happy ending. He combined several early bedside successes with a public pledge to speak no evil of Dr. Powell. With honor as his tactic, Jobe soon pulled patients to him; his rival packed up his medicines and left for California.[24]

The import of Jobe's story is that a novice doctor's ability to persevere, and to do so in a way that reflected his steady, moral character, mattered more than anything else, even his learnedness. Once he gained a toehold, it was up to some mixture of skill, honor, and fate through which a new practitioner would struggle to balance the kind of care people wanted (or were used to receiving) with the kind of professional he wished to be. Tennessean William Moody, like most other young doctors, worked out his moral stance at the bedside itself. Commencing practice in 1840, he almost immediately was drawn into a consultation with a senior man. Moody was put off by the brusque way in which his older colleague approached the patient. So, Moody wrote, "[I] gently passed my hand over his [the sick man's] face, stroked his hair back," and carefully took note of symptoms but otherwise stayed in the background despite his doubts about the older man's therapy. A day or so later, the patient surprised Moody by asking him to take over his case. Although delighted, Moody felt a "great delicacy" in revising the older doctor's prescription even though the patient "insisted that I should." Hoping to avoid the enmity of the older man but also determined to hold on to his new patient, Moody decided on a therapy that deviated only a "little from the former prescription," and, fortunately, the patient recovered. Thus, like Abraham Jobe, young William Moody balanced honor and self-interest with a shrewdness that bespoke a long future career: he did what he thought best, consonant with what the patient wished, and did it in a way not to embarrass his senior colleague.[25]

For the neophyte, then, the encounter with an established doctor was a lesson that summed up many of the difficulties of starting out. Making the transition from school to practice was about standing one's ground and seizing the opportunity. It was about honor, as well as chance, and about the many ways a community held the decisive power to choose its healers. It opened the new man's eyes to how the warmly collegial nature of his schooling had lulled him into a too-easy equation of school and the broader southern community. Indeed, the mean-spirited senior practitioners that so many young men encountered—and later, as senior men, pointedly recalled—suggest a crucial weakness in grassroots professional relationships among M.D.s in this century. Not able to call upon the corporate resources of a band of brothers, the doctor starting out was forced to fall back on his individual character as the moral center of his claim to practice good medicine. The "profession" scarcely existed as an arbiter, or even as a buffer, in this world of practice. In the social texture of each community was the locus of influence and patronage from which a new doctor had to shape his own vision of knowledge and moral purpose.

FIRST PATIENTS, "MONSTER" DISEASE, AND "INWARD SATISFACTION"

In these ways, new doctors calculated the terms of material success and struggled to define a relationship with the powerful community. It would not be the last time they made these calculations. But it was an especially revealing time, a suspended moment of sorts, and many men imagined their calling in new, dramatic terms, believing themselves uniquely on display. They also began to think about the ways disease took shape as illness—as something not coolly tracked by science but rather as a fearsome monster who came to destroy. Both of these concerns mirrored a new sense of falling headlong into people's troubled lives. In doing so, the physician encountered his own subjectivity as he sized up the subjectivity of others, and many men wrote about the disturbing possibility that this aspect of actual practice might diminish rather than enhance the satisfactions of orthodoxy.

In light of all this, a man's "first patient" was the grail of his initial days of practice. Waiting for the first call was to be placed in a harsh spotlight of public curiosity and gossip. Because many practitioners had laid hands on at least a few patients during apprenticeship or schooling, the fact that one's own first patient was such a major event testifies to the importance attached to starting out in solo practice. It was a rite of passage that combined a man's fear of failure with his fantasies of triumph into a potent mixture of dread and suspense. Samuel Leland had only been in practice two years when he sat down to write a recollection of his first days as a full-fledged doctor. His resources had consisted of "a Bed, a trunk of clothes, my horse (paid for), and a few bottles of medicine. No money, but plenty of credit." Then began the torment of waiting "in silent expectation for a '*call*,' but no call would come. . . . I would read until books became a weariness; and my medicines disgusting." Weariness, and intense urgency besides. When Henry Clay Lewis wrote as Madison Tensas, he affected the voice of an old-timer; but his actual youth broke through when he spoke of waiting desperately for his first call, wanting, "with all the pruriency of a young neophyte," to get his hands on somebody: "white, black, old, young, maid, wife, widow, masculine, feminine, old bachelor, or Indian, I cared not which; a patient is what I wanted." He set up his books in his office, put out a sign in front. Sometimes he felt calmly professional, but then he would feel as if he were desperately setting a trap, "constantly upon the lookout for some victim approaching the bait."[26]

The first "victims" probably reminded new men of apprenticeship; they often were not patients who enjoyed autonomy, stability, or a happy history with caregivers: slaves with "minor" complaints, boatmen off the river, travelers of various kinds. Usually the first case was a modest piece of work. "I had a case of gonorrhoea, Sumner (stage driver)," J. M. Richardson noted with relief in his diary in 1853. "I charged him 75 cts for prescription. The first money I ever made professionally." Another recent graduate prescribed an emetic for his inaugural case, a robust young woman, in order to "dislodge a supper of beef" causing her abdominal pain. But though he tried his best to persuade her, she told him "she 'wouldn't take a puke'" and left his office. "A small beginning, this," the young doctor wrote ruefully. A first patient finally came to Samuel Leland, too, after his days of anxious waiting. It was "Frank, a servt. of the estate of James Henry. Disease Hemmorrhoids. I gained some reputation from this case." His second call came five days later, at night, a young white woman and a member of the same wealthy Henry family. Leland believed that he responded well this time, too, and in fact was told by the Henrys shortly thereafter "that I would be their Dr. in the future." His practice was under way.[27]

First failures, too, especially first deaths, were vivid episodes, often memorialized in doctors' later writings. James Hundley wrote to console his brother, who had "lost" a patient for the first time, telling him that "Physic cannot prevent the will of the Almighty. Be attentive to your patients & read every day." New doctors thus began to realize how limited and particular the school's vantage point on caregiving had been, how tilted toward objective disease and toward patients who were either anonymous or seen through the scrim of apprenticeship. Now that his skills were to be the hope of his neighbors, illness—not disease—took center stage. At least some young doctors began to understand that a physician's life, too, was altered by another's illness, by the terrible time when sickness "attacks an only son, on the threshold of manhood . . . or . . . fixes on a favorite daughter, in the midst of bloom and beauty."[28]

In a small community, the moral cast to a man's initial work thus gave it a sharp public visibility. Gossip about the new doctor's personal style reverberated through the community in a way that caught many young practitioners off guard. Despite the intimacy of the bedside (or, in another sense, because of it), the community as a whole eagerly tracked a man as he responded to each demanding moment, hearing about what he diagnosed, judging him by what he prescribed. Francis Porcher discovered to his dismay that the breadth of the learnedness he had worked hard in school to achieve was of little import. People expected "*only* and *precisely* what is necessary to the present relief of the sufferer." There was no deferring the reality that "knowledge is demanded of you *daily* and *hourly*—and in a thousand various ways; on occasions, too, when no warning, no time for preparation is allowed—the Physician must *go forth* to meet the emergency, however full of peril." Sometimes the young doctor responded exactly as he hoped he would and was glad that people were watching. An exalted J. Marion Sims wrote to his fiancée in 1835, "I have had the glorious consolation of knowing (to a certainty) that by a very simple operation I have saved one man's life." It was a personal triumph, but hardly a private one; immediately, young Sims heard that "in his [the patient's] neighborhood the people believe in me." Not only one's own public image but others', too, were wrapped up in the moment. Sims, for example, was somewhat startled to learn how quickly what a doctor saw and said at any particular bedside spread through the community and "may involve the reputation of a respectable citizen or family, and even lead to disgrace." Indeed, as another practitioner put it in 1851, each time a physician determined what needed to be done and then did it, he "must either sustain himself, or be publicly disgraced."[29]

It was a lesson in the force of rumor and the instability of reputation. It also raised fresh doubts about just what the orthodox man could or should do to stress the advantages of his orthodoxy. Interestingly, some physicians concluded that being on public display might be managed by using it as an opportunity to instruct patients. They imagined themselves mentors of sorts and tried to control what was said about their work by providing a didactic—and, they hoped, final—word on it, directing the curious community to look beyond particular outcomes toward the general benefit of medical science. No outcome was certain, these men argued, but orthodox medicine's sheer breadth of learning should be part of the reason to choose an M.D. over other kinds of healers. Because "remedies of some sort will constantly be given by somebody, by the patient himself or by his friends," the question people *should* ask, Algernon Allan reasoned in 1846, was not whether the M.D.'s remedy was successful in each and every case but whether, in general, "it is better to have medicine in the hands of the ignorant or intrust it to the scientific." People needed to understand that a physician's knowledge was not a dark mystery but "highly interesting to all mankind," as another neophyte observed. "For although by this [medical] knowledge men may not all become adept in the art of healing, they may yet be enabled to guard & defend themselves against much disease & misery." Thus, some young doctors sought to turn the unnerving public visibility of their practice into a public lesson informed by their schooling, hoping that in acting the mentor they might close the gap between a graduate's image of himself as a schooled professional and whatever new image practice would bring.[30]

More frequently, however, the new public display of their skills and their first patients' fates led men to take a more heated, conflicted view of their orthodoxy and disease—one tilting sharply toward the subjective experience of illness. There was so much at stake, so much that was differently framed by one's own practice among neighbors who had their demands and secrets, that the image of disease was difficult to hold within science's cool linguistic restraints. Although they continued to speak of "process," "expectancy," and "clinical evidence," young M.D.s also revived and enriched a popular language of warfare and enmity between healers and disease. Only this language possessed the weight and texture equal to the threat of sickness in a community, permitting the doctor to inscribe great arcs of words beyond what was necessary to description. "He goes forth to battle against disease which is repugnant to his sight," as one man wrote of the M.D.'s mission. The word "repugnant" held something more horrible than anything schooled language could suggest. Such language possessed strength because it went beyond the observed surface of things—beyond behaviors and symptoms—to acknowledge the emotional power of illness to confound prediction, as well as hope. The doctor's struggle in practice was less an effort to understand nature gone astray than it was an all-out attempt "to protect the citadel of life . . . , to frustrate, the . . . dreaded secret wiles, which the insidious and treacherous foe is ever ready to practice." The greatest reward of bedside work, as another man learned, was not in the school's style of learning, in which small, new experiences were added slowly to the old, but a popular style based on heroic action, in which "the wild career of the fell monster has been impeded."[31]

This language and the sense it conveyed of dramatic struggle was not used by younger physicians alone, of course. But it appears more frequently and urgently in their writings and in the writings of older men seeking to impress them (and people in general) with the complexity and finality of a physician's everyday work. In this context, the rhetoric of monstrous disease had a double effect. It addressed the painfully public nature of a doctor's efforts by binding him to a common dread of illness shared by patients. At the same time it heightened his own subjectivity—his sense of personal risk and urgency—as he made the transition from study to giving care. That is, through images of monsters, enemies, and battle, the new M.D. faced the power of disease to kill his patients and ruin his every effort. As we will see, this subjective engagement with sickness was deeper and more far-reaching among physicians than a young M.D. could know at first. It would be a constant counterpoint to his role as a learned man of science, a staple of a country orthodox style founded on the reality that practice encompassed not only physical but moral events. To be sure, this subjective approach might easily become self-indulgent: the ripe rhetoric of lone-scientist heroism underwrote physicians' fantasies of being far more sophisticated than anyone else in the community. Or it might set up a man for ridicule; the excesses of young doctors gave new life to the parody of self-important physicians as "knights of the pill-box." And yet the insight toward which young men strove should not be reduced to either self-promotion or self-denigration. More important, practitioners' sense of being on public display in a battle against a monster was a way to imagine themselves as fully worthy men, serving the community while also serving self.

Even so, tensions continued to abound as many new practitioners clung to the conviction that orthodoxy was unique despite growing evidence that it was completely situated within local needs and wishes. In particular, many men held on to the image of the physician as first of all a learned man, despite the social risks of being seen as someone isolated from others by his exotic knowledge. Convinced that the intellectual life nurtured by school must be kept alive, novice physicians and sympathetic senior men encouraged each other to continue in their mastery of empiricism and synthesis. Even in the midst of worrying over livelihood, first patients, and failure, "a physician should endeavour to learn every day more and more of his profession, and to add something more to the general stock of knowledge for the advantage of posterity," as South Carolinian S. Carswell Ely resolved in 1834. Indeed, another new doctor reasoned, there was a silver lining to the small number of patients he had so far seen, for, "if we reflect properly, it is to our greatest advantage that we become not merged in heavy practice at once, for then we should be precluded from study."[32]

The image of the physician as a man of intellect—taking bedside notes and studying them, reading far into the night after his rounds—was not the same thing as the image of the mentor-doctor who instructed his community. The lonely man of intellect was a problematic figure, in some sense a counterimage of the involved, community mentor, who continued to cherish the idea of orthodoxy as a world beyond ordinary ken. Young physicians struggled with this contrast, and while unwilling to let go of schooled habits, they feared that continued study would have no place in small, southern communities. As one graduate said in 1856, even though the physician knew the value of study with regard to the "almost insurmountable difficulties" of sickness, "he finds it very difficult, to convince the world of this important truth." More bitter was the advice James Gage received from an older practitioner friend who singled out the South as an especially difficult place for the man of mind. It was a waste of time, Gage was told, to strive to become a man of intellect in southern medical practice, "for here science and mental cultivation weigh not a feather in the scale of reputation. Nay they even act deleteriously than otherwise." The only consolation was in "the inward satisfaction . . . of feeling superior to . . . ignorant pretenders and unblushing quacks."[33]

All told, it was a disquieting image of what practice would bring: a man of mind isolated from the community that denied him the intellectual life that might benefit everyone. Moreover, the physician was doomed to face this reality with few real brethren and without a professional structure for the fellowship that would keep his mind active. Taking "inward satisfaction" bereft of a group of like-minded colleagues was not the expectation created by the school's fraternal world. Nor in the practical-minded, limited society of a rural neighborhoods was inward satisfaction clearly a route to a successful career. Instead, indifference or suspicion on the part of neighbors might force the doctor to make a choice between study and community. Medicine construed narrowly as a "trade" beckoned the young doctor away from his profession because, for most of his neighbors, a trade "is deemed a little more respectable and lucrative" than the pursuit of high-flying and incomprehensible professional values. So the young doctor gives in and fits in, and before he knows it, as another new practitioner expressed it, the "halls of public entertainment [become] more inviting than the silent study." The light of intellect goes out and the graduate resigns himself to mediocrity: treating new cases on the formulae of the old, measuring out his advice and drugs according to people's prejudices, and otherwise taking his cues entirely from the local scene.[34]

Struggling with these misgivings led at least some new physicians to the brink of an even darker moral prospect. Stripping him of his intellect, solo practice took the practitioner below the social surface of life into people's ugly secrets and self-deceptions. That some people were secretive about their intimate lives only added to the new doctor's sense of being a stranger; that others relished self-disclosure had a different but equally isolating effect. The exposure or confession of a patient's worst secrets was a moral jolt to a novice doctor. For some, at least, there was no better example of how the supportive fraternity of the school was missed, and no surer instance of what the school had not prepared them for. As one young physician expressed it, nothing had prepared him for "that hideous sight a naked human heart." Under attack from disease, people's courage failed, morality shattered, faith collapsed and blew away. And, to their alarm, new physicians discovered that in putting their hands on these patients they joined themselves to malady. In Francis Porcher's stark phrase, sufferers viewed the physician and the disease together as "the *destiny* which has awaited them."[35]

Porcher was telling graduates to take courage. But the image of the physician as the instrument of fate was deeply troubling. Sick people, fearing such a doctor, clung mutely to their secrets or invented transparent lies; their bodies betrayed their immorality, and they told feckless or shameful tales in trying to make it all fit together. A practitioner might easily become demoralized himself and seek merely to profit by others' misfortune. He might decide to feed a community's predatory appetite for "sordid views," as one graduate realized, by using his authority to search out and reveal peoples' personal secrets. There were, indeed, as Albert Bachelor wrote to his sweetheart, "fearful privileges" in a medicine "so fraught with responsibilities, 'so capable of good if rightly used, so full of evil to ourselves & to mankind if administered ignorantly or unfaithfully.'" The abuse of a doctor's authority was not just in betraying confidences or spreading rumors, though these were bad enough, but in the greater evil of "abus[ing] by Quackery" people's bodies; taking advantage of how easy it was to fool patients with double-talk and drugs. Indeed, driven by malice or lust, a physician might be tempted to "the commission of many secret crimes, and the unprofessional world would never detect or even suspect that such crimes were ever committed." Against such temptations, would "inward satisfaction" be enough?[36]

∽

It may seem surprising at first to hear new graduates imagining such dark "what if" possibilities for immorality in everyday healing. But remembering that these men now were without the enclosing familiarity of mentors and friends, it is not so strange that a vision of predatory power should be the bedfellow of their wavering dreams of success. They saw that practice might in multiple ways detract from orthodoxy, not enrich it; they feared not knowing how to balance failure with learning, power with knowledge, and, perhaps most important, solitude with community. There is no way of knowing how many new physicians quickly decided that the practice of medicine was not for them. But the men who did persist realized that, somehow, practice would have to leaven learnedness just as learnedness focused practice. If he understood this, even vaguely, the new physician glimpsed the career-long challenge of doctoring: as substantial as his orthodoxy was, it was not something he brought whole to his neighbors from the school but something he *made* by integrating himself and his special knowledge into the community.

This near paradox was in essence a moral one, calling for a man to serve his neighbors by espousing not only the correctness but also the goodness of what he knew, and at the same time releasing his exclusive hold on it. He thus asserted his professionalism by staging it in the moral terms of manhood and character. This is the dynamic that underlay the complex, personal authority individual practitioners accorded something they called their "experience," the quality at the heart of country orthodox medicine. Neophytes grasped at the hope that in gaining experience they would combine school and community, intellect and practice, and be proof of the ultimate unity of these things. Holding on to this hope, they would have agreed with the benediction that the novice Virginia physician John Hundley received from his brother in 1849: "Read your works, study hard, & be attentive. You are now a man." They would have agreed, too, with Charles Hentz, who wrote in the first weeks of his backwoods Florida practice, as 1848 turned into 1849, that he was "at times wearied, at times satisfied with my calling—Tis new." Above all else, he resolved "to discipline myself for a much higher sphere of action, than that in which I have been compelled to launch my bark."[37]

PART TWO

DOING MEDICINE

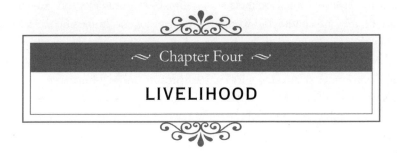

Chapter Four

LIVELIHOOD

In the early afternoon of November 27, 1873, someone in the G. Wilson Efferson household in Springfield, Louisiana, asked neighbor Washington King to carry a message to Dr. George Colmer. Sometime later, probably the same day, Colmer wrote this entry in his daybook:

> Nov. 27 (Thursday) About 2 P.M. Washington King arrived at my office with a request to go to Efferson's house and relieve Mrs. E of an afterbirth. She sent word that she was "just as she was before," and therefore instead of going out, Rx.

Just below this entry, Colmer added:

> 28—Visit to residence—fetched by   Efferson (Wilson's brother). Started at 10½ A.M., got back about 5½ P.M. Went in Louis Shenk's vehicle, drawn by Louis Shenk's horse, and driven by [Winfield?] Christmas. Removed retained placenta and drew off urine with catheter. Child (a boy) born the day before.

Removing a retained placenta was a risky procedure, and Colmer charged the Effersons thirty-five dollars for effecting it, a hefty fee. In fact, it may have been a tense scene at the Effersons'; on top of everything else, Colmer charged Mr. Efferson a dollar for a bottle of "medicinal whisky" prescribed, it seems, for Mr. Efferson himself.[1]

George Colmer turned sixty-six years old in 1873, and the Efferson case was typical of how he responded to—and recorded—hundreds of other calls during his thirty-year practice.[2] His daybook notational style, though more detailed than most, is nonetheless typical of the informal, time-driven, heavily peopled notes made by other physicians. Indeed, notes of this kind do not change in any significant way throughout the midcentury years, comprising one of the key texts that made for continuity in a physician's sense of his work. Meant for his eyes only, daybook notes are terse and minimally reflective. By the same token, however, they are candid and wonderfully unapologetic, imparting a clear view of this chapter's concerns: the fundamental economic and social realities of southern community medical practice that shaped, and were shaped by, the everyday routines of making a living. Part profession, part business, the physician's pursuit of his livelihood sketched with broad strokes his domain as he strove to lead, but also learned to follow, his community in matters of health.

Drawing on daybooks, as well as on correspondence and other personal sources, the focus of this chapter is on the basic social and economic conditions of country orthodoxy: the essentials of making a living, the variety of patients and the influence of their views, and the way in which everything a practitioner perceived was shaped by making neighborhood rounds. The aim is to see this framework of everyday practice as having more than its material significance, however. It is to see it as doctors wrote about it, as a dynamic combining economic survival with moral purpose, making the physician into a certain kind of public figure. In this way, practitioners gained a new purchase on the desirable quality they called their "experience." As his schooling suggested, a man's sense of his experience was a coveted but problematic thing, richly subjective and personal, and yet something recognized by everyone. Although physicians thought of their experience as something they acquired, here they are seen as subjects shaped by the experience they created in the routines of making a living. And although there is much here that is distinctly southern—especially the social relations of slavery and the continuing reality of a biracial setting for medicine after emancipation—there is much in this wide-angled view, too, that tells us about the livelihood of orthodox doctors elsewhere in rural America.[3]

As he recorded his routine in his daybook, a physician steadily wrote himself free from many of his early fears and wishes discussed in Chapter 3. He logged satisfying lists of people seen, recording their prescriptions and fees; he experimented with his eye for detail and context, which he would later develop at greater length in his bedside notes and case narratives. Daybook entries record surprise and happenstance, too, in his shifting personal relations with patients, thus opening up a glimpse of a practitioner's moral bearings as he compiled what amounted to a rough dossier on the well-being of the families under his care. Consider again George Colmer's notes on the Efferson case; more is going on in this terse account than it might at first seem. In telling what happened in this single instance, Colmer also inscribed something of the larger routine shaping country medical work. First, it is notable that Colmer had not been called upon to attend the birth of the Efferson child. Like most rural physicians throughout the mid-nineteenth century, Colmer did not do much obstetrical work, assisting at fewer than one birth a month throughout his long career. It was the retained placenta that led the Effersons to call on Colmer, and even then he did not immediately go to them. Instead, relying on Mrs. Efferson's own self-diagnosis that she was "just as . . . before" (a reference, Colmer indicates in a bottom-of-the-page note, to a retained placenta in an earlier childbirth), the physician simply wrote a prescription: "instead of going out, Rx."

Colmer's daybook notes also reveal how wide was the social circle of a single case. There is a considerable number of people whom Colmer thought mattered enough to include in his account: Mr. and Mrs. Efferson, of course, and the child (whose sex Colmer records); the messenger, Mr. King; Mr. Efferson's brother; the wagon driver, Christmas; and even the owner of the horse and wagon. Colmer doubtless included all of these people, as did other practitioners, as a context for recollection should he ever need it. But such details also reveal how a single call inescapably implicated a doctor in the social relationships of his patients. In small, rural communities, few cases were, or could afford to be, more "private" than this one.

Like many other physicians, too, Colmer regularly returned to his book to add new information to a household's record (whether or not he was present) about births and deaths, who was down with what affliction, and who assisted him. In the November 28 Efferson entry, for example, Colmer left a space for the name of Mr. Efferson's brother. By the same token, Colmer occasionally included details that had little or nothing to do with caregiving but were important in his community generally: who moved in and out, who married whom, how the crops appeared to him as he rode through the fields. No informal text better reveals how a physician helped shape social life, directing events where he could, watching them when he could not, trolling his community's potential for sickness and health. He fashioned his livelihood from deep within his community and yet, at the same time, recorded his neighbors' ways from a certain remove, becoming a peculiar combination of actor and witness. In this way, a physician redefined orthodoxy as a claim on local means, local respect, and a sense of belonging.[4]

LOGGING PATIENTS, SEEING RACE

As an immediate means for translating what a doctor did into something he wrote, daybooks look much the same in 1880 as they did in 1830, plotting a remarkable continuity of everyday practice. Daybooks braided together a markedly orthodox style (M.D.s were more likely than other kinds of doctors to keep written accounts) with an intensely personal one (every daybook reflected its author's individual habits of notation). This meant that physicians could live up to their professional obligation to collect ever-changing medical information while adopting a personal style of expression that rarely changed, becoming, in fact, a kind of commonsense that resisted critique. Moreover, even though utilitarian daybooks might seem to stand outside ideology, their unselfconscious practicality and their baseline medical judgments gave them an essentially ideological power to reinscribe and naturalize fundamental social relations. With these considerations in mind, then, we begin by looking at how a physician typically took note of his routine activities and typically bundled patients into groups, thus sketching something of his community, as well as something of his own subjectivity.

We know about the slow and conflicted course of therapeutic change in orthodox medicine during this era, largely in terms of innovations or reforms in urban or institutional sites. The daybooks of rural physicians, and the routines of vernacular medicine they inscribe, add an everyday dimension to the conservative nature of ordinary practice, suggesting how and why these physicians' deeply personal style of practice resisted amendment. For instance, many if not most physicians' daybooks include only minimal notes on procedures and medicines. Physicians noted only that they dispensed "sundry medicines" or "prescribed" for this or that patient. Although serving as economic records, daybooks clearly were intended to be medical records, too, and the lack of specifics suggests that certain details (the type of "medicine," for example) either rarely varied or were simply not important enough to recall. Such minimal notes tended to leave the particulars of daily orthodox regimen locked up in each practitioner's head, where they were not open ot review or change.[5]

In another implication of this personal style, some daybooks include notes on the doctor's daily doings, comprising a kind of rudimentary diary that suggests how easily he tied his work to his personal life and how firmly his style of practice was rooted in his identity as a man. Dr. A. Armstrong, for instance, practicing in Georgia in the 1840s, included among his clinical notes recipes for medicine, some poetry, autobiographical notes, descriptions of parlor games and puzzles, and an occasional account of his dreams. Similarly, Thomas Davis, a planter-physician in Franklin County, North Carolina, noted his doings throughout the 1830s in a typical, linear way that gave equal weight to everything: "June 17—Went to see little sick Negro at Mr. Griffins. Found him very ill; also to Lebanon, heard an excellent sermon by Brother Dye; killed a squirrel today." This style, accepted as wholly appropriate by orthodox men, underscores how professional standards of record-keeping were built on foundations of personal expression steeped in individual experience. It vividly suggests how the basic routine of medical work was so saturated by a man's life that it would likely change only as the surrounding context of his life changed.[6]

Inevitably, physicians mapped aspects of the local social order in their daybooks. Practitioners almost always grouped their patients, slave and free, under the name of the head of the white household, thus reinscribing the male-headed, white family as the primary social unit. Gender emerges in other ways, too, as a central organizing aspect of a doctor's practice. Patients' names almost always revealed gender, and when they did not, many physicians made it a point to identify the person's sex next to his or her name. Occasionally, doctors indulged in more pointed social observations, as when Thomas McCarty ironically noted "Miss" by the names of certain pregnant women he encountered on his rounds. Unlike gender, the age of patients seems to have mattered only in the most general way. The exact age of anyone, even young children and the aged, was not important enough to determine; most practitioners used terms such as "young child" or "old man" well up to the end of the century.[7]

Given this style of logging in patients, the great emphasis antebellum southern physicians put on race and bondage is striking, suggesting how deeply physicians were implicated in the racial order of southern communities. Indeed, nowhere in the lecture and clinical notes of a man's schooling was there a text that so clearly used race and bondage as an organizing system for patients. Daybooks thus suggest the power of ordinary practice to focus, and to some extent modify, the vague racial pedagogy of medical schools. As in the school, but much more clearly, doctors' daybooks show how the details of medical work with slave patients were shaped by the institution of slavery rather than by the more abstract notion of race. At the same time, however, aside from the particulars of everyday doctoring, race emerges as the more fundamental category for putting patients in their broad social place.

This said, race and bondage are not always noted in ways that we might think of as stereotypical. For instance, despite the fact that physicians often lumped their slave patients together anonymously, especially during epidemics, many sick slaves appear as individuals, too, in daybooks, suggesting that patienthood was a category that could sometimes override the anonymity imposed by slavery. Most commonly, slaves emerge as individuals slowly, over a succession of visits, as the very sick children Lenah and Moses do here:

[February 27, 1844]: To visit and medicine negro child
[February 28]: To visit and medicine little negroes
[February 29] To visit and medicine negro children . . . to visit and medi-
cine negro boy (night)
[March 4]: To 2 visits and medicine negro child Lenah
[March 5]: To visit and medicine Lenah & medicine (Moses)
[March 7]: To visit and medicine Lenah, prescription Moses[8]

In this regard, there are unintended ironies in what physicians took for granted as they inscribed masters and slaves in daybooks. For instance, the very prominence of a slave owning, white family might lead their physician to neglect noting their names in his daybook. And yet at our historical remove, this makes members of the wealthy family less individually sharp than many slave patients whose names were recorded.[9]

Despite such ironies, however, and despite the fact that the category of "patient" in some ways cut across racial lines, physicians relentlessly relied on race to segregate people. Thus, "Negro," not "servant," was the term most often used for slaves in daybooks, sometimes in rapid-fire, shorthand form—"N.W." for "Negro Woman" or "N. George"—suggesting how subtly a "natural" category shaped a mnemonic device, which then, in turn, contributed to the general social power of "race" to denote and divide. In this regard, practitioners employed widespread white usages that linked gendered and racial language; the blunt term "woman," especially, denoted only slave patients. Thus in Dr. Robert Butler's notation under Mrs. M. J. Ellis's account, "Operation, woman Lucy," and under Judge Guion's, "visit & prescription for woman," there can be no doubt that these women were slaves and that race and gender were locked into a commentary, one on the other. Identifying a patient as the "woman Lucy" did not better describe her as a woman than simply calling her "Lucy." The object of the gendered term is to underscore Lucy's status as a slave and, unmistakably, to divide black women from white by suggesting that each possessed a peculiar kind of femininity.[10]

Most doctors flagged their mixed-race patients as well, fixing them in their books and in their minds by the single characteristic that made them most physically and socially distinctive. Under the account of a household head oddly identified as "E. Dalby alias Sharpe," an Augusta doctor recorded a visit to a "N[egro] W[oman]" in late October 1845, and was careful to note her "mulatto child." George Colmer noted the birth of a boy to a slave woman, Eliza, in April 1862, and in a July visit he gave "advice for Eliza's child (white boy)." Similarly, many physicians specifically highlighted free African Americans. Sometimes the doctor's logging device was simply to append a note of the person's free status to the usual first-name-only identity given to slaves. For example, patient "Sally" has "Freewoman" written under her name in one physician's journal. At other times, doctors recorded free blacks' surnames, but almost invariably underscored their race in other ways. Thus, John Knox referred to a seamstress as "Mary Mobley (coloured)," and even the wealthy African American William Ellison appears in his doctor's book as "William Ellison—colored man."[11]

This record-keeping style permitted physicians to help patrol relations between the races, strengthening the powerful double meaning of race as both a social and a biological reality. This was so even though daybooks reveal that racial considerations alone did not determine either the type or the quality of treatment in the antebellum years. Slavery, and especially a master's willingness to intervene, more clearly structured the actual provision of medical care. Physicians charged the same fees per visit, whether the patient was black or white, and slaves whose masters were willing to pay for it received costly care. Although most masters put a financial cap on overall medical care for their slaves, they often spent considerable amounts on a slave who was especially valuable or well liked. Dr. Thomas Cox, for example, called on Abner Ellis's "boy" Floyd nineteen times to dress a serious wound in late 1848, charging Ellis the sizable fee of $59.50. Peggy, a slave in the wealthy Wilkinson household in the Georgetown District of South Carolina, went through some sort of life-threatening crisis lasting six weeks in 1848 that brought in E. Belin Flagg for almost daily attendance and ended with her recovery and a fee of well over $100. As with other doctors, Flagg's mode of recording his prescriptions did not vary with his slave patients, either, no matter the irony of his dosages measured by dessert spoons or by "half a wineglass."[12]

In sum, then, daybooks make it clear that in any given case the social relations of slavery most obviously structured which individuals in bondage came under a physician's care, and when. At the same time, "race" and its social divisions structured the broader organization of everyday practice. Race was so unquestioned as a way of remembering and locating patients that it became fundamental to clinical vision itself. In this sense, the most ordinary daybook terms—"Negro Man," "the boy George," "small Negroes"—employed over and over, unquestioned, as was so much else of practice inscribed in daybooks, gained a taken-for-granted force that drove race deeply into a white doctor's sense of his daily work.

Daybooks also introduce the world of physicians' fees and income, and, along with it, a sense of how physicians' livelihood defined their problematic desire to belong to their communities in an integral yet "special" way. Until the very end of the century, many physicians used the terms "my practice" and "my business" interchangeably. And yet a man's livelihood had more than a material significance. Many country practitioners, scattered across the South, recorded the economic facts of life in ways that refracted but did not dim their allegiance to the orthodox ideal of a schooled profession in pursuit of the general good. To be sure, as we have seen in terms of novice physicians, the "profession," as a corporate body, had scant presence in rural M.D.s' lives. Nevertheless, it mattered to many of them that they sustain both a livelihood and an imagination of professional virtues; how to fit in but also be superior. Physicians therefore sketched the arc of their professionalism broadly to include a moral dimension to their fees and services.

Daybooks clearly capture how difficult it was for most physicians to maintain a steady income throughout the midcentury decades. Good health in the neighborhood brought a whiff of poverty; in private, doctors were unguarded about decrying "distressingly healthy" times. On the other hand, sickly times meant that some families would move out of the area, thus threatening a doctor's income in another way. Worst of all, a doctor's skills might fail and his patients abandon him. Circumstances varied from place to place, of course, but broadly speaking, the income of a typical midcentury rural practitioner—measured in terms of the fees he "booked" or billed his patients for—seems to have been in the range of $500 to $2,000 a year. A successful city doctor with an established practice might expect to book twice as much, and a handful of wealthy physicians made up to ten times the country doctor's income. In any event, booking fees was one thing and collecting them another. Most physicians felt they were doing well if they collected half of their booked fees, either in cash or in kind, each year; the remainder, like all other goods and services in this era's economy, was put on credit. All told, the actual income of rural doctors was not greater than that earned by many skilled craftsmen, or by lawyers and clergy, for that matter.[13]

Off and on, local physicians joined together to publish fee bills denoting charges for common procedures, in order both to regulate their own competition and to advertise the orthodox man's commitment to fair dealing. However, fee bills were unenforceable and famously unstable. Indeed, any given fee bill included strikingly elastic guidelines for some procedures: pulling a tooth (which daybooks reveal as the most common procedure) was fixed at two dollars; but obstetrical visits were listed at ten to thirty dollars, and an "opinion as to the soundness of a negro" ranged from five to twenty-five dollars. Moreover, daybooks reveal how practice modified fee bill generalizations. Actual fees, for example, clustered at the lower end of fee bills' range. These charges were remarkably consistent for the entire century throughout the South, although fees fell somewhat during the war and then inflated immediately afterward. Still, it is not unusual to find a physician charging the same fees in 1880 that he did in 1850, mostly the "visit and prescription" calls at two to three dollars each. Fee bills to the contrary, it appears that country doctors did not charge for mileage unless called upon to travel well beyond their normal riding range of fifteen miles or so a day. However, some practitioners added a relatively modest surcharge for "rising at night," or "noct." calls (which fee bills recommended), and although fee bills did not mention it, some doctors charged for certain patient requests they found annoying, such as being asked to put oral directions into writing. In practice, physically demanding work or discomfort justified the most common surcharges. Typically, physicians like George Dunlap, in Lancaster District, South Carolina, charged up to 50 percent extra for cases he noted as "attention strict" or "6 hours vigilance." Bad weather merited special mention in daybooks. Virginian Philip Southall charged one to two dollars extra for visits denoted as "a very rainy day," "visiting in a hard rain," or "visiting in a considerable rain." Josiah Hawkins appears to have charged more than five times his usual fee for a call he noted as "Alexander Carpenter V[isit] P[rescribe] & M[edicine] to [him]self & staying all night & getting wet & cold."[14]

Although there were variations in this pattern of income, and different ways of supplementing it, orthodox livelihood was firmly centered around this household-by-household, visit-by-visit core, where fees reflected the doctor's particular work habits and preferences rather than, as they would later, the cost of procedures or drugs. This was the context for the moral cast physicians gave to their work as they struggled not just to make a living but to justify it as a calling that rose above economic calculation. Seen from the ground level of practice, such an effort was contingent on each doctor's moral standing in his community, which, among other things, included how he went about one of his most prosaic tasks: collecting the money owed him. This vexing aspect of work runs throughout doctors' daybooks and spills over into their correspondence. The various methods of dunning and scheming reveal the markedly dependent— though inventive—position of solo practitioners. The punctilious South Carolina physician James Spann, for instance, tried to put his finances on a contractual basis in the early 1830s, proposing that patients sign promissory notes to pay within three days and to pay interest if they did not. At the other end of the continuum, and far more numerous, were practitioners like George Colmer, who improvised patient by patient, according to what he knew of his patients' lives. He frequently noted making "a proposition" to a patient who owed him money; indeed, he seemed to relish coming up with yet another ingenious means for getting his due.[15]

Every account of money owed or received inscribed anew a pattern of favor and responsibility between physician and patient, or its opposite. "I enclose $100.00 Dollars which you will please pay yourself for your visits to the Plantation in [18]51," began what must have been a welcome letter to Dr. Gerhard Muller from his patient James D. Trezevant, who, like many patients, paid once a year. Nor was it only the well-off patient who paid. In the accounts of Joseph A. Eve, for example, may be found working-class households like that headed by M. S. Kean, who owed Eve $114 for twenty-one visits following a difficult childbirth in 1866. Eve "discounted" $14 at the outset, and, as far as the extant accounts reveal, Kean still was paying off the bill in small amounts three years later. Nevertheless, physicians were more likely to write about neighbors who did not pay, revealing much about the moral axis on which their livelihoods turned. "A physician goes from chamber to chamber, dispensing light and hope and comfort," Dr. William Holcombe complained. And yet when the time comes for him to be paid, "Alas, what a falling off [is] there." Nonetheless, he resolved to help "the entire genus homo . . . pay or no pay, gratitude or no gratitude." Frank James, unhappily practicing in Oceola, Arkansas, resolved to do the opposite. "A doctor's bill is the last one that these people will pay," he wrote angrily in his journal, adding that he would have to cut back on his visits "if some of these damned yahooes around here don't pay up pretty soon." Throughout the South, daybook accounts resound with the staccato of lost income. "Gone to Savannah," Joseph A. Eve wrote across the page for the Coggins family account, who left without paying their twenty dollars. "Dead Loss," Robert Ryland wrote at the bottom of the McDaniel account for 1850. "Ain't worth shucks," was his summary note for the Gibbons household, and, among the deadbeats he notes "Gen'l Zach Taylor," in arrears for an unspecified amount, of whom Ryland remarked, "[He] may be put down for nothing, as I have never received the first cent of it."[16]

Patients' reasons for not paying often only deepened the tension between money and moral obligation as, for example, patients implored the doctor to make an exception for their suffering. Mary Peterson had promised to pay John Young Bassett what she owed him—"you have acted like a gentleman and a father to us"—but she was at his mercy, she told him, because her husband "continues to drink and neglect his business." Each practitioner developed his own means of cajoling, embarrassing, and otherwise attempting to pressure patients to pay. Stewing over his uncollected fees, Frank James was not the only practitioner to see that, "with a little combination between professional men here, all this could be changed." But, like so many physicians, he was fiercely protective of what he saw as his autonomy, though this individualism only exacerbated his economic dependence. The unusual—and futile—proposal of Dr. G. F. Steifer, of Abbeville County, South Carolina, to organize his fellow physicians in 1870 underscores how physicians conflated their economic and moral purposes. Writing to colleague John A. Robinson, Steifer proposed publishing the names of delinquent patients and then organizing local doctors to refuse to treat them. "We must make a change in our Profession," he asserted. And yet the subsequent correspondence between Steifer and Robinson suggests why such efforts usually failed. Although pushing for collective action, Steifer did not come up with a specific plan for organizing it. Instead, his letters dissolve into mere complaints ("Samuel Shaw is the only Shaw that will pay a Medical Bill"), which suggest that personal insult was at the heart of not being paid. Robinson's careful reply to Steifer, too, suggests the personal scale of practice embraced by most men. Although he also "felt keenly the tardiness" of late payment, Robinson believed that publishing a list of debtors would simply be a way of predetermining "who will not pay their medical bills" in the future, and, in any case, withholding care would frighten the majority of "honest" patients. For men like Robinson, each physician properly made individual decisions based on his relationship with "my patients" under a broad canopy of mutual honor and obligation, rather than on accounts receivable.[17]

Like most other physicians, then, Robinson saw the relation between doctor and patient not only as fundamentally ethical but as irreducibly personal, reflecting on his character, as well as theirs. This may be seen in another sense in doctors' eager attempts to make the cash-poor southern economy work for them. Everyone had a scheme for economic success, and everyone had a story that revealed their character and powers of judgment. For instance, in Springfield, Louisiana, in 1874, W. Hugh Caldwell had not paid Dr. George Colmer the twenty-five dollars for treating his fractured leg. Colmer, noting that the fee had been discounted once already, devised some "instructions for collection" in his daybook: "If Mr. C. pay $10 in full *on the spot* the remainder will be remitted. If he does not pay the $10 ask him to sign the blank note for $25. If he does neither, give the account to T. M. Akens to sue on. . . . P.S. If Mr. C. will have me credited, *at once*, with $10 on the books of Settoon and Dearing, it will do as well as the cash." And here is the Reverend Alexander Campbell's plan for reimbursing his physician ten dollars: "If by any means you could collect the $10 due me in the hand of Justice Field, that together with the $25 due from Mr. Moon would reimburse you for the excessive remittance of $10 which you made, and also meet the demand of Crutcher & McKavin."[18]

This house-of-cards language of debt runs throughout all types of mid-nineteenth-century business transactions in the rural South—a masculine language rife with passionate schemes and the stuff of reputation. Appearing in doctors' daybooks, such language also captures life on the edge of sickness, becoming over time a discourse of hopefulness, displacement, and regret. It suggests how deeply rooted physicians were in the assumptions and appraisals of their many-layered local communities, something that took yet another turn when patients paid not with the preferred cash but in kind. Daybooks all through the century reveal a thick texture of in-kind exchange; patients and doctors constantly weighed a medical procedure—the pulling of a tooth—against, say, a basket of fruit. One patient paid Dr. J. H. Davis in 1829 for medicine and venesection "by weaving," for example, and a Natchez doctor was given "a small grey horse" in payment for surgery. Samuel Henning spent a couple of days digging a hole worth the nine dollars he owed Dr. Robert Ryland in 1850, and the Traylors evened their account with George Colmer with a bag of wool, hauling wood and pine knots, and having Mrs. Traylor mend Colmer's socks. David Weeks was paid by various people in 1827 with a horse, bacon, twelve barrels of sand, and, in a sort of coals-to-Newcastle twist, two bottles of "Swain's Panacea," a patent medicine. About one-quarter of Robert B. Pusey's patients gave him payments in kind during the years 1863 and 1889, including whiskey, many bushels of corn and oats, "fixing buggy wheel," a ton of hay, shoes and boots, fruit, timber hauling, a thousand boards, and untold chickens.[19]

Such exchanges suggest how a doctor's livelihood was inextricable from other face-to-face relationships between neighbors. In exchange for mending their neighbors' bodies, physicians consumed the fruits of their neighbors' daily labor and took into their homes artifacts made by neighbors' hands. It was a process of sharp calculation but also of intimate knowledge. Practitioners dealt with their poorest patients by developing a sense of charity—Christian and otherwise—first experimented with on the hospital wards. Moreover, there was an ancient tradition of pro bono community work among M.D.s, and although southern physicians rarely invoked it, their local "charity" in a sense reinvented the tradition daily. Most physicians discovered, however, that the relationship between a given patient's good character and charity in the community more broadly was a much more complex matter than it had been on the wards. But when it worked, charity practice instructed a man's "experience" by transforming economic disappointments into moral acts. "Cr[edit] by friendship," Joseph A. Eve wrote in his daybook under the 1866 account of Mary Ansley, erasing the money she owed him in the name of his fondness for her.[20]

Nevertheless, as many physicians had learned on the wards, the quality of charity was soon strained, and doctors' generosity, like that of any other mid-century philanthropist, was colored by who was deemed "deserving." Without ties of personal friendship, especially, charity became another term for being taken advantage of. "Do you have to do much charity practice?" North Carolinian William C. Wright wanted to know in 1846 of his brother practicing in Georgia, complaining that "I have had more this year than any other year before." Most physicians, like Samuel Leland, were relieved to see nonpaying families move away; their absence, he wrote, "will lessen . . . my *labours* considerably without affecting my income in the least." With regard to "undeserving" people, most physicians had no qualms about shucking off the burden of their charity, and, as with others who undertook philanthropy, the ambivalence of charity as a language for both morality and economics became clear.[21]

By thus framing the most prosaic aspects of their livelihood with larger moral concerns, physicians attempted to bridge a tricky gap between their ideal of overarching professional values and the actual practice of making highly personal judgments. The drudgery of assigning fees, dunning one's patients, and formulating conditions for barter, along with the difficulties of defining who was worthy of charity, needed to be placed on an honorable professional stage that enhanced a practitioner's estimable character. "I made warm friends, but little money," is the way Florida physician Charles Hentz summed up the balance of charity and income in his career, with irony but with satisfaction, too. An experienced, professional man was a man who *chose* to see his work as a moral theater. William Holcombe struggled with his "charity" and his self-image in exactly these terms. Though frustrated by the discomforts and chancy income of his practice, Holcombe strove to live an ethic of benevolence and self-sacrifice. He attempted to see every day, every decision, as reflecting his moral capacity. He wrote in his diary in 1855, "Reproved myself tonight for getting impatient and petulant at pauper calls. A truly philanthropic spirit *works* and *works* and *works* for others without a hope or wish of reward." He reminded himself that a "doctor who rejects a needy supplicant for his professional blessing is as mean as a preacher who should refuse to pray for a poor sinner."[22]

Looking at how physicians defined the values of their work as they tallied accounts, bartered with neighbors, suffered bad weather, and otherwise put together a living brings up the importance of the broad, popular consensus on the nature of health and sickness. By this consensus I mean the fundamental ideas and assumptions shared by most southerners—including physicians themselves—that made up a deep common sense of what signified and preserved good health. Working in accord with this common sense was an essential condition for a physician's successful livelihood, and a key component of the country orthodox style. By definition, popular consensus on health was self-evident, but it required frequent airing in what might be termed the "health talk" of ordinary social intercourse. In their personal letters in particular, people regularly offered brief commentaries on their health and the health of family, friends, and community, free and slave. Such "minding" of bodies, drugs, seasons, and weather was a modest but indispensable way to keep important obligations and relationships fresh. And it fashioned a context for a doctor's acceptance into the community. When practice went smoothly, this consensus was invisible to the physician; he simply had the sense of possessing the "experience" he needed.[23]

Children of literate southerners learned to speak of the health of their neighborhoods and families as a part of their mastery of letter-writing and its inscription of social and emotional life. Learning how to talk about health was part of learning how to speak like an adult, to converse easily on the surrounding world. More broadly, news of a community's health was an epistolary theme that expressed much and persisted largely unchanged in its basic form throughout the years under consideration here. Health talk was, at one stroke, a practical report on general well-being, good gossip, and testimony to the unchanging instability of life itself. News of good health was a kind of summary of personal contentment: "Friends are all in good health & with courage persuing their different forms of industry," David Campbell wrote to his sister Maria. Conversely, when malady entered a community, talk of it comprised the essence of anxiety, imparting a sense of life's riskiness and of the need for watchfulness, inquiry, and faith. "I heard also that Mrs. Folk was about to die," Jane Barr wrote to her brother and sister in 1854. "Our family are not very well—they are all up this morning. John was in bed all day yesterday with fever in him & Billy has had it for some time. Frances Bowers is lying very low at this time." Health talk addressed both the impermanent body and the everlasting God's mysterious ways. Elizabeth Bell wrote to her friend, "Thank god for his goodness to me so far my health is very good but [Mary?] and Harriet has had the fever and Ague. . . . Poor Mrs. Patton has had the cholick for four Days but is some Easier to day. . . . I am sorry to hear Mrs. James Ewert is so unwell as to have to go to the north . . . but the Lord is all sufficient and do what seemeth [to] him good."[24]

From 1800 to the 1830s, as letter-writing style became less formal, broad characterizations of an entire community's health became somewhat less common; people spoke less of a general well-being and more about an immediate circle of family and friends. But most of health talk's themes remained constant: God's overall plan, his mercy, and the joinery of faith and fate; the familiar yet mysterious—and always fascinating—flow of disease into and out of the community; the recuperation of some people and the demise of others; the overarching importance of eating well, sleeping soundly, and being mindful of shifts in the weather.

Southerners spoke of good health in terms of balance; equilibrium, not energy, was the key measure of health. When health talk was taking its more personal turn by the 1830s, people increasingly scrutinized their own habits and physical transformations in their letters. They sized up their bodies in terms of how "fleshy" they were (a good sign) and how often they suffered irregular bowel movements or headaches. If anything, talk about the body in the midcentury decades tended to move further into the body's interior and become more specific. "I am so far . . . quite well—except a little soreness in my teeth & headache from want of sleep & costiveness," a man wrote his wife in 1880. People wrote of the actions they took to stave off ill health in order to recommend them but also simply to acknowledge the common sense of proper living: riding in the fresh air, drinking a tonic before sleep, wrapping up in flannel and protecting against changes in the weather. Health talk was spatial and architectural: people sank or rose in health; they climbed heights or fell to the depths. Thus one man who had worked for years without regard for his health "has sunk under the labor, & laid the foundation of a sickness which terminated his life."[25]

Next to the body and personal habits, a person's age summed up what was important to know and do about health. To a certain extent, gender figured into this, too, though not as prominently as age; in this particular, popular health talk reversed M.D.s' emphasis. Childhood and old age were equally vulnerable, and people spoke about young children as being in their own way close to the grave as the aged. Parents described their healthy youngsters physically as if loving images were a charm; no bodies are portrayed as closely as the bodies of small children. In Tennessee in 1852, for instance, Virginia Shelton wrote home to family in Virginia about her toddler David, "He is more like a fat wren or partridge now than anything else & the bloom in his cheek is the clearest rose tint." Mary Henderson's one-year-old son Richard, growing quickly, "is very fat and rosy cheeked, you would scarcely know him except from his sparkling black eyes." She added with terse satisfaction, "I have had no use for medicine." Somewhat less vividly, people wrote of aged family members as if doing so might also keep health stable. One woman told her father to "take particular care of your health, as you begin to advance in years. A small neglect . . . might be attended with fatal consequences to one past the meridian of life." Elderly people themselves often expressed physiological decline in the spatial terms of journeys and descents, a common language over the course of the century. After an illness, a Virginia man wrote in 1851 that he had not realized "how fast I was becoming an old man. I now feel it and know that I am fast approaching the foot of the hill of life."[26]

Again, letters earlier in the century sounded a deeper tone in some ways. A letter-writer before the 1820s tended to write with an awareness of a watching world, something that gave a certain public heft even to intimate letters. As expressive conventions changed, growing more subjective, and as the culture of family life generally became more introspective and oriented toward the expression of personal emotions, epistolary conventions of family health news became less gravely portentous. Thus, when Daniel Grant began his letter to his son in 1791 with the words "We are all still alive," he was employing a familiar convention that pronounced a sense of expansive well-being, grateful and calm. The same words, however, if used to begin a letter a half century later, would imply that the writer had barely escaped some catastrophe that he would now go on to relate. Similarly, earlier in the century, a person would write of illness as if from a height, to "let you know that, through the great goodness of God I am still in life . . . a few small complaints excepted." Fifty years later, it was close, domestic (and physiological) detail that pulled the reader into health talk: "Well here we are all just snuffling and coughing and crooping about with the very worst spell of influenza I ever saw in the family." In sum, sickness later in the century was more likely to have a name, be described in terms of its personal, physical symptoms, and become, if no less a threat, then something unique to the individual's personal life.[27]

At times, midcentury health talk slipped into a register that raised anxieties instead of quelling them. Health talk easily was colored by a sense that small events might signal life's fateful turns. A North Carolina man wrote, as did many people when separated from family, that whenever he traveled he worried excessively that they would become sick and "fear[ed] that some evil may befal one on whom my happiness is staked." Family members at home replied in like fashion.

Anna King's long correspondence with her frequently absent husband in the 1840s and 1850s constantly wove her physical symptoms of ringing ears and short breath into her expressions of longing, disappointment, and, sometimes, deep frustration at being left alone. Health talk thus became charged with deeper, unresolved aspects of personal relationships. Words about health might conceal or mislead: "Sister Fanny writes in a very lively strain," Virginia Shelton told her aunt in 1850, "though sister Margaret says [Fanny] had not been well."[28]

In the South, these themes of health talk were complicated by powerful but unexamined notions of race and by the practices of slavery that led whites to view black people as simultaneously property and persons, ordinary and alien. Owners of large numbers of slaves, for instance, routinely took note of the general health of their workforce in an impersonal way not dissimilar to the way they noted changes in the weather. At the same time, certain African Americans appear in some whites' health talk as individuals; in a sense, health talk was one of the clearest ways whites acknowledged African Americans' humanity. Blacks were seen as liable to the same general risk of disease and were perceived both as sources of cross-racial sickness and as victims of it. Whites and blacks were spoken of in the same breath, and if most whites uncritically took slavery for granted as a "natural" condition for blacks, they did not necessarily highlight race or give it consistent weight in their health talk. In Lucila McCorkle's hasty summary of her sick household in 1847, for instance, Laura and Sophy, who were slaves, simply are part of the generally unhappy state of affairs: "My dear boy was very unwell. . . . Laura is down with scurvy or scrofula—& Sophy complains of hard work & weak back. Mr. McC. is often feeble & I am not of much account." Occasionally, however, white writers did highlight race, etching it as a fundamental social divide as sharply as any doctor's daybook. "[W]e have had a verry sick family," a man wrote to his son in Georgia. "Your Mother is the only one of the whites that have escaped and but a verry view of the blacks and some have been sick two or three times." In 1842, Adaline Evans reported to her brother that there was "more sickness with our negroes than we have had in five or six years—Mickel was down five weeks—he has done us but little service[.] yet our white family keep well except Mr. Evans." In this kind of white talk, "the blacks" or "the negroes," whatever their proximity, are a distinct caste.[29]

Because letters written by slaves to each other are hard to come by, their health talk cannot be heard as fully as whites'. Some slaves are audible in conversation with their owners, however, as individuals whose work included reporting on plantation affairs. This health talk, on its surface, is much the same as that between whites, although there are nuances that betray the interests imposed by slavery. Lucy Skipwith, a slave belonging to John H. Cocke, wrote regular reports to him over several years, sketching by way of health talk the well-being of Cocke's family and neighbors. "Mrs. Carter has been very unwell since you left," Skipwith wrote, typically, in 1856. "Her baby is five weeks old. . . . the doctor came to see her a few days ago and said that if she is not very carefall she would be in bad health all of her life. she sends her love to you." Skipwith's reports on her fellow slaves' health, couched in much the same terms, nevertheless carried an extra dimension of meaning. Skipwith assumed her owner's sympathy, and yet she was careful to total up how many hands were unproductive as a result of sickness. Similarly, her occasional mention of her own health was in one sense standard health talk fare; and yet, because of her bondage, her personal well-being always was in the shadow of her owner's interests: "I have been quite unwell for the last day or two. . . . I Am not geting along with my busness very well at present. so much sickness is seting me back." Countless such exchanges reinforced for everyone—M.D.s included—the view that slave patients' health was properly a part of the master's calculations.[30]

Moreover, even though slaves and masters talked in much the same way about the broad, practical means to good health, there were certain sharp divergences in understanding as well. As with other aspects of African American culture, slaves' understanding of health derived in part from African sources, which shaped a sense of it as rooted in realms of power and faith not completely divorced from white understandings but having their own distinctive contours. Here modern ethnographies have something to suggest. A respect for the power and abundance of Nature has been an abiding tradition among African Americans. One twentieth-century African American woman, telling an interviewer about folk remedies, at first contrasted them to "*medicine*, real medicine." And yet she went on to claim equality for the folk remedies: "Why, there's a lotta *weeds* out there *now*; why you're walkin' over *medicine*!" This sense of a provident Nature equal to the threat of disease, in a way not unlike physicians' sense of "expectant" treatment, often was joined to a distinctively African American sense of a spirit world whose array of amulets and rituals might be conjured for either good or ill health. Most fundamentally, "conjure" yielded a sense of disease as being not merely at large in the cosmos but related to individual lives and to specific antidotes. Strikingly, slaves and former slaves rarely expanded on "voodoo" or conjure in writing or in interviews, doubtless wary of white ignorance and disapproval. Indeed, in interviews collected in the 1930s, most former slaves seem reluctant to talk about sickness at all. "Twasn't much sickness back in slavery days," Lizzie Williams recalled, for example, and, according to Rachel Santee Reed, "Niggers didn't get sick so much in dem days." Such responses may be clouded by forgetfulness, by implicit differences in defining "sickness," or they may be deliberate efforts to avoid talking about this entire realm of conflicted experience. "I don't believe in them Hoo Doo doctors neither," former slave Smith Simmons told an interviewer. "I don't pay them no attention." While this doubtless was true for some people, other such respondents, as in "slavery times," may have been evading white curiosity about the spiritual powers at black command.[31]

As for the role of white physicians, former slave Frank Jackson recalled that under slavery local herb medicine would be tried first, either at the master's direction or at the slave's initiative, and "if the misery leaves dat's all dere is to it, but if it don't he calls the regular doctor from town with his pills and stuff." In a way, Jackson's recollection is a trim summary of all health talk. "Misery" comes and goes; when it comes, you might come under the care of a physician, but you might not. Everyone acknowledged the weight of popular wisdom above all, relying especially on the belief that Nature repaid respect and would reward a healer's careful work with useful substances and signs. Everyone acknowledged a sense of a healer's "experience" as the key to good medicine, and many individuals of both races implicated well-being in religious faith or spirituality, as well as physicality. If an M.D. embraced the consensus, he might more easily find compliance and success. But the consensus was risky, too. Immersing himself too thoroughly in popular views, he would cast off too many skills and ideas dear to his orthodoxy, and his self-esteem would depart along with them. And if he resisted the consensus at too many points, clashing with what he saw as a weak fatalism or an unjustified disrespect for his medicine, he ran the risk not only of seeing his livelihood suffer but of finding his moral image of himself dismissed as so much grandstanding or greed.[32]

ROUNDS

The most ordinary and the most inclusive: fees and business; the variety of patients; popular ideas about health and the things that supported and defined it. These were the broad conditions under which physicians made the everyday practical calculations that underwrote—and to some degree justified—their mode of practice. Now we need to see these basic conditions put into motion, so to speak, by a physician's rounds through his community. Of course, such rounds have been at the heart of a sentimental vision of nineteenth-century doctoring, with "horseback" physicians portrayed in the hardy pioneer mode. Here, the emphasis on rounds is as most doctors wrote of it—its rote character, its taken-for-granted drudgery, as well as its satisfying moments of mastery. The allusive nature of doctors' writing on rounds—terse, sometimes ironic—is itself a key to how rounds indirectly but surely gave a broad pattern to a practitioner's most cherished possession, his "experience." Rounding gave particularity and character to the common stuff of livelihood. It became part of each man's individual identity in a subtle way, not through self-conscious reflection, but as a background rhythm to the medical events of the bedside and beyond described in following chapters. Listening to what physicians said about rounding thus lays a foundation for us, as it did for them, for how "experience" was channeled by the most humdrum aspects of their work. It reveals, that is, how rural physicians fashioned a mobile, country orthodoxy from the pattern of moral and material encounters in community practice.

There are few better ways to grasp how sharply the daily routine of physicians has changed since the mid-nineteenth century than to realize how thoroughly medical work was outdoor work. It was work in which weather, topography, horses, and the hazards of travel not only were calculated as part of a fee but also shaped in myriad ways the tenor of each day's labors—not to mention the fates of patients. Rounds gave an ironic twist to medical school lectures on the beauty and power of Nature; here was a Nature of mud and flies that worked against seeing patients and collecting fees. "As the roads are mirey & the weather cold & unsettled, [I] declined going to see my . . . patients today," a Hertford County, North Carolina, doctor wrote in his diary in 1825. Were these words written easily, as a matter of fact, or did the doctor wince at letting his patients go unattended, hoping that none of them slid closer to the edge? Charles Hentz, summing up a day's practice in his diary, typically stitched events together by writing of travel in bad weather, in the "pitchy dark," or of being called in the middle of the night "from my warm bed" to ride many miles to a patient who might turn out to be fine or, like one slave, "sick unto death." Conditions of weather and terrain were more than punctuation; they were among the bedrock conditions of everyday work and a central way doctors assessed their obligations and character. As Samuel Leland wrote simply of one call in October 1854, "It was very cold, and required a great deal of resolution, for me to leave at the dead hour of night."[33]

Cold, rain, and dark were offset by times of delightful travel. "Give me a bright, bracing day, a fine road and a lonely one, an active, stirring horse—and a certain mood of mind, and nothing is more pleasant," wrote William Holcombe in 1855. He sometimes composed poetry or "drew out a train of medical or theological argument" as he rode along. Often he sang, taking pleasure that "my knowledge of songs and hymns has thus beguiled many a wearisome hour." Dr. Hentz, after the shock of leaving his warm bed, sometimes delighted in "the glorious moonlight" or marveled at the fog-wrapped dark that the lantern on his sulky did little to dispel. "Oh! the lone starry hours give me love / When still is the beautiful night," a Louisiana doctor wrote in his daybook. The beauty and power of nature, the familiar yet always changing road itself, worked to sustain and calm, placing whatever was about to happen at the bedside into a frame larger than any particular need or effort.[34]

So, too, were horses an essential part of whatever was accomplished in a day. Doctors sometimes had more than one mount—one on each side of a river, for instance—reasoning along the lines of a Tennessee doctor who calculated that each month "you can do thirty dollars the more worth of riding for having three horses as you can [with one]" because no matter when the call came "[you] have a fresh well fed one ready." Only in later nostalgia does the midcentury doctor's horse ride free from criticism; doctors themselves usually wrote of their mounts as flawed and prosaic beasts. In fact, it is impressive that so many physicians held on to the ideal of having a beloved or renowned horse while going through a large number of mediocre ones. The perils of horse-trading and the boggling peculiarities of individual mounts were key topics among doctors. "Bought a Gray horse, or rather a mare . . . *said to be 7 years old*," one doctor noted warily. Of his new horse J. A. Reedy said only, "she looks better than I expected." Charles Hentz paid more than $200 for his first horse, taking a ribbing from his parents for this extravagance, only to find out the animal was a poor swimmer—something that put Hentz at a disadvantage during the spring flooding. Hentz went through a large number of horses (and one mule) over the years, mounts with names like Jack, Mike, Tom, and Charlie, and he was always in search of an animal of good habits: one that would walk swiftly, given its own head, and one that would wait without being tied when the doctor had to dismount in haste. Often, though, he and other doctors ended up with horses that unaccountably balked or started at nothing, or came down with horrible afflictions like the "blind staggers" or "big head."[35]

Snakes in the road, hidden nests of yellow jackets, falling tree limbs, and unhelpful or even dangerous people punctuated doctors' mounted travel. The southern countryside never looked so inhospitable as it does in physicians' accounts of rounds. "I have been all day down in 'The Slashes,'" William Reedy wrote of a local swamp in 1883, ". . . the mosquitoes and sand flies have nearly eat me up today it is just terrible on both me & horse." Henry Ravenel practiced science by collecting botanical specimens on his rounds, though it led him "among the Snakes & red bugs," and John Knox discovered after one outing through the underbrush that he had somehow lost his lancets and pencil case. He looked for them back along his route, failed to find them, decided to stop for dinner, and then, just as it was growing dark, returned once more to find them "under an apple tree." There were inexplicable misadventures, as in Frederick Weeden's experience when, out on a river and losing his way to a new patient, he "hailed a fellow on shore, ask'd him a few quisical questions, & he very deliberately discharged his gun at me loaded & dis'h the 2nd time as though shooting people was a trade with him." More commonly, people met along the way merely confounded the practitioner in need of help. Charles Hentz, who asked a young, poor white boy directions at a crossroads, was puzzled at the youngster's unintelligible reply until he realized after a while that the boy was asking him for a chaw of tobacco in exchange for information. The days were made up of such things, ludicrous or near fatal.[36]

Along the way, doctors met rivals of various sorts. Alternative healers— Thomsonians, hydropaths, and botanical healers of different hues—were everywhere and equally in hot pursuit of medical livelihood. One itinerant botanical doctor chided his indecisive partner in 1843 by reminding him that the South was uniquely hospitable to men "*determined* to *get rich*," adding, "we must *skin* these lazy Georgians. . . . The *opposition* to our [botanical] system *in Maine* is more formidable than it is here. . . . You would be a quack there." In some rural neighborhoods, there was competition as well from black doctors, including, in the antebellum decades, a few talented slaves who made rounds as a source of income for their owners. Former slaves frequently recalled fellow bondsmen and bondswomen as healers, and doubtless there were other doctors like Frederick Cousins, a free black practicing "on the Thompsonian [*sic*] principles" near Lynchburg, Virginia, in the late 1850s who was so well established that he retained an attorney to make a claim against a white man's estate.[37]

Still, when physicians wrote of meeting other practitioners on their rounds, they were more likely to comment on fellow M.D.s than other healers. A brother physician became one's toughest rival when patients narrowed their choice to the orthodox style of medicine. Moreover, because physicians considered only each other as true peers, competition and collaboration among individual M.D.s went deeply into what "experience" meant, touching self-esteem, as well as the pocketbook. Such rivalry also revealed, again, how the corporate "profession" was a kind of fiction in rural locales, where what counted most of all were the personal relationships among individual doctors. In asking for a consultation, then, M.D.s were careful to praise their peers and at the same time not to seem too needy. One physician requested, for instance, that a colleague "advise with me" on a case, a nice turn of phrase that permitted the writer to be an equal rather than a supplicant. In praising their local colleagues, physicians often used language that evoked medical learnedness, but only in the most general way: an experienced man was one with "excellent medical acquirements" or "considerable talents & acquirements." Personal qualities of character, on the other hand, were sharply described and, significantly, derived in large part from patients' esteem. An experienced colleague was a man admired for his "prudence and strong patronage" and one "ably patronized, popular & successful," with a wide variety of patients. Conversely, the undesirable colleague was more often characterized by his moral transgressions or social disapproval than by failings specifically related to his orthodoxy. Thus patients' views of a given doctor, indirectly at least, were factored into his colleagues' professional assessment of a man's "experience."[38]

In all of these ways, doctors' daybook and diary accounts of rounds suggest how their everyday work was shaped into a local brand of orthodoxy by each man's personal routine. Sometimes medical labor was inscribed only on the margins of a day. Samuel Leland wrote in 1856 of a day of trees and surgery, with surgery as the afterthought: "Today has been one of hard work. I planted out 15 trees down my avenue. Some one in after time will enjoy them, unless the place shall fall into the hands of some utilitarian vandal, who would make but little ado in cutting them all down, should they happen to shade a little corn, or cotten. Just about sunset, I cut a large tumour, from a woman, growing just above the umbilicus." At other times, though, medical work swallowed up everything else, and practitioners' notes take on the quality of hurried bulletins. Courtney Clark thus recorded the sheer range of afflictions lying in wait for a practitioner: he extracted a bean from a child's nose ("done with forceps"), attended Mr. Woodly in his fatal bout with peritonitis brought on by the "kick of a musket," treated Mr. Green's slave girl for syphilis, attended Mr. Young's son after the boy's arm was "torn" in the gears of a cotton gin, and medicated a slave woman belonging to Mr. Scott for hysteria caused by painful menstruation. Sometimes doctors echoed the health talk of their patients, wrapping both of them into a single world of closely watched anxiety and timely action. So Wilson Yandell took a minute to jot down the calls that had tumbled into his lap over two days in 1825: "Pleasant Childress up the river . . . exposing himself on Saturday . . . frothing at his mouth & delirious. James Gibson juvenile's oldest daughter so burnt from her cloths [sic] taking fire the day before yesterday that she had an ungovernable vomiting & the river so high they could not cross till last evening. Wm. Vaughn Esq. epileptic again from drink." After a day in May, 1855, that included rising at daybreak to three "severe cases" before noon—including scarlet fever and cholera infantum in children—William Holcombe attended four "obstinate cases of dysentery" in the afternoon, and then found himself "out since supper twice, and promised to call at one place again between one and two o'clock in the night. Afternoon nap interrupted. Wife sick in bed. Thermometer 90° in the deep shade. Dust almost insufferable. A little indisposed myself—*Finis*."[39]

A man's routine took its temper in turn from the elements, the animals, and the pace of medicine through patients' veins. It was not so much plot but portent that runs through these accounts of rounds; they were the seeds of the stories later written into lecture anecdotes and the more substantive case narratives to be considered later. But perhaps the accounts of rounds themselves best reveal how a man's sense of his practice was grasped on the move, inscribed as a kind of itinerary through a landscape to a crisis or, more often, to something indeterminate. So in August of 1883, J. A. Reedy sketched the place—it was no place in particular—to which his day had brought him: it was Sunday and he had hoped to be in church, but instead, "I am in the drugstore waiting to see the effects of a dose of morphine which I gave to a man in Eady's Hotel. . . . It is well perhaps that I have little to do as I am suffering from Rhumatism in my knee and Howard has my horse." There was something essentially elastic about this style of practice. There was no consistent pulse of tasks, no institutional place from which the physician organized his resources in a uniquely orthodox way. Rather, orthodoxy followed channels cut by each practitioner's livelihood, and the "experience" that marked him as a worthy man grew from the addition of day upon day. Orthodoxy therefore may be seen as a local phenomenon spreading widely and shallowly through the myriad personal habits of physicians. Beneath the surface similarities in their collective labors lay an almost unfathomable web of idiosyncrasies. Taking strength from these individual variations, and yet at the same time wishing to put them together into a unitary body of work and knowledge, practitioners grasped at "experience" as the beneficial outcome of their jumbled daily work.[40]

In these sketchy accounts, patients are portrayed mostly in terms of their afflictions. Their fates and feelings are secondary to the story of travel, arrival, and getting back on the road. Even so, peoples' exposed lives clung to the rounding doctor. Indeed, part of gaining "experience" by way of rounds was learning how to be the bearer—if not the reporter—of people's mistakes and secrets that so unnerved many young physicians at the beginning of their careers. John Knox's case notes include a typical cascade of accidents to which a doctor was privy: "I visited Sarah d[aughter] of M. Walker, who was climbing over the fence & fell & a large pole fell or rolled over her head." A man was "accidentally shot"; an "old negro woman" was struck on the head by the falling limb of a tree; Frank G. "got his leg broke by a Horse falling with him"; and W. Wilson "has had his eye badly hurt in splitting a pine knot." It was the stuff of people's health talk, difficult to keep confidential. Whether to traffic in the misfortunes and secrets of their patients was a decision left for individual practitioners to make on their own. What goes around comes around, as everyone knew, sometimes with destructive effect on an incautious doctor's own practice. But it was hard to keep mum. We can wonder whether many country doctors would have deferred passing along the news that Wilson Yandell received of a "deplorable disease," clearly sexual in nature, that struck a neighbor everyone had thought respectable. Sexual stories were available to every physician, in fact, and each doctor had to decide how much he wanted to be the source of stories that would amuse or horrify his neighbors. Consider Dr. William Reedy's predicament. He was informed by one of his neighbors (who was asking Reedy to intervene) that a medical colleague, a Dr. Simpson, "has taken Sudie Bairel away from Calvin Dillinger's to a little old cabin.... If she does not get a home she will be certain to go to a whore house and I believe that is what Simpson is trying to force her to do, so he will have an excuse to drop her." It is not clear what Reedy did about this, if anything; but since the circumstances involved not only sexual misadventure but also a fellow doctor, it is safe to assume that Reedy thought twice about it. Or consider the choices facing Arkansas physician Frank James, called to treat one of the "lady riders" of a circus, who was accosted by a townsman who wanted to have access to her. "I lied like a tombstone," the doctor told his diary, but "I see from his actions that he will not be satisfied until he runs up against her cartwheel."[41]

James wrote about being sexually tempted himself. Few doctors did so, but the experience must have been common enough. Women disrobed and confided in them; they were seen while unconscious or in emotional distress. If a woman was attracted to a physician, inviting him to her home was a good opportunity to act on the attraction. Of one young woman's breasts, James wrote in his diary, "They are simply glorious and roused all of the old Adam that was in me." Another woman in James's practice, a "Miss H.," one day "threw herself on the sofa by me [and] almost smothered me with passionate kisses. She lay against me and on me in perfect abandonment and I was in Hell" for resisting her. Two days later, James confessed, "The tempter came and I fell! The first time I have allowed my passion to get the better of my personal vows." Richard Arnold was similarly tempted in 1832 while examining a "pretty female patient this evening, who is on the town. She was en deshabille, and as she really has a beautiful pair of breasts . . . I was near falling a victim to the temptation. The eyes of this girl fairly sparkled and she imprinted on my lips a voluptuous kiss which shot through my system like electricity."[42]

Not only sexual opportunities but charged episodes of other kinds drew rounding physicians into neighborhood conflicts, sometimes as part of official investigations as coroners or witnesses, most notably in cases involving violent or sudden death, mental competence, or crimes involving slaves. In their day-books, and even in letters to each other, physicians spoke only minimally of such matters, suggesting their unease at the mixture of professional expertise and sensationalism. The scarcity of commentary on slaves involved in violence, for instance, either as perpetrators or as victims, is especially striking and seems a good index of physicians' wariness of being the possessors of volatile informa-tion. Wilson Yandell cautiously confirmed to his son "a rape having been com-mitted on a daughter of the Rev'd John Wiseman by a negro," adding tersely that the accused man "has since been executed." J. A. S. Milligan wrote to his father, also a physician, of a man who "held his wife & made his colored mistress give her a whipping." Samuel Leland officiated in an 1853 case of a deceased slave who sometime earlier had been "punished rather severely for forging a pass." Leland, examining the body, concluded that the whipping had not been "severe enough to cause death or even sickness," although he could not say what had caused the man's death.[43]

Such testimony in cases involving slaves, cases in which a master's power and reputation were at stake, were especially touchy. Investigations of anything having to do with fatal violence by or against slaves often were kept informal, thus bolstering the power of masters by giving them great flexibility in defining due process. Everyone in the white community had to play his part, and physi-cians knew that if they misread or deviated from what was required of them, they might create a loaded situation that put whites' racial control into the balance against their professional self-esteem. Give one's testimony and leave seems to have been the expedient course for most doctors. Only occasionally did doctors publicly stand up against a gross misuse of a master's power. Several Virginia doctors, for instance, apparently joined together in 1856 to testify against a slave owner whose slave had died from punishment; the owner was convicted of second-degree murder. But most physicians, who doubtless saw much more of this kind of abuse than they recorded, avoided having a salient role to play. If pressed, they might dissemble in an attempt to hold on to some part of their own self-esteem. While a slave, Charles Ball was accused of attack-ing a white woman and arrested. Ball recalled that a doctor was called in by whites for the purpose, they said, of skinning Ball alive. The doctor, doubtless wanting no part of that assignment whether or not it was a bluff, told the whites present that Ball was too "full of blood" and thus not a good candidate for a skinning. The doctor might have been willing, Ball feared, to bleed him to death if the other whites had insisted. But it did not come to that.[44]

In such ways, highly charged or otherwise, doctors' "experience" arose from the fact that rounds took them to the turning points of other peoples' lives. Secrets were revealed, weaknesses exposed, and the hidden or damaged parts of neighbors' lives came into view. "Experience" in this sense became the catch-all term for a unity of effort and meaning doctors strove to find in their itinerant work on the roads of the rural South. They prized this sense of "experience" as combining into a single, moral entity the patient's good, the community's good, and the doctor's own benefit. And yet the everyday meaning of their routine often was more circumscribed and ambiguous than this. In call after call, the profoundly individual bent of their daily work distracted them from the broad, social significance of what they saw. The health of whole classes of people, especially the systematic abuses suffered by slaves, found no record in the way rounds were written.

LIVELIHOOD, SUBJECTIVITY, AND
THE COUNTRY ORTHODOX STYLE

Throughout the century, as other scholars have shown, physicians only slowly adapted to the "modern" innovations in their practice initiated by schools and elite reformers. Ordinary doctors' slowness to respond to change has been seen as a failure on their part, and yet the context of their response has not been a matter for much historical curiosity. Seeing physicians from the ground level of everyday livelihood, however, suggests that what is important to understand is not best seen in terms of their "failure" to embrace modern changes in professional organization and values. Rather, it is the appeal of a profound continuity in the local context of practice—summed up by the sense of "experience"—that needs understanding. In the wide-open, rounding style of practice, being judged a man of "experience" was more satisfying, and more immediately useful, than being a "modern" man. The solo nature of practice led physicians to search for meaning in the fine grain of their own particular habits and personal history. Their self-focus then was turned outward to become the essence of orthodoxy with its moral claims to being superior. Thus, rural physicians found themselves moving in two different directions that, as we will see, also shaped the particulars of their bedside work: though attracted to an ideal of orthodox medical knowledge as something that transcended any one individual, physicians continued to embrace an ideal of local practice based on a man's personal, individual style as something irreplaceably valuable.

This tension in orthodoxy percolated through its local setting in the South as physicians strove to see their work not simply as scratching out a livelihood but as a test of character—an economic but also moral contest in which each man pitted his sense of orthodoxy against the vagaries of community life. Evidence of his success in this struggle was his recognition as a kind of public figure. Thus, a Georgia practitioner welcomed the fact that "the doctor is manifestly a public servant—and his office a common rendezvous for everybody. His patients of course have a right there, [and] others have the right to see him and talk with him." Moreover, many doctors gave this more-than-a-livelihood definition of doctoring a preeminently southern cast. In southern communities, a physician "cannot screen himself behind the Yankee placard 'call upon a man in business only on business,'" as James Milligan told his son in 1846. Rather, a good doctor willingly observed the local "law of custom" that made him available to all and gave him a special, public status. In return, the public servant physician was given much more than "business." He was given the love of the people he served. In short, being available when neighbors needed him "will make a man of you," Milligan told his son. "It will moreover endear you to the people for whom you are denying yourself. . . . You must not measure everything by dollars and cents." Seeing the essence of daily rounding as a moral dynamic of self-sacrifice and self-esteem, with the consequence that a man was not only respected but loved, was one of the deepest wishes binding physicians to the routines of their work. It was an interpretation of doctoring that allowed an M.D. to say, despite long hours and hard work (indeed, because of them), "my enthusiasm in my profession . . . remains unabated." To have a sense of being an instrument of a community's well-being led more than one practitioner to declare himself "devoted to the practice of medicine. [I] love it better & better."[45]

But this powerful wish, when thwarted, shaped an equally passionate rebellion against the limitations of an orthodoxy shaped by rural distance, scarce cash, and ungrateful patients. All of these were signs that, in seeking people's embrace, the doctor gave over some measure of his orthodoxy to the people and to rural life. In a city, one rural doctor imagined, a physician could "enforce his plan of diet and temperature better than it could be done by a country practitioner. He could more readily see the patients . . . at the critical moment." A country doctor had a harder time at everything; critical moments came and went unattended, time for study contracted, books were hard to obtain. E. W.

Thomason loved the rural South, but, all told, "I cannot say that I like a country life as the work is hard and the associations are not near so pleasant as those in the city." In their discontent, many rural doctors blamed their patients; in one man's mind in 1843, patients lined up in several disagreeable types: "pusilanimous [*sic*] patients, tight patients, those who believe in medicine, and those who do not, docile patients, the Silent patient, the Loquacious patient, the prejudiced patients and the patients half Physician." Interestingly, the shrewd, "half-physician" patients were the worst because, like doctors themselves, "they never say what they feel, they are not satisfied by receiving good advice" but always want drugs. They reminded the doctor that the breadth of his knowledge did not count if patients chose not to accede to *his* definition of "experience." And when they did not, the physician's predicament was that he could neither prove their ideas wrong nor easily admit his own limits. As Dr. Sanford Chaillé observed, because a doctor needed his patients' fees and needed to live among them, he "is often forced either to keep silent, or to pander to their nonsensical prejudices."[46]

There was yet a further kind of personal cost to rural practice, one measured by a man's separation from family and other moral centers of community life and by the public scrutiny of his behavior. Martha Battey told her aunt in 1857 that her physician husband was "very busy all the time. I see very little of him[,] less than I ever did. . . . I feel very lonely sometimes." Dr. William Anderson wrote in this vein to his sweetheart in 1881 about what to expect if she married him and his "inexorable Public." He wondered if she could accept, as he had, that "you can never feel secure in calling any hour your own. Such is a country Practitioner's life. Would you like it?" Half-bantering (or maybe not; they never married), Lydie McLure similarly wrote to her sweetheart, "I don't see how I am going to become reconciled to being a physician's ——. You'll belong to everyone more than to me." Complicating such exchanges was the sense among physicians that they were held to a higher moral standard than most people, although here many men were kicking against the consequences of their own desires. Nonetheless, Richard Arnold was dismayed in 1838 at being subjected to public scrutiny at the scene of an accident after having drunk, he admitted, "too much wine to render me a cool & safe adviser." Arnold wisely withdrew when another medical man appeared, but the damage had been done. The "next day it appeared to me that everybody knew it. . . . How dangerous then for a medical man . . . to subject himself to the chance of such an exposure." Alabaman Josiah Nott agreed that rural communities knew altogether too much about doctors' private lives and was happy to leave the country for Mobile. In the country, "I knew everybody & many were portraied as friends, who expected me not only to give Physic, but to devote a great deal of time to them." In Mobile, to his relief, "it is a mere money transaction. You give your pills & put off just like a tailor would after taking your measure."[47]

~

To conclude, as did Nott, that tailors had more desirable relationships with their customers than rural physicians had with their patients—less insistently personal, less demanding—went to the problematic heart of the identity physicians struggled to make from the daily pattern of their livelihood. Nott's desire presaged a certain kind of modernity: the detached physician and the cash nexus. But most of his contemporaries sought something quite different. They hoped through their rural livelihoods to stand both inside and outside their communities, superior in knowledge to their patients yet beloved for being one of them. They aspired to be the moral men their neighbors wanted. And yet because they witnessed their neighbors in times of intimate and desperate need, and then dunned them to pay for it, doctors were a far more edgy and difficult presence in their communities than they wished to be. "A physician's life is a very uncomfortable one to say the least of it," James Milligan wrote to his sister Margaret in a fashion common to doctors during the entire span of the century. "The responsibility, anxiety, obstinacy of patients, & ingratitude of a large proportion of those whom he has been instrumental in saving when ready to perish, all considered, render his path a thorny one—& a very crooked one too." Moreover, as we will see in terms of the bedside, as physicians fit the imagined breadth of their orthodoxy to the close quarters of the sickroom, a general anxiety about the uniqueness of orthodox medicine emerged from the particular anxieties of each case.[48]

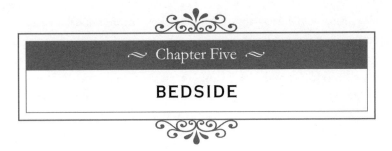

Chapter Five

BEDSIDE

The solitary rides, the rainy nights, the advice of colleagues, the money owed—all emptied out at the bedside where waited the sufferer. Malady waited there, too, a protean, lively thing, part invader, part nemesis. This chapter seeks to illuminate the everyday diagnostic and therapeutic means physicians employed to make the bedside an orthodox place, and how these efforts in particular shaped the medical and social meaning of local practice. This means looking first at people medicating themselves and their reasons for summoning the physician in the first place. Then we will look at the physician undertaking his diagnosis and initial therapy in terms of a key dynamic that shaped nearly every bedside to which he traveled: his sense of "good" medicine collided with the varied, unpredictable, and often unruly social context of domestic sickroom care. Arriving at the bedside, he found his skills and knowledge—his "art"—flowing immediately into the larger stream of caregiving devised by patients and their families. He thus became not only an actor in the drama of suffering and healing but also a witness to it. He had to inhabit both roles as he sized up the sick body and named the disease and then set about transforming with his therapy the terrible bond between the two.

The focus here, then, is on the immediate, initial performance of a physician's medicine as he brought it into play under circumstances that were not simply his to control. Being summoned and undertaking care was an important moment in doctoring for several reasons that shape the argument of this chapter. Physicians themselves talked of it as a crucial time; each new sickroom entered, each new performance of their skills, was an edgy moment remarked even by established doctors. Indeed, the achievement of a country orthodoxy followed directly from how physicians imagined a personal style of doctoring with enough complexity and flexibility to respond to each new situation. It follows that by focusing on the doctor initiating his care, we can refine our understanding of the distinctive way ordinary practitioners tied their overall means of diagnosis and therapy to community bedsides. Specifically, diagnosis—the doctor's effort to identify and name disease—appears to have been more important to midcentury physicians than we have supposed. Moreover, the route taken to name disease and counter it, often portrayed as chiefly a matter of power and negotiation between patients and physicians, lay within a common social world that included more than power struggles. It was a world that embraced imagination and emotion as well, further shaping a country orthodoxy rooted in the cherished continuity of a caregiver's personal style. Finally, bedside drama has lived on in sentimentalized accounts of "frontier" doctors, a mixed image in which physicians are portrayed—with reference to twentieth-century medicine—as both heroic and ignorant. Here, the attempt is to tell a story in which neither heroism nor ignorance sufficiently describes the physician's bedside world. Nor did this world simply impede the emergence of the "modern" bedside. Rather, it was a world where a physician's bedside work—inextricable from his character— created a complex balance of science and morality that in some ways pointed to a different configuration of the "modern," rich with its own satisfactions.[1]

As we will see, the challenge for the physician in initiating his care was to establish himself as a man with the moral authority to direct what was, in fact, a composite of vernacular and orthodox ways to counter sickness. To be sure, orthodox ideology was manifest in the sickroom; physicians eagerly asserted their schooled reasons for being the "best" bedside attendants. But even more important than ideology was what might be termed the phenomenology of bedside practice—the timing, staging, and social rites of establishing care with individual patients. As we have seen, their schooling and their search for a place to settle already impressed physicians with the fact that their "experience" was something they could not dictate but had to create from the surrounding community. The bedside compressed the scale and heightened the intensity of this reality. It showed the physician that his "experience" was not to be found in controlling the events and people in the crowded sickroom; few physicians even came close to that. What the bedside revealed was that the heart of "experience" was not *control* but *performance*. A physician had to enact the worthy doctor he admired and wished to be.

Before the physician arrived, the bedside already was a place for the social staging of illness and caregiving. It was a place given over to many voices, littered with past experiences, wishes, fears, and hope for recovery. It was littered, too, with corresponding powders, amulets, ointments, and other substances that mobilized the household—and, in another sense, surrendered it—to the struggle with disease. Rural southerners, like other Americans, watched the body and plied it with drugs, charms, and prayers. But there was a southern accent to the bedsides considered here: free and slave patients and caregivers attended each other on a regular basis, and they, like physicians, believed in the existence of distinct southern ailments and medicines. From childhood, southerners learned that the world might turn against them; the special heat of southern summers, sudden changes in temperature, and shifts in the wind might portend something malign and personal. Like countless other southerners, Sallie Price wrote to her friend, "How I dread the summer. I almost imagine myself shaking [with fever] now." A Mississippi woman saw autumn's "sickness and distress" waiting in the wings of early summer and wrote to her sister, "We must expect attacks from the invisible enemy, but I pray our share may be light." Personal risk was not the only thing to be dreaded. The social chaos of epidemics was greatly feared as well, one woman recalling her community overwhelmed by cholera, with "the bursting of coffins—the indecency."[2]

When southerners felt themselves becoming ill, they felt their bodies breached and imagined disease seating itself within; they felt "exposed" and "reduced." Throughout the century, they consulted the women of the household and domestic health-care books, and they examined their own and each others' bodies. Skin temperature and moisture, the head, the teeth (in children, especially), and the gut caused the greatest concern as the chief sites for fever and congested blood; if blood backed up within the body, a person became vulnerable to all sorts of ills. People took medicine preventively, believing that the body in fact thrived on a certain amount of medicine. Not content with a tea tonic or a glass of port wine before bed, many dosed themselves with full-bore drugs such as quinine (especially after 1850) and the purge calomel, with the practice of preventatively "taking a vomit" not an unusual occurrence. Women, slave and free, dusted children's clothing with crushed cinchona bark to ward off the fever in the air, and youngsters stood naked over hot coals every evening so that seed ticks would jump out of their hair and into the fire. Slave women, especially, hung packets of camphor and asafetida around the necks of their children to fend off harmful atmospheres. Harriott Pinckney was enthusiastic about plum jelly, a few spoonfuls of which "is excellent for the throat. . . . [I] send three mugs of it." Children of both races grew up tied to amulets and drugs as something prudent and desirable. The fundamentals were simple, as one health book urged: "Keep your body open, your feet dry and warm, and your head cool!!"[3]

When preventive measures failed, southerners poured on the medicines with even greater energy. A dislike for M.D.s' harsh allopathic medicine has been seen as the reason many patients avoided physicians; but, clearly, many others defined a good medicine by its thumping impact on the body. Conscientious women throughout the South pulled down bottle after bottle from the medicine shelf, brewed up one decoction after another, poured them down their charges' bodies, and waited for the change. As Fannie Moore recalled of her childhood as a slave, the children would try to avoid taking medicine, "but twarnt no use granny jes git you by de collar hol' yo' nose and you jes swallow it or get strangled." Agnes MacRae, bedridden with a bad cold in 1879, wrote to her brother that he "assuredly would have pitied me" as her relatives laid on with "plasters, camphorated oil, lemon and sugar, glycerine and whiskey, cream of tartar and paregoric—I never received a greater variety of doses in my life." A body shaken with the chills and heat of fever had to be strongly seized by a therapy its equal. And so although it was unpleasant—even daunting—most people thought it quite proper, as one South Carolina woman put it in 1832, to feel "the good effects" of being made "an invalid" by medicines themselves, and to attempt, like Zillah Brandon, to counter "the prostrating power" of her illness with the "thrilling effects of sugar of lead."[4]

Slave and free met each other in the heat of self-care, at times establishing a greater closeness between the races than other social encounters under slavery allowed. At other times, however, sickness revealed the alienation between the races. Slaves and masters struggled over the very definition of disease and therapy. Though sharing the use of many of the same teas and poultices, care-givers on both sides of the racial divide had scant knowledge of (and even less respect for) each other's explanations of sickness. Whites were especially impatient with, and sometimes fearful of, African American belief in the power of conjuring. One slave owner, a physician himself, wrote in typical exasperation that his slave Isaac "is gone today to see a negro doctor, 16 miles in the country, to get medicine 'for poison that a negro gave him in Gibson four years ago'!" Although scornful-amused at such a diagnosis, the doctor "thought it best to humor his superstition" since Isaac was determined to pursue his cure. Partly in response to white unbelief, slave doctors appear to have segregated their therapies by race. Victoria Thompson's father, a slave, was recognized as a valuable healer by his master, who called him "Doc" and deferred to his prescriptions. Doc dispensed certain remedies to the white family but reserved certain others for the exclusive use of black people. For the whites, various teas. For his fellow slaves, "he made us wear charms. Made out of shiny buttons and Indian rock beads. They cured lots of things and the misery too."[5]

Owners and slaves also brought the broader struggles of slavery into the sickroom. To be sure, some former slaves, when asked, remembered white doctors favorably, and former owners' recollections of admirable slave caregivers, like Susan Smedes's memory of Maum Harriet, are set pieces of Lost Cause literature. But these memories are more than offset by antebellum accounts showing owners and slaves trafficking in the bitterness of slavery, as well as illness. Mary Henderson, grieving over the death of her young daughter in 1855, blamed her slave nurse—"old and experienced but selfish and lazy"—who "neglected my precious little lamb . . . and overfed her I fear with tea and bread *too much sweetened.*" Lucila McCorkle "left orders for Lizzy [a slave] to stay at home" with McCorkle's sick son Gamble in 1847. "[B]ut when I returned from S[unday] School she was not to be found or heard of and did not make an appearance till 11 o'clock. My feelings were very much roused but I endeavored to defer anger till Monday." At times, however, the sickroom refracted the usual organization of white control, throwing masters' authority into odd relief if not actually limiting it. Caregivers of both races laid hands upon each other in ways that caused pain or relieved it, pushing aside modesty. Slaves and masters bathed one another, spoon-fed each other's children, forced down the medicines. When Maria Davies was sick with a severe sore throat, both her sister and her slave Bessie "have been treating my throat with caustic." Davies sat in a chair, her sister restraining her, while Bessie, forcefully holding her mistress's head, swabbed her painful throat.[6]

People eagerly attached names to what they suffered, drawing upon a vocabulary of diseases heard about, seen before, and diagnosed by doctors, family, or friends. Names were a gesture toward control, implying that malady was a known thing with a predictable "course." So one man was satisfied, if not exactly relieved, when he decided that the growth on his face was "what is called a tumer." Louisa Muller determined that her mother's "severe pain in her side" and rash "is what is called Shingles," and another woman decided, after talking to friends, that she had "something of the Erysipelas on her Feet." In another sense, though, naming diseases added to their disruptive power. To evoke "the Scarlet Fever prevailing about the country," to travel in order "to keep from the ravages of the scarlet fever," or to say of a city that "Scarlet Fever is there" imparted new life to the disease each time the name was uttered. One South

Carolina woman's 1830s notebook compiled antidotes for an array of ailments that, despite being arranged in neat lists, suggest the terrible disorder inherent in nameable afflictions: consumption cough, whooping cough, bowel complaint, spasm in the stomach, worms, indigestion, scarlet fever, pleurisy, dropsy, obstruction, piles, sore nipples, and "what is termed *death mould*." The sheer proliferation of names implied that protean malady could be fully caught by no one's word or deed—no one's "experience"—including the physician's. One woman was certain, for example, that "neglected ulcerated sore throat terminates in consumption," another that a head cold had transformed itself into "a turn of intermittent fever." In the Boulware family of up-country South Carolina in 1867, malady can fairly be seen ricocheting about the room in the father's diary report on his three daughters: "Lulu took a chill & had a hard spasm. Mary Jane sick all day. Lulu clear of fever tonight and very lively. Mattie took a violent headache from the excitement caused by Lulu's spasm."[7]

This widespread vision of pervasive malady greatly foreshortened the distance between the natural and the moral, something novice physicians glimpsed in their image of "monster disease" as they began their careers. There were moral lessons aplenty in the texture of a person's affliction. Whether or not a person drank or ate to excess, and whether or not she was foolish in getting a wet head or venturing out into the sun too late or too early in the day or the season—all reflected on the quality and weight of her judgment and thus on her character, shaping her health into a moral edifice, inevitable and revealing. Physical and moral language flowed together easily, extending malady's scope and power yet again. A Presbyterian minister, in describing crucial differences between Methodists and Baptists in matters of belief, relied on the physical language of humors: Methodists were more sanguine, while Baptists "have more Phlegm in their temperament." A father in Mississippi in 1855 advised his daughter to strive for faith the size of a mustard seed and then told her "when the weather is cold . . . take *mustard seed constantly*."[8] People's accounts of sickness and caregiving often became small devotional tales, enlivened for many by the broad language of Christianity that allowed the idiosyncrasies of personal suffering to flow into lessons of courage and moral character: "Poor Mrs. Knox is drinking the cup of affliction—Little Rosa is doubtless a corpse. The whooping cough is going through the village. My Heavenly Father—for thy dear son's sake deal mercifully with thy servant & handmaid. Thou knowest what is best for us & we submit. The disposal of ourselves our lots—our all to thee. But deal not with us according to our demerits."[9]

This sense of illness amounted to a near paradox that implicated M.D.s as well as others: people responded with an active submissiveness, an aroused watchfulness. They made illness an urgent puzzle to be solved while suggesting at the same time that disease was in the world to instruct people about their characters. In much of this, the physician was more or less a marginal figure, sometimes a figure of fear. One day in 1852, Maria Davies sought relief from her worrisome symptoms by "lying on the floor" but decided against calling a doctor because, "teeth pressed tightly together in the imaginary suffering of pain," she realized that what she feared most of all was "Dr. Carradine hurting so."[10]

Letters summoning the physician give a sense of how and why people turned to him, despite their fears or doubts. These letters, minimal and rushed, precisely capture the ambiguous and uneasy intersection of domestic caregiving and the physician's particular knowledge and skills. Many people called on a physician because he had seen more ailments, or because he would do unpleasant things they were unwilling to do for themselves. Or they called him simply because he had more medicines on hand. A neighbor wrote to Dr. J. S. Copes in 1836 merely to obtain the pink root tea requested by a sick slave, along with "directions for giving it." An Alabama man whose small daughter was vomiting did not ask for J. M. Heard to come out and examine her but rather asked him to send "a small quantity of magnesia, or whatever you may think will answer my purpose." Such requests imagined an M.D.'s experience as merely an extension of the domestic: he was a man who shared in a common sense of healing and who most likely had the drugs. Somewhat differently, troubling symptoms not before seen moved some people to call upon the physician. One alarmed patient sent a note to J. S. Smith in 1833 to say of his body that "it appears that something comes down and turnes inside out and then I have to try to get it back before I can get any ese. . . . My mouth & tongue will be constant drye and no spittle on it." Some people summoned the physician only after sickness had torn through all their measures and now, suddenly, threatened the very life of the patient. Extreme need scarcely could be more evident than when A. B. Johnston implored physician Beverley Jones in 1854: "Dr. Sir, I send for you in a case of emergency. I want you to come as soon as you can get here. My wife cannot live 24 hours without relief. . . . I do not know anything I can do. I now call upon your skill."[11]

Thus, a physician was summoned not because of the deeply wrought orthodoxy he himself prized but because he would be one more fresh hand at the bedside. The language of letters summoning him—terse or rambling, vague or alarmed—suggests that when he began his treatment, a rural doctor's grasp on his "experience" depended on his ability to take in and judge a wide range of persons, moments, and expressive styles rather than reducing them to a few uniform "complaints." In more ways than one, then, his neighbors clearly placed the physician wholly within the spectrum of vernacular wisdom; it would be up to him whether or not it mattered to assert the uniqueness of his ortho- doxy. In this regard, summonses described intensely social bedsides. Sometime in the 1870s, for instance, the mother of a young South Carolina boy named Georgie wrote Dr. James Chapman in a passion—her handwriting shows her haste—about how the boy "has had constant fever, color more of a corpse than living mortal. His only desire is water, water. Dr. S. has been attending but I see no improvement. His little pulse this morning alarms me. A few beats very free and this same length of time very dull. Mrs. S. thinks I [am] alarmed, but I know he must have help soon. Have given him calomel until I think it time to stop (enclose a powder for your inspection). . . . If you can't come I ask you earnestly would you trust Georgie in Dr. S's care any longer[?]" She already had been doing much of what an M.D. would do, reading the pulse, giving purges. Others were advising her, including another doctor and his temporizing wife. Now the mother turned to Chapman for something more. Her voice is both alarmed and certain ("I see no improvement"), and there might be an echo of the boy's voice here: "water, water." She wants the physician's assessment of everything, all at once—medicines, Dr. S., Georgie's symptoms, her own caregiving. For her, this is what Chapman's experience meant.[12]

Summonses from masters to see sick slaves rarely had this intensity, although they do include similar self-diagnoses, requests for drugs, and often a sense of emergency. Such calls vividly suggest how the vernacular context for sickness and care tapped into the cultural forces holding slavery together. For one thing, it is important to appreciate the significance of the fact that the summons came from the master not the slave. This fact underscored all of the other ways a master controlled certain options in a slave's life and inevitably made the white doctor one more agent of the master's power. Lucila McCorkle, for example, was typical in allowing certain slaves care for themselves but withholding such permission for others. She sent for a physician to treat her slave Laura's sick child, for instance, because she believed that Laura was not a good mother, "too sleepyheaded to have the care of an infant." Physicians had little choice but to accept such decisions and little inclination to do otherwise, although sometimes they chafed at masters' double standards. It was axiomatic among physicians, for example, that slave owners waited a longer time—sometimes too long—to summon a doctor in a slave's case. As one physician wrote, critically, these masters lost slaves to fever because they thought they could handle matters themselves; yet when their own "wives or children become sick with a similar type of disease . . . they must have a physician immediately."[13]

Moreover, some masters called on physicians not because slaves were sick but as a further means of coercion. So, in the spring of 1859, South Carolina physician Joel Berly received a call from a planter named Thomas Holloway, who was supervising his slaves' work clearing "cloddy" swamp land. Holloway's angry-ironic request regarding a woman named Pricy implied that the doctor would simply fall into step with a master's purposes: "Dear Doctor: Pricy flinched today from the cloddy bottom—she complains of a slight pain in the head, and says she had a chill today *after dinner*. I suppose a dose of pills like Dr. Epting gave me once Poto—can't spell the name—or something that *will* make her sick enough tonight to put her in good flight for the clods in the morning. . . . If you know of anything to cure Belly's, prevent puking, or in short, to entirely make an old negro young, send it along: I want medicine of the right gut without *hesitation*."[14]

Here was medicine as the lash. Although there is no evidence of how Berly responded, it is clear that Holloway cared little for orthodox or any other standards. Doctors and their hard-to-name drugs were interchangeable. Reading such a letter, a physician would have to juggle a number of considerations: his livelihood, a local slave owner's power, his own self-esteem, and, perhaps, his own future bedside relations with slave patients.

Brief requests for services from slave owners to John Peter Mettauer, an M.D. practicing in Prince Edward County, Virginia, in the 1830s and 1840s, suggest the destructive influence of slavery in more subtle ways. The requests reveal how slavery twisted the terms under which the doctor was summoned and thus misshaped the very heart of caregiving: trust, sympathy, and the patient's best interests. For one thing, even as they asked Mettauer for help, masters frequently noted being skeptical of their slaves' complaints. One neighbor sent an unnamed slave to Mettauer because the man "has been deseased [*sic*] for a length of time"; that is, the master added, "at least he thinks himself so." This kind of summons, found only with regard to slaves, engaged the doctor in looking for and exposing deceit at the outset of giving care. Moreover, many masters openly made the cost of a slave's care central to their summons. Though hardly surprising, the power given to the dollar over human well-being is never more baldly seen than it is in the thousands of small decisions that made slaves' health a subset of owners' finances. James Neal wrote Mettauer, "I have sent Old Bob to come & see if you can do him any good—if you can without too much expense you will please afford him relief." Monetary interest was taken to be so central that owners who wished to downplay it had to say so. James Fretwell emphasized that in sending "my man Washington" to Mettauer that his sole aim "is the benefit of the negro" and the doctor should not stint on therapy.[15]

Even masters who wrote anxiously about certain slaves used language that mixed genuine concern with self-interest. Nancy Jeffress, for instance, wrote Mettauer in 1839 about "my woman Sally," down with scrofula. Jeffress singled out Sally as a "favorite negro," adding, "please do for Her the best you can . . . I am very much distressed about her." The emotion seems real; but what did it signify? Words like "favorite" when referring to a slave frequently had a twisted, double meaning. Jeffress might have used the word, as masters often did, to allude to Sally's monetary worth; then, again, she might have meant "I am fond of her regardless." Either way, at the very moment of the summons, the slave patient's subjectivity was objectified and subsumed into the master's interests. The summons became a distinct genre of calls for help, one that doctors referred to as a "Negro call." As such, it distorted at the outset of care not only the concrete things a physician might do in a given case but also what he might observe and discover about African American patients generally. Accepting such terms, making them a part of the moral landscape of practice, physicians helped root slavery all the more firmly in the order of things.[16]

And with all patients, slave and free, the physician almost always arrived midscene and on a tangent to other measures already tried. The summons barely touched the surface of what awaited him. Mary Henderson recalled in 1854 her decision to summon a physician—who is nearly invisible in her account—as the last of a series of terrible misjudgments on her part in the fatal sickness of her young son Edward. It was morning, she remembered, and she was in the dining room with her sister and her slave Polly. Little Edward

came to the dining room door whilst we were at the breakfast table, told Polly to get his breakfast and amused us all with his brightness and playfulness. . . . [A]bout 11 o'clock Polly walked through the passage and he bothered her fretting very much she said to him I know you are going to be sick babe for it aint natural for you to be so fretful. Hearing this I arose immediately [and] went to him and as I always [do] when I suspect fever placed my hand upon his forehead and found it burning hot. . . . I told sister he had fever and really was so shocked I became appalled, lost all presence of mind. . . . I became completely unnerved and beside myself— we had water put on, a tub brought in, mustard and everything preparatory but Sister begged me to send for a doctor—[17]

And so, finally, she did. The physician arrived and dosed her son, but to no avail. The boy died. Henderson, looking back, believed that she had failed all through that fatal morning, failed in her reasoning and her in spirit. Not she, the boy's mother, but her slave had noticed the first symptoms; Polly spoke as one who knew her charge's ways, and Henderson recalled the woman's ordinary words as a kind of terrible forecast. And when Henderson's sister pushed for bringing in the doctor, Henderson failed again, able to do only "as I always [do]," resorting to her medicine cabinet, by then already too late. The physician, a latecomer, seems a shadow, the harbinger of her son's death.

SEEING BODIES: THE PHYSICAL AND THE SOCIAL

Stepping into sickrooms, physicians hoped they would avoid the fate of Mary Henderson's nameless doctor. Their aim was to take charge of the patient's body and to roll back disease. But to do so, they had to organize and direct the often fractious social bedside. Physicians strove to do both of these, first, by *seeing* the patient's body in a distinctively close and dramatic way and then by intervening to *change* the body in ways that threw off malady. This section concerns the former, how physicians typically visualized the stricken body and initially put their visualization into words; in the next section, we will look at what they did to alter what they saw by choosing a course of therapy. Physicians braided these together into a style of healing and a phenomenology of sickness.

Ordinary, rural physicians were more eager to "diagnose" or name disease than either their schooling implied or historians have since appreciated. To be sure, a modern style of diagnosis—using clinical techniques to systematically rule out possible diseases on the way to a "positive" identification in the pathology laboratory—was not possible or even well-conceptualized through most of the century. Nonetheless, in the sickroom encounter itself (though, interestingly, not later when they logged accounts) rural physicians clearly desired to put a name to an affliction. They wanted to do this, in part, because of the orthodox imperative "to dive into all the hidden mysteries" of the body and thus reenact science each time they exercised their art. But the diagnostic desire arose even more powerfully from the physician's role at the social bedside. The physician manipulated the body in order to better see it and to witness disease in it. But as he worked with others around the bedside, his efforts to uncover the objective entity *disease* inevitably uncovered the subjective force of people's *illness* as well. The immediate predicament of his "experience" at each bedside grew from this double vision that both inspired and distracted him. Naming disease helped him bring both into focus.[18]

Thus we must try to see the bedside as the physician saw it, as a place ripe for his particular expertise and yet a place belonging to others, too; coming to this place was the immediate test of whether his "experience" would serve to fold his personal insights into the larger body of orthodoxy, transforming both. The sick body before him was an imbalanced body, toppled in some way by malady's influence on "natural" physical and chemical harmony. The midcentury physician laid hands on the sick body in order to discover the ways in which disease had made it "excessive, and what [ways] deficient; what functions are too active, and what suspended." At each bedside, the physician's task was to match "the force of the disease [with] the strength of the patient" by discovering specific physical signs of disease—lesions, malformations, fluids—amid the blare of symptoms. Significant changes in the physician's diagnostic means occurred during the mid-nineteenth century, with certain techniques becoming more systematic by the 1840s. But there were important continuities as well. Indeed, at the very outset of his intervention, the M.D.'s methods rehearsed overlapping traditions. In one sense, his diagnostic actions followed schooled orthodoxy's most esteemed forefathers, from Galen and Hippocrates down to the Paris clinicians. At the same time, as we have seen, many of these same actions (taking the pulse, for instance) mimicked—albeit with greater variety and nuance—those employed by women and domestic healers, who were themselves influenced by the ancients, whether or not they were aware of it. Thus, a physician might prize his schooled orthodoxy as the source of his diagnostic means, but at the bedside he scarcely would be unaware that at least some of these means were broadly vernacular ones that daily reinvented ancient ways within local communities.[19]

Working from within this matrix of ideas and techniques, many physicians initiated their care by sizing up—and describing in writing—the whole sick person. The long view, the view from the sickroom doorway, so to say, was a first, objectifying view: the patient's posture in bed, how her skin appeared in terms of color and moisture, and whether she was quiet or restless. Then, if possible, the physician spoke with her in order to assess her "intellect," meaning her mental state. By taking this overall view, he aimed to discern what doctors called her "habit," the combined assessment of the patient's present state and her "constitution," that is, her characteristic openness to certain kinds of physical and emotional responses. Habits were described in broad, covering terms, drawn from ancient humoral insights, which maintained a remarkable continuity through the nineteenth century: full, nervous, plethoric, relaxed, delicate, intemperate.[20]

Simultaneously, in terms of the social bedside, assessing "habit" focused attention on the physician, creating, he hoped, a distinctive space for his work. Then he took the body in hand in ways not radically dissimilar to patients' ways, though the particularly close study he gave to stool, the tongue, and, especially, the pulse, marked him as an orthodox man. He asked about frequency of bowel movements and any change in the stool's appearance; he asked patients to save samples for him. Emerging from the gut, bearing the marks of the struggle within, stool was the closest he could come to the intensely desirable, but impossible, feat of seeing inside the body. Because stool was something even healthy individuals monitored, patients were able to give the doctor information about it—its color, consistency, and odor: the clay-colored stool of yellow fever, the blood and mucous of dysentery, the "stinking" bile that signaled a recovery from intermittent fever.[21]

The tongue was scrutinized, too, as an organ especially alive to mutations and afflictions within. An easily visible organ (lying at the vulnerable point of the mouth), the tongue signaled changes vividly seen and recorded, in terms of shape (described as flat, swollen, pointed), color (red, white, brown, black), and texture (dry, moist, velvety, glazed, coated, furred, cracked, spotted with raised papillae). The meaning of its appearance might be fairly clear; a thickly coated tongue was closely related to the many fevers of the southern countryside, for instance. But other tongues challenged a practitioner with their alarmingly broad significance—a "cracked, spotted" tongue, for instance, might indicate "decayed teeth or syphilis."[22]

No sign was as esteemed as the pulse, however, and no part of the doctor's body-work so richly combined his objectifying intentions with the sheer power of his own subjectivity. Unlike stool, which many people monitored even when feeling fine, the pulse was largely "absent" in the normal, healthy person's awareness. Not the muscular action of the heart but the body's supply of blood—its movement and consistency—was what the pulse revealed. The amount of blood and its fluid quality were thought to change drastically during sickness, and in the throb of the pulse there seemed more prognostic power than in any other single sign. Indeed, to "take" a person's pulse was to grasp the very essence of the body's closed, coded nature. Terms for different kinds of pulses far outstripped any other diagnostic vocabulary, in terms of both number and imagery. Pulses were described as hard, slow, soft, frequent, small, quick, corded, feeble, undulating, depressed, thready, shallow, weak, jerking, bounding, tense—and more. Many of these terms were Galenic in origin, and they thrived and multiplied in mid-nineteenth-century practice, appearing in every kind of text employed by physicians, from hasty notes to published work.[23]

Taking the pulse was not like inspecting the tongue or stool; the pulse depended on a relation between bodies, the caregiver's and the patient's. The depth of meaning a physician found in the sheer number of pulse words suggests the personally compelling nature of using his own body to read disease. The *doctor's* body and senses tied him to individual patients and, in the very act of using his body, he asserted his control of the bedside. His language testified to his discriminating touch. A feeble pulse, for instance, during the diastole, or contraction of the heart, is one that "produces a weak impulse against the finger." A soft pulse was "when the artery appears to be filled, and yet offers no resistance, vanishing by slight pressure." The physician's touch and the surrounding world of metaphors became more vivid and complex with experience: a corded pulse, "when the artery is felt firm under finger like a tense cord"; a shattered pulse, which "feels like a shattered quill under the finger." Physicians many times combined several terms, feeling through their own bodies not just a type of beat but the very presence of malady at work. Thus, a depressed pulse, "small and apparently feeble and occasionally quick," signaled a serious "internal venous congestion." A hectic pulse, "quick, tense, small, hard, vibrating," indicated rheumatism, and there were typhus pulses and typhoid pulses as well.[24]

The terms aimed for technical precision, of course, but they are far more striking for their subjective, even dramatic, energy. Taking up the patient's body with his own, the doctor experienced the vitality and contour of disease, felt it as it "creeped slowly along its channels," and thus he sized up malady's power in subjective terms, as illness. That is, a pulse suggested malady's capacity for harm, for wiliness. A deceptive pulse, for instance, one "not standing at one thing four hours together," would "from its full and frequent beat, induce the careless observer to imagine the inflammatory type or element to be in the ascendancy; yet . . . its compressible character—entire want of firmness and vigor—would clearly indicate that such was not the fact." Over time, certain pulses became like well-known voices or signatures, sometimes outstripping the empirical urge to describe them. Alfred Boyd, for instance, was convinced in 1856 that during his practice he had discovered "a certain indescribable vibration of the pulse [by] which I have . . . been able to prognosticate with much certainty wheather [sic] my patient would die or not." In thus taking the pulse, and in engaging with the sick body in a literally sensational way, the physician intended both to exercise and to develop his professional authority while at the same time making a place for himself at the social bedside. A man's "experience" at the heart of his country orthodoxy grew from the twining of these two desires.[25]

These broad purposes obtained when practitioners examined black patients as well, though it is important to remember that doctors' sense of a "Negro call" exaggerated their skepticism and limited their sympathy. Nonetheless, the physician's fundamental inspection of black bodies similarly seized upon stool, tongue, and pulse. Physicians typically singled out only one aspect of African American patients for extra scrutiny—the skin. J. E. Smith's 1857 note on his slave patient's recovery is typical in its emphasis on the "healthier hue" of the skin as a key indicator of a black patient's recovery. Another doctor believed that in certain kinds of sickness African Americans' skin "presents a paler hue than natural; or, if the subject is a mulatto, an ashy white." Many physicians thought it important to record the palate of tones they saw in these patients: yellow, reddish, full black, ebony, tobacco, mulatto, coffee colored. Their gaze was wholly superficial but concerned to discover unseen worlds by seeing the surface especially well. By singling out skin in their black patients, physicians exposed their willingness to see African American sickness as perhaps different in kind and to generalize about race, however tentatively, as did one Tennessee doctor in 1855, who, after careful observation, thought that "Negroes who are healthy have a peculiar softness and apparent moisture of skin" while those who were sick "have a scurfiness, or branny, or mealy appearance." Thus white doctors' bedside vision bolstered the sense of race as something as "natural" as a heartbeat.[26]

The persistence over the century of these diagnostic means, and the way they required the physician to imagine disease in the opaque body and to engage his own senses with those of his patients, shows how deeply physicians' experience was shaped by the bedside not simply to confirm orthodoxy but in fact to create a local version of it. Inevitably, a man's experience included the subjective power of illness, as well as his knowledge of objective disease. It was precisely this grasp of the intersection of disease and illness, not an unthinking resistance to the "modern," that caused many M.D.s to reject the use of certain instruments that interfered with their physical connection with the patient's body. The stethoscope was known to some rural doctors by the 1820s; many ordinary practitioners knew about urinalysis by the 1860s and about the oral thermometer by the 1870s. But very few doctors saw reason to adopt them. No doubt some practitioners were simply incurious; but many clearly disliked the physical disengagement that instrumentation entailed. If disease roamed about the body unmediated, so must the physician. "The *fashion* of consulting the thermometer as a *correct* index of the gravity of a case should not be allowed to supersede any other symptom," was how one doctor expressed it as late as 1878. And so doctors continued to put their ears to people's chests, apply with their own hands various ointments, and thrust down people's throats the pills they had just rolled. A Georgia physician, searching for a spinal tenderness he associated with a certain kind of fever, sat astride his prone patient and "press[ed] *with an equal amount of force*, directly upon each spinous process, calling the attention of the patient forcibly, to the degree of uneasiness . . . and begging him to compare these sensations together." Here was the heart of the bedside's dramatic shaping of "experience." At its core was physical engagement with patients' bodies, a sense of meeting malady on its terms as something itself active and embodied. It was a satisfying thing to use one's own body in the apprehension of disease, its sheer physicality offsetting the tedious travel of rounds and times when he was forced to merely witness the work of disease.[27]

When this combination of witnessing and acting worked, then, the M.D. became the person at the bedside who was esteemed not because he did esoteric things but because he did familiar things better than anyone else and, often, with a heightened sense of performance. The experienced physician realized that there were two kinds of bodies to manipulate with techniques—and with words: the patient's body and the social body of the sickroom. One young physician's breakthrough discovery, he told his friend in 1875, was to learn to take charge of the social bedside by controlling not only what he said but how and when he said it. He advised his friend not to be distracted by the fact that "people will expect you to name the malady at your first visit." The key to taking charge of the sickroom was to control language and its timing. In agreement, Dr. Lewis D. Ford argued that while a few important diagnostic facts might be picked up by listening to a patient's—and his family's—"long story of aches & pains," it was even more crucial to realize that listening was a means to shape the social bedside to his purposes: "You will . . . obtain [the patient's] confidence which exerts a material influence in the cure of disease."[28]

Even so, paying attention to the vernacular was not just a tactic; physicians often *preferred* to use everyday language. They frequently departed from their close accounts of stool and pulse to speak in a way as familiar as anyone else did around the bedside, using plain words to weave a country style of orthodoxy from the social setting of care. "He lay with his mouth open, his tongue dry as a board, and covered with a thick brown coating; his eyes shut, and breathing with a snore, or a kind of snort." So Dr. W. R. Sharpe's fevered patient appeared to him one afternoon in 1860. Sharpe characterized pulse and stool in professional language, of course, but his image of the open-mouthed patient would have been legible to a broad audience of observers. Such images are everywhere in bedside accounts, published, as well as unpublished. Indeed, the simple focus on the colloquial, visible body often became the focus of the physician's most deeply felt descriptions of malady. To so describe a person robbed of her normal, healthy appearance was less a way to track disease than a way to gesture toward the full social and personal meaning of its fearful effects; that is, to describe illness. Here the afflicted body is not coded into obscure signs but rather alive with flagrant display. The "red, muddy eye, continual motion or winking, [is] unfavorable," wrote William Galt of a patient. "Forehead dry and wrinkles, complexion pale or livid—very unfavorable. . . . Voice—a sharp or quick tone of voice, bad." A Tennessee doctor noted in 1860 how a delirious patient "grasps [as] if he was trying to catch something and trying to pick up something off the quilts." Benjamin Musser found his patient in pain, "moving himself about the bed . . . by placing his elbows under himself and in this way raising & throwing himself from one side of the bed to another."[29]

Colloquial figures of speech likewise served physicians as a particularly satisfying language for malady, a metaphorical language, visual and textured, keeping the physician attached to the sufferer and both of them attached to the everyday social world. Bloody vomit was likened to "a mass of wet gunpowder," a splintered bone to a "broken stick of tough, straight-grained wood," a woman's rigid cervix to "an ivory ring," and infected glands to "that decayed portion of honey comb usually called bee bread." Physicians easily used many blunt, vernacular terms for how patients appeared or felt, words patients themselves used: "reduced," "right smart," "diminished," "on high ground," "sinking," "laboring under disease," "taking a bad turn." Indeed, patient voices sometimes break into physicians' words. A slave woman being treated by Charles Chester in 1847 uttered "the most distressing cries—my *head*! my *head*!" A Virginia doctor recorded in 1859 that fevered patients implored him with "Oh! how weak—how weak I feel doctor" and "If you will only give me something to strengthen me, I will soon be well."[30]

As such language integrated the physician with others around the bedside, it also troubled M.D.s' sense of their uniqueness by giving others license to speak with similar authority. Tapping into vernacular talk, the physician risked becoming completely undistinguished in the sickroom, something that especially weakened his authority when the time came to pronounce what ailed the patient. The act of giving a particular name to illness illuminated precisely the point of tension where orthodox training met the social bedside. On the one hand, as we saw earlier, the desire to name disease derived from the schooled imperatives of science that drove a physician to pursue the foe past death into autopsy. When Charles Hentz's slave patient Sam died, for instance, Hentz undertook a postmortem in which his desire to see disease was inextricable from his desire to name it. He began at the throat ("nothing wrong up there") and continued to the thorax. There, "oh, my!!! such tremendous disease— unexpected developments" of tumors and pockets of fluid that he felt compelled to name. On the other hand, the desire to name sickness also arose from the patient, his family, and the pressures of the social bedside. Many physicians, like Hentz, wrote in ways that showed them excited by naming's public drama of exposure. Thus, after working for days to save a patient, one doctor, like many others, experienced his diagnosis as an intense moment created by the disease itself. Pursued, the malady had "now thrown off its last mask, and stood there in the form of *Diphtheria*." "Old fashioned *violent* bilious fever" was all the more dangerous, said another doctor in 1857, because, once cornered, "at any moment, it may turn to typhus." In describing such ailments as tertian intermittent fever as having the ability to "personate with great exactness a phrensy, pleurisy, hepatitis, lumbago, or rheumatism," a physician marshaled names as testimony to his personal, public struggle against a foe.[31]

This struggle to identify disease amid the mysteries of illness thus led many physicians to wonder whether their medicine was significant because it belonged to them alone or, rather, because it tapped into a shared store of knowledge allowing them to belong to their communities. Although daily making use of it, increasing numbers of M.D.s were concerned by the 1840s that the mixture of popular and orthodox names and descriptions was a sign not of a principled country orthodoxy but of an indecisive, diluted one. If science was to be extracted from the bedside, some physicians pointed out, names should be uniform. Yet all physicians knew that, in practice, names, especially orthodox names, could be frustratingly imprecise. Physician R. L. Scruggs was troubled by the fact that "typhoid" "may be used simply as a name (arbitrarily if you please) or to express a condition," that is, as a noun or an adjective. Many M.D.s distanced themselves from certain names even as they used them, making for a stark division between the ideal of uniformity and the actual variety found at the bedside. For instance, physicians often qualified their diagnoses in their notebooks as "something like pneumonia" or "something like dysentery." An Alabama physician, in an 1849 article on congestive fever, put his finger on the heart of the problem of straddling the schooled and vernacular worlds of diagnosis: "Although I use the term [congestive fever] myself, from custom, I believe it inappropriate."[32]

Such widespread uncertainty about names and disease—it is found throughout published, as well as unpublished, medical writing—must be understood not simply as a sign of physicians' simple premodern "ignorance," as it often is, or as mere missteps on the way to modern diagnosis. Rather, the uncertainty must be seen as a complex dilemma growing from the bedside collision of two compelling versions of orthodoxy. One was based on an ideal of scientific naming fashioned apart from popular ways. The other grew directly from the realities of sickroom caregiving and the productive likeness between a physician and the people he served. In putting names to afflictions, then, the physician stepped to the edge of a personal and professional choice with implications for his identity as a healer. He might intentionally stay away from the vernacular—speaking jargon, acting mysteriously, looking for science at every bedside—and run the risk of going unsummoned. Alternatively, he might fully embrace the vernacular and gain support but risk giving up the quest for a comprehensive, systematic knowledge. So it was that many M.D.s looked for a third way that recombined these choices into another route to success at the bedside—reifying a man's personal "experience" as the heart of an orthodoxy suited to southern practice. This sense of experience, as we have seen in other contexts, claimed a basis in broad knowledge that nonetheless was appropriately configured by each individual practitioner in his work. How such "experience" was called upon at the social bedside is no better seen than when the physician moved from diagnosis to the prescription of his medicine.[33]

CHANGING BODIES: "EXPERIENCE" AND THE CHARM OF DRUGS

The therapeutic moment—the point at which the physician translated his view of body and disease into discrete measures aimed at effecting a cure—was a defining moment in a practitioner's caregiving. In most cases, the moment called for some kind of drug, tying the doctor's sense of his "experience" to his ability to persuade, cajole, or coerce patients to ingest some unpleasant substance that would then have the predicted effect. The therapeutic moment thus brought into sharp, material focus the recurrent tension between orthodox learning and community ways, daunting malady and equally fierce medicines, and the doctor's moral place as both witness and actor in the drama of sickness.

In particular, the therapeutic moment raised basic questions of timing and expertise at the center of a man's "experience." Despite the fact that prescribing drugs was an utterly routine aspect of medical work, it remained for most doctors a signal turning point in which everything he represented was put on the line. His training aside, the bedside reality was that certain drugs worked mysteriously—or, worse, mysteriously failed to work. Indeed, the finer points of pathological and therapeutic theory, though much debated in the pages of medical journals, seldom gave physicians a purchase on their immediate therapeutic challenges. A diagnosed disease many times implied no single remedy. "In a pathological point of view," wrote one practitioner, "there may be propriety in the division [of fevers] into intermittent, remittent, and continued. . . . [B]ut in a therapeutic point of light, the distinction is inadmissible" because the fever types "so often pass alternately into each other" during treatment that making meaningful distinctions was impossible. In other words, when it came to medicating, the science of pathology was next to useless. The key was not pathological or pharmacological theory, therefore, but bedside timing. The therapeutic moment reconfigured everything—the embodied nature of disease, its name, the very self-image of the physician—in ways that were impossible to control but might be channeled by medicines given at just the moment when things hung in the balance. One theoretical stance that did in fact matter at the bedside, then, was the notion of "expectancy," which is revisited here as a genuine bedside issue of timing, not least because it shaped the terms of trust between the patient, her family, and the doctor.[34]

Earlier, we saw how the debate over whether to be an "expectant" doctor prompted medical faculty and students at midcentury to think about the troubled relation between specific medicines and the larger scope of pathology and physiology. Should medicines be thought of as attacking disease or as assisting the patient? Was Nature a field to be explored or a force to master? How can waiting to intervene be justified? These matters took on their full, phenomenological meaning only at the bedside when the time came to prescribe. Indeed, looking at the bedside reveals that expectancy as a theoretical issue carried a charge mostly because of the bedside's intense valence of fear and trust. That is, its urgency as an issue must be seen not only as trickling down into ordinary practice from hospital study or anatomy clinics but also as bubbling up from the dilemmas of countless sickrooms.[35]

Seen from the bedside, then, the expectancy debate was essentially a moral debate about the social context of medical practice—in effect, a debate over how a practitioner might bring his orthodox principles into alignment with the trust and hope his community invested in him. M.D. opponents of expectancy, as noted earlier, believed that expectancy breached physicians' traditional allegiance to the "active" measures that exposed disease. As important, though, was the sense that expectancy violated the trust between a physician and his patient. Opponents pointed out that many patients trusted a physician to use aggressive therapy to "take the disease out of the hands of nature." In this view, the moral character of allopathic medicine was less a sacred legacy than it was an agreement between a doctor and his neighbors, reaffirmed at every bedside. This was the view that accounts for the strong emotional language of men like John Esten Cooke, who declared in 1828 that expectancy thwarted the best medicine and that "I should hold myself criminal not to give such do[s]es as . . . in my best judgment I believe will succeed." A practitioner's therapeutic choices grew from the pattern of his own experience among neighbors and rival healers, not from abstract principle. " 'Letting a patient alone,' " J. A. Eve wrote scornfully of expectancy, "is . . . too often only a subterfuge for ignorance, a resting place for indolence."[36]

On the other side of the debate, expectant physicians also understood the issue in terms of timing and trust, but they cast therapy and the community of patients into a different pattern. They argued with equal passion that expectant medicine was legitimate because it best united orthodox science and popular wisdom. Expectancy arose from the bedside wisdom that a sick person lived in a world of great social, as well as pathological, complexity. Waiting meant more than simply standing by; it meant working with families for consensus based on trust. Francis Porcher, for instance, argued that a careful, flexible expectancy combined watchfulness with consultation to arrive at "a judicious administration of remedial agents." By sensitively waiting and watching, the physician would be able to gain a family's trust by harmonizing his own "administration of . . . tonics, porter, ale, wine, iron, etc.," with theirs. At the bedside, there was no better definition of valuable experience than this: to know how to get patients to agree to the medicines one thought best.[37]

From the vantage point of the sickroom, then, expectancy was about much more than Nature-trusting; it was a means for strengthening the emphasis a practitioner put on his own personal experience—and his personal morality—as the bedrock of good medicine. Moreover, being expectant allowed physicians to pay tribute to the commonsense, domestic caregiving he met up with each day. Doctors recounted instances, often with a nod to commonsense wisdom, in which simply waiting for nature to act proved just the thing. A Louisiana doctor in 1856 approvingly told the story of a wise patient who, accidentally swallowing his false teeth, reasoned that "nature had made a way for the getting out of whatever could get in," and was proved right, making the doctor's intervention unnecessary. Similarly, in the case of a man who inadvertently swallowed a half-dollar, a medical journal affirmed that this was a case "where the very best practice was to *do nothing*." Restraint, the journal pointed out, not only was consonant with a scientific grasp of the unfortunate event ("Nature being fully competent to relieve it"), it also gained the goodwill of the patient, who was pleased that "no interference was required."[38]

Still, the difficulty was in knowing when this watchful mode of practice crossed a line between an appropriately flexible orthodoxy and a flabby lack of standards. Often, it seems, a practitioner's personal attachments to his own favorite drugs guided him to an answer. Physicians' emotional tie to their favorite medicines—their eagerness to combine, trade, and advocate for them—was a striking feature of everyday practice. Indeed, as we saw with regard to southerners' health talk, the century-long continuity of widespread, unregulated medicines inspired a general willingness to embrace favorites. Historians have both pitied and criticized nineteenth-century M.D.s for working with crude and ineffective medicines. And with hindsight, of course, it is easy to see why most mainstream allopathic medicines were bad therapy. Not only were they frequently misapplied (by modern standards), they were fearfully toxic. Like nineteenth-century critics of allopathy, later historians have focused on the appalling consequences of "heroic," poisonous dosages: acute diarrhea, vomiting to exhaustion, and elevated temperature. And these were only the visible surface of a deeper physiological distress wrought by such drugs, ranging from impairment of nutrition to rapid dehydration, shock, and, over longer periods of time, the buildup in the body of harmful minerals, not to mention the risk of addiction to drugs such as morphine. Although historians have acknowledged the few major therapies now thought to be beneficial—among them quinine for the symptoms of malaria, digitalis for regulation of the heartbeat, vaccination against smallpox—they tend to linger over the spectacularly ill effects of most of the allopathic pharmacopeia.[39]

But the use of powerful, toxic substances should not imply, as it often has, that they were valued for their simple, bludgeonlike force. To the contrary, bedside practice suggests the extent to which ordinary physicians studied, combined or modified, and, most important, personally identified with what they considered to be not just powerful but also subtle medicines. Most physicians did not prescribe by rote but studied dosages, strove to keep medicines fresh and uncontaminated, and regulated the dose to the standards accepted for the age, weight, sex, and race of the patient. They knew that ever larger doses of some medicines had to be given over time (in response to what is called a patient's "tolerance" to medication) and that opium and morphine, among other drugs, were addictive. Negative features of certain drugs did not deter mid-nineteenth-century physicians from using them any more than modern doctors are deterred from using their "aggressive" drugs. What all of this adds up to is that even though physicians frequently were mistaken about much of the physiological and pathogenic effects of their medicines, the "ignorance" of the era's physicians is not the key point in considering the long continuity of this style of medicine. More important is understanding how practitioners' allegiance to certain drugs was rooted in a deeply felt, personal constellation of perceptions and decisions tied to their very identity as healers.[40]

For instance, physicians admired certain drugs for being easily portable and amenable to different forms (as pills, draughts, ointments). Favored medicines also were those readily available throughout the South; except during the Civil

War, physicians almost never complained about difficulty in obtaining their mainstream medicines. Above all, a medicine was prized for being wonderfully flexible in multiple combinations, permitting the physician to match the power of the medicine exactly to the strength of embodied disease, in *this* body *now*. A useful remedy, well combined and well timed, was the one that seized each sick body and held it in a unique way, producing a vigorous "operation" or "working" that indicated a successful engagement with disease on the body's interior landscape. Only a novice doctor focused on the power of this or that drug in isolation; what impressed the experienced man was the wonderful complexity and suppleness their medicines possessed. More than other kinds of healers, M.D.s wrote about medicines as forming a grid of therapeutic action and of casting up the sick body (or, by the 1840s, all of physiology itself) against this grid. Chief among the two dozen or so most often mentioned categories of drugs were the cathartics (enhancing the action of the intestines), emetics (exciting vomiting), stimulants (arousing the action of an organ, especially the heart and kidneys), diaphoretics ("opening" or promoting exhalation of disease through the organs, especially the skin), tonics (strengthening the body's general organic processes and energy, especially through the stomach), narcotics (affecting the brain, either sedating or stimulating), analgesics (reducing pain), and expectorants (augmenting secretion, especially of saliva and mucous).[41]

This basic field of drug actions was extended and deepened when the doctor orchestrated the size of the dosage, the sequence and timing of its administration, its combination with drugs of the same or different agency, the form in which it was administered (as a tincture, for example, or a pill)—all with an eye to the likely course malady would take. Here physicians saw further dimensions to be explored. The agency of each drug—some said its very character—changed in response to embodied disease. Each drug or combination of drugs was seen as more or less "direct" or "indirect," elastic terms denoting not only the time elapsed before drug and disease collided but also the physiological route taken by the medicine in the body. All of these levels of activity were further influenced by the habit or constitution of the patient, and finally spiraled outward to include the surrounding topography, the weather, and the season. Under some conditions, a medicine might jump categories; given as a stimulant, it might act as a tonic, that is, less dramatically and less quickly, necessitating a shift in the doctor's next move. A substance given as a diaphoretic, for example, if administered "when the capillary action is in a state of exultation from disease," would not act to open the veins but instead "retard . . . the transpiratory process." Even in the most ordinary circumstances, then, medicines appear in doctor's writing as shimmering substances made volatile by a powerful matrix of forces and qualities.[42]

In short, the power and attraction of heroic medicine as visualized by physicians is not best described in terms of its harshness or hammerlike effect but rather in terms of possibilities—possibilities commanded somewhat differently by each astute man of experience. In this way, the orthodox impulse in therapy further deepened the intensely personal nature of practice. Hearing physicians talk about prescribing is not like reading through the dry pages of the *United States Dispensatory*. Physicians' drugs were their companions and servants. Writing to and for each other, in medical journals, as well as in private correspondence, many doctors rehearsed their most esteemed measures as they reported each new case. Everything in a physician's experience came down to the "dispensing of the articles of Materia Medica," as one practitioner reminded his colleagues, "so as to relieve pain, mitigate suffering, and assist nature in throwing off diseases." Throwing off disease; being "under" disease and struggling to get on top; "lifting" the patient—a language of physical effort runs throughout accounts of therapy. There was an epic—and gendered—cast to much of this talk, figures of speech that placed the doctor's personal efforts into a setting of great travail, where the manliness of the task was central to its importance. Many saw the drama in nautical terms, the doctor as a navigator entrusted with the "barque" of the body amid the dangers of shoal and storm, his drugs relied upon to "guide this ship to a safe harbour." This was the language not only of neophytes but also of older men who had been to many sickrooms in the backwoods and yet still wrote of themselves as captains and warriors. The therapeutic purpose, the very essence of being a physician, said one twenty-year veteran of practice, was to "keep off the enemy as far as possible from the Sanctum, keeping inviolate as far as possible her inner courts."[43]

This kind of language fused the larger moral potential of medicine to the personal pride of each man's everyday prescribing. When a sudden attack of "inflammation of the brain . . . struck terror to the neighborhood" in which he practiced, a North Carolina physician felt it with the force of a personal affront. He was "shocked and confused with the first few cases which appeared as sudden and overwhelming as an avalanche," and the sheer violence of the disease "aroused me, and caused me to adopt the very active treatment" that he went on to describe. At other times, the beauty and power of his array of medicines suggested not warfare but rather charm and fancy. Rolling a new supply of pills one evening, a young Alabama doctor mused about how each one soon would be swallowed up by its own crisis, and he speculated how each small, waxy sphere carried its own small measure of hope out into the world of sick people. He thought how interesting it would be to write "a history of the adventures of each [pill] . . . in a *physiologico-romantic* style."[44]

If the skilled manipulation of medicines both delicate and muscular thus in some sense reinvented a man's medical experience each time he prescribed, then the style of his prescriptions over time became a badge of his moral, as well as material, practice. A practitioner's prescriptions arose from his character, where skill should be matched by an equal measure of sympathy. Like many other practitioners, E. B. Flagg of Charleston wrote prescriptions that rehearsed the act of caregiving itself; more than lists of substances, they are small, sharp *scenes* that convey a sense of the bedside relationship of doctor and patient, and the way that the proper prescription created a moral setting for giving care. Consider one such prescription (interestingly, the patient was a slave) that reveals the typical sense of therapy as multiple and complex, almost fragile in its hoped-for precision, sensitivity to timing, and dependence on the trust between the doctor, his patient, and other caregivers. Flagg prescribed a quinine mixture, directing the caregiver to "give half a teaspoonful 3 times a day in a little molasses. Increase the dose should the bowels not act at least once a day and diminish it should they act oftener than twice. Rub the back and shoulders every night and morning with turpentine and sweet oil in equal parts. Let him have meat once a day, and warm baths at mid-day once a week. . . . Once a fortnight apply a blister as large as a man's hand between the shoulders and dress it with lime water & sweet oil."[45] These actions were utterly ordinary but nonetheless inscribed an ideal of therapy—conscientious, informed, tender—against its opposite potential for disorder and harm. At the same time, such prescriptions skated over social tensions by portraying all patients as equally willing, and able, to act on the best advice. In particular, such description floats above issues of slavery and race, avoiding the question of whether anyone on a given plantation would follow through with so attentive a course of treatment for a slave.

Thus, the way in which M.D.s conceived of their medicines as varied, supple, and inescapably subjective uniquely defined their sense of "experience" as intensely personal and essentially moral. In this way, through a succession of therapeutic moments, case by case, physicians tightened the link between orthodoxy and their identity, giving each man's practice precedence over a more generalized view of therapy. This, in turn, meant that criticism of orthodoxy was easily taken to be *personal* criticism—criticism of a practitioner's character, as well as his means. As with his diagnostic measures, but more dramatically, the link between therapeutic choice and a practitioner's identity made it more difficult for the doctor to change his basic therapeutic allegiances—and therefore more difficult, too, for orthodox medicine to change.

Important consequences of the fact that physicians served a wider orthodoxy by being loyal to their own bedside measures arose when doctors were faced with the need to improvise. Although professionwide precepts may be seen shaping many of their measures, they were shaped just as surely by the "experience" of others who happened to be present at any given bedside, and by the emotional tenor of the moment. Again, far more than strict orthodoxy would allow, practice was configured by *performance* as well as precept. The bedside was a stage for acting out good medicine—a social place where the morality of medicine was as much a feature of practice as its materials. Thus, for good reason, medical histories have highlighted the "sectarian wars" of the mid-nineteenth century, seeing orthodox modernity taking shape through its struggle against competing ideas, as well as practices. And yet a close look at everyday medicine in the rural South suggests a more complex dynamic—less a matter of ideology ("allopathic" vs. "botanical," for instance) than a phenomenology achieved by mingling a wide array of drugs and means in which everyone's therapy was borrowed, experimented with, and, in some cases, imposed by violence.

At the bedside, despite the disclaimers of professional leaders and many teachers, a savvy physician fully expected to improvise. "Experience" in this sense meant having a sharp eye for a new medicine, as well as a catholic sense of what counted as an orthodox medicine; it meant a willingness to think of orthodoxy as something creative rather than authoritarian. In this regard, remedies, African American and white, served to knit together allopathic and domestic pharmacopeia in a way that blurred the line between them. A good example is castor oil, a mild cathartic with some antibacterial action that was a staple of households, slave and free, and widely used by M.D.s as well. Other such medicines—to name only a few—included turpentine (in the form of an oil locally distilled from pine trees, administered internally as a remedy for colds and topically for rheumatism); sassafras (used as a tonic by whites and, similarly, as a blood purifier by blacks); camphor (used internally as a narcotic, externally as a liniment); digitalis (used to regulate the heartbeat); ergot (a fungus used as a muscle contractant and abortifacient); poke root (a kind of hellebore, much in use by slaves as an emetic and adopted enthusiastically by many M.D.s in the 1850s in the form of the cathartic veratrum viride). Even "straight" allopathic remedies such as laudanum and quinine were found in many households. In their recipe and prescription books (those descendants of the almanacs and books of secrets of earlier centuries), southerners moved easily in and out of allopathic territory in recording various wisdoms and formulae. Axioms, puzzles, moral tales, calendars, and recipes were thrown together into a homey, potent mixture. Planter Joseph Dupuy's book, for instance, compiled in the 1840s and 1850s, blends between its covers cures for diseases in cattle, horses, and people; it includes notes on individual slaves and their ailments, planting times for various crops, recipes for paint, the "Chinese method for making cloth waterproof," boot blacking, vinegar, and "good & cheap beer." Dupuy transcribed formulae for medicines derived directly from allopaths (Cook's pills and Pancoast's cathartic pills) side by side with local women's formulas for cough syrup, a body rub, and scrofula paste. He made similarly eclectic notes on the value of cod liver oil, calomel, Epsom salts, and morphine.[46]

In many instances, then, the domestic medicine chest was so familiar to everyone that, in the heat of bedside practice, physicians could choose to ignore the ways in which it was *not* orthodox and adopt what they liked. Nature, after all, was the great supplier of all remedies, and the widespread popular use of a substance might simply be Nature's way of bringing it to light. Physicians kept their own notebooks of new therapies picked up on rounds, testimony to their unembarrassed borrowing. Dr. Albert Bachelor's 1873 treatment for scarlet fever employed the latest orthodox drug therapies, but he also included the note to himself that "old physicians wet the whole surface [of the body] with fat bacon. May do good." About the same time, R. W. Rea also noted the bacon-fat therapy, which he credited to "women," and noted, too, another folk recipe that could be used as a substitute, "sweet oil mixed with Bay Rum or Cologne or cream and Rose Water." A Georgia doctor in the 1840s recorded that blood drawn "from an artery in the back part of the little finger" relieved epileptic fits—"this is an old woman remedy, however I have tried it several times and never failed." Along with bacon fat, physicians frequently took notice of other ordinary items such as pure water, ice, and flannel as having multiple therapeutic uses. And a Louisiana physician, after trying other remedies for "local inflammation," discovered that making an ordinary batter cake and applying it to the skin "appears to have a happy effect; it has not only the effect of causing moisture and elasticity of the parts, by local diaphoresis, but it appears to impart nutrition also." The pancakes "should be made soft, and as one is removed, another applied."[47]

The image of an M.D. making pancakes and carefully placing them on a patient's body is an image of nineteenth-century orthodoxy worth thinking about. Some of his colleagues would have laughed at him or seen the pancakes as heresy. But most would have understood that therapeutic moments inevitably were made from such collaboration. No one's measures could be rejected outright, and, indeed, happy results were eagerly recommended to colleagues, both privately and in orthodox publications, in terms of their social acceptance. One doctor frankly praised a remedy in 1821 because it found favor "amongst the citizens," as well as among local physicians. Another recommended a decoction of honeysuckle as a remedy for dropsy, observing that he had tried it simply because "I heard a countryman urging the claims of [it] and became convinced of its merit." A man's bedside esteem arose from the fact that he was trusted by his neighbors to reliably weave together all useful therapies and give a persuasive, conversational account of them. So L. B. Anderson, practicing in Hanover County, Virginia, in 1856, enthusiastically recommended to his colleagues table salt and egg yolk as a cure for cancer. Although he admitted the mixture was, strictly speaking, unorthodox, the story of how he had come to use it served as sufficient professional grounds for recommending it. A "woman patient" had told Anderson's father, himself an M.D., of the mixture, and the father had used it successfully several times. Though skeptical, Anderson subsequently tried and approved of it, and he passed it along to a "sensible and talkative old lady" in his neighborhood who had since reported back to him that it had worked satisfactorily for her, too.[48]

It is striking that even orthodox textbooks discussed prescriptions in ways that invited such individual experimentation. Clearly, therapy was so locked into a physician's personal experience that textbook authors found it impossible to generalize very far about drugs and dosages. The influential author John Eberle, for instance, almost never recommends exact dosages, typically qualifying his therapeutic information to the point where bedside experiment becomes imperative. Speaking of childhood diseases, for instance, he recommends purgatives but only "under judicious management"; emetics "deserve . . . much more attention . . . than they appear at present to receive." His words are cautious and moral, respectful of any "experienced" man's prior knowledge. Opium, tobacco, and other medicines he acknowledges with approval but only "under certain circumstances," of which he gives not a hint. Blisters? "Blisters will sometimes do considerable good . . . but I have often known them applied without any perceptible advantage." Ipecac? "Some speak very favorably of it." Eberle's recommendations imply that only those with bedside experience could possibly know what he means and that such experience could not be defined in general terms.[49]

By definition, then, the bedside demanded medical experiment, not in the sense of the systematic, "clinical trial" procedures of the twentieth century, but in immediate, case-by-case, interactive trading and innovation. To be sure, physicians and patients agreed on broad (though markedly vague) ethical limits on a wide-open, let's-see-what-happens approach to therapy. And physicians' codes of ethics portrayed the doctor-patient relationship as one that bound the physician to be certain that each of his measures was for the patient's benefit, not for the sheer satisfaction of curiosity. Nevertheless, it is striking how often the bedside borrowing and combining of medicines blurred this ethical line. The therapeutic moment gave so much priority to chasing down malady and reversing it, and even "expectant" prescriptions entailed so many unknowns, that a practitioner had considerable ethical license for trying almost anything. So we find practitioners readily owning up to the experimental reality of their orthodox practice, seeing a course of medicine applied in a mysterious sickness as, necessarily, "a lick in the dark," as one South Carolina doctor told a colleague about his prescription for a Miss Singly's hemorrhaging in 1848. After prescribing an antimony treatment for Mrs. Semmes, an Arkansas doctor added, "I am curious to see how it will act."[50]

Borrowing therapies and experimenting with them, physicians at bedsides throughout the century thus further defined these elements of a country orthodoxy that privileged an individual's "experience" over all else, raising personal practice to the status of a doctrine that turned criticism aside. Doctors like J. A. Reedy in 1884, coming up against their limits in a case, made an innovation in therapy and then "push[ed] it and watch[ed] the effects." Many like Reedy, and like William Holcombe in the 1850s, found such routine bedside experiments over time to be the most intellectually exciting aspect of their work. Reminiscing about his first experiments with homeopathy, Holcombe portrayed himself, interestingly, as both predator and innocent. He recalled his willingness to experiment as being like "the unquestioning docility of a little child," and yet, once he got used to it, he recalled waiting for "my next patient like a hunter watching for a duck." When one pair of anxious parents asked Dr. William Turner for his diagnosis, he did not tell them that he was stumped but instead stalled them with "recourse to technicality." He knew this was morally questionable, but the goal of making a new discovery at the bedside justified his fudging, and he "was determined at all sacrifices to hang on to the case which was so interesting, so puzzling, and to see its termination."[51]

Turner's phrase "determined at all sacrifices" suggests how the excitement of pursuing an experiment might cross over into coercion or even violence. Physicians' coercion of patients was (and has remained) a matter of controversy. Alternative practitioners decried it as allopathy run amock, and historians have cited it as central to orthodoxy's premodern abuses. Both criticisms have merit, but they do not explain why coercion made sense to physicians—and even to some patients. Indeed, blunt, physical force was a part of any M.D.'s routine practice. Logically, aggressive physical means followed from the conviction—

part trope, part tenet—that medicine was warfare against disease. A certain amount of physical pain was part of the battle. Moreover, pain was accepted by nearly everyone as an index of a patient's ability to rally against disease and, in many cases, as itself contributing to recovery.[52]

Physicians were candid about the orthodoxy of violence. Indeed, the many calmly written accounts of violent struggles at first belie what actually went on in the room. In 1878, Frank James twice injected caffeine into a patient who had overdosed on morphine and then "used a wet towel to whip him with"—a standard procedure—until the man was alert enough to protest the beating. In many instances, doctors interpreted patients' resistance to coercion or abuse as a therapeutic turning point in a case and a guide to further treatment. Samuel Dickson, among the most thoughtful of physicians, believed that the manic violence of a person suffering from delirium tremens had few equals for sheer terror and desperation, and, he warned, such violence *must* be brought under control by using equal force. Not only was alcoholic mania—the screaming, cursing, and destructiveness—a threat to the patient, it also challenged the doctor's efforts to create the social bedside he needed; the out-of-control patient can "constitute the most embarrassing complication which we can meet with" in therapy. And so, Dickson wrote, the manic patient must be forced to the bed, stripped of his clothing, and subjected to cold water poured upon his head "from some height," followed by bleeding, vomiting, and enemas, in spite of his screams and terror; the enemas, especially, must be administered repeatedly and "at intervals of no great length." Other therapeutic measures aside, the memory of being physically dominated, Dickson suggested, would add to the patient's chances for recovery after he sobered up.[53]

This being said, however, there is little doubt that some practitioners became caught up in abusive measures for other reasons, often in cases where the patient did not respond to increasing levels of violence. For these physicians, therapy and experimentation had to force some visible outcome, often with horrifying results. One day in 1856, for example, Maryland physician W. Chew Van Bibber and one or more colleagues were summoned to revive a six-year-old girl who had passed out after drinking alcohol. Thwarted by the girl's stubborn unconsciousness, which became, in Van Bibber's view, a kind of entity in itself, the doctors engaged in a series of increasingly extreme measures aimed at rousing her. Although at first it is possible to see something of the girl in Van Bibber's account, his avid effort to get "results" soon leads him to write only of body parts—of "the mouth" and "the head": "neither whipping, pinching, pricking with pins, nor scratching the cornea" got any response from the child, nor did the "fluids poured into the mouth" cause her to vomit. "All efforts to arouse having failed, a stream of cold water was poured upon the head for an hour and a half continuously," though this resulted only in a "contraction of the pupil." This was just the beginning. Van Bibber and his colleagues proceeded to blister the girl, inject acetate of ammonia into her stomach, administer a turpentine enema, and force her to ingest calomel, castor oil, beef broth, and more— three days of this sort of thing. She convulsed one time; and once, the observant Van Bibber noted, she gestured as if "to try to drive a fly from her face." Otherwise, nothing much changed until she died. Death came "about 83 hours after the ingestion of the poison," Van Bibber observed, as if it were the alcohol alone that had killed her.[54]

In such instances, clearly, violence assumed its own momentum and rationale, pushing physicians to borrow and experiment in ever more aggressive ways. If deliberate enough, physicians could rationalize violence as anything but the slow fall into panic that it frequently was. Of course, some physicians were wary of such reasoning because they shied away from violence under any circumstances or because they feared patients might be driven away. But no working M.D. could entirely avoid such times or the way they illuminated the special quality of his medicine as bold and radical and his persistence as honorable. That is, forcing the issue through aggressive means made bedside doctoring seem larger than life and thus personally heroic. "[I]t seems that my presence and my pills are incompatible with any disease in these parts," exulted one doctor in 1861. Not only had his forceful means saved his patients, it had produced results "in every way flattering to science." The language of bedside success was assertive and masculine, configuring bedside violence in terms of warfare and reputation. Doctors wrote of experiencing a "hard struggle but victory finally perched on my banner," of going "full blast with the Veratrum Viride," and of using closely packed, multiple medicines that "broke up disease entirely," persisting in it "until the disease yields." Practitioners praised the "noble effects" of their favorite drugs. The power of beloved remedies sometimes seemed to go beyond even science. "These means had a magical effect," George Grant wrote in 1836, in awe of his fortunate choice of therapy.[55]

Thus, with therapy feeding on such an open-ended rationale, and with so much of their own identity invested in their prescriptions, most practitioners urged on their patients to greater sacrifices. What they saw in their drastic measures was not a story of a patient's pain and a doctor's coercion but a story of their united courage and inventiveness. A Mississippi physician, during an outbreak of erysipelas in 1845, cupped and bled his patients, following up with hot mustard baths, blisters, calomel, and opium "in large doses"; but, "in spite of every rational resource, we were destined to see our patients . . . snatched away by the relentless hand of the scourger." And yet this outcome diminished neither his faith in his drugs nor his sense that his patients fully supported his measures. In the very violence of the treatment, in the avid desire to try *everything*, physicians' personal passion for their therapy framed it as orthodox and thus insulated it from their own self-criticism.[56]

THE SHADOW OF BEDSIDE PRACTICE

As the physician examined the body and began with his drugs, each bedside became a kind of personal theater for his knowledge, skills, and, ultimately, his sense of himself as a moral man whose bedside labors were inextricable from the trust placed in him by his patients and community. If the ideal of a broad, schooled science excited a man's intellect in his pursuit of disease, the subjective realm of the bedside excited his visceral desire to subdue illness. And thus the theater of bedside work revealed the significance of everything orthodoxy took from the surrounding flow of popular ideas, remedies, and the social flux of each sickroom.

In particular, this style of undertaking care—this purchase on "experience"—was a powerful force for the continuity of a physician's medicine. It privileged the individual practitioner by encouraging him to see a variety of bedsides as "his," marked by his particular insight and personality, and thus not to be changed lightly. At the same time, it was a style that sustained the belief that in every case a physician might contribute to a general science. This possibility further invested a man in preserving the continuity of his work by giving him an intellectual purpose that rolled over non-M.D. critics and even elite M.D.s, who, after the 1880s, were developing a vision of a different kind of science, one located in standardized protocols, urban institutions, and money. So it was that one rural physician in 1850, typical of hundreds who wrote up their bedside discoveries and got them published in medical journals, told excitedly of his discovery of a remedy for infant tetanus. His experience was that many afflicted infants were found lying on their backs. Thinking that perhaps pressure on the back of the skull might be a factor, he turned one symptomatic infant over on his stomach. The baby recovered! A single case, a moment of personal insight, was sufficient for him (and the medical journal) to make an enthusiastic, universal recommendation that infants sleep on their stomachs. In the same eager, experimental vein, another doctor reasoned in 1849 that because chloride of lime worked around the farm to decompose animal wastes and filth, saucers of lime set out in a room might counteract harmful vapors in the air. He tried it in his own household, setting two saucers of lime solution on the mantle; no one got sick for months. He recommended dishes of lime solution wholeheartedly. Medical journals are filled with this personal-scale science throughout mid-century. Each new sickbed was an equal opportunity to rehearse the continuity of orthodox medicine and its benefits.[57]

In this way, coming to each new bedside enhanced physicians' traditional ways of subjective insight and medicine's standing as an "art." It is not that practitioners necessarily resisted looking toward the objectifying kind of modernity that would come to define the bedside in the next century. But they were more quick to embrace a different kind of "modern" view, an essentially Romantic vision that configured what was "new" in personal terms that highlighted a man's individuality and linked him to his like-minded neighbors. Southern physicians, then, doubtless like their counterparts elsewhere in the nation, shaped an almost paradoxical bedside identity. They hoped to participate in a medical science whose shadow would grow to cover more and more of the unknown. But at the bedside it very often was the *practitioner's* shadow that grew larger. In their much-cherished individual habits of diagnosis and prescription, and at the social bedside where they became both actors and witnesses in the drama of sickness, it is evident how this style of practice hallowed a man's personal sense of what orthodoxy was. This resolutely personal mode of practice, despite times of openness to change and collaboration, ultimately bonded orthodoxy to the experience of individuals in a way that made any attack on orthodoxy an attack on a practitioner's personal reputation and character. And in a republican, southern setting, especially, challenging a man's character entailed a risk for any critic. The following chapter explores further the significance of this link between the personal and the professional in terms of orthodox medicine's peculiar blend of empirical and subjective means for inscribing the patient in case notes, and the resulting confrontation with families over the terms of co-attendance.

PART THREE

MAKING MEDICINE

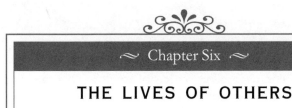

Chapter Six

THE LIVES OF OTHERS

As physicians continued their treatment over time, they were drawn into the lives of others. Simultaneously, they were drawn more fully into the ways the sickroom configured their "experience" into something that was both orthodox and yet intensely personal. Malady's surprises, the array of therapies, and the social bedside continued to shape everything the physician said and did in a case. To an important extent, as this chapter shows, the physician created continuity from these pressures by keeping a written record of what he witnessed, flexing his experience against disease, the patient, and whoever else was in the sickroom. As the physician did this over the course of treatment, case by case, he wrote not only his confrontation with disease but also his engagement with illness, inscribing with objectifying purpose what was nonetheless a powerful subjectivity. His bedside notes thus may be seen as richer extensions of his brief daybook notations of calls and prescriptions considered in Chapter 4. They also were the raw material—that is, less "public," less consciously autobiographical— for the central orthodox text: the full case narrative looked at in Chapter 8.

In particular, bedside notes combine the schooled impulse to record medical observations with a sense of how the doctor reshaped this impulse in order to perform his everyday work. Here we will look at the notes of three midcentury physicians for what they reveal about the doctor's purposes and self-image, seen especially in the way notes featured the M.D. and excluded others. As a context for looking at these notes, this chapter begins by characterizing the sickroom world in terms of the conflict that often erupted there. Although the views and labors of families and physicians overlapped in many ways, as we have seen, there were sharp tensions as well. A doctor's bedside notes must be read as texts created in the heat of this conflict or its potential, in which he asserted his vision against both disease and the social bedside. One important consequence was that good medicine defined not only a man's skills but also his character as he met malady as a personal challenge.

CO-ATTENDANCE AND CONFLICT

In caregiving over time, as in other aspects of his doctoring, the physician's schooled orthodoxy shaded into the vernacular world. Rather than seeing this process as something that detracted from the advent of "modern" medicine, however, the view here is that practice in rural communities is best understood not as a drag on change in some absolute sense but as a stage on which physicians and patients together explored possible medical futures in the context of their immediate needs.

We have seen how southerners' health talk, their tradition of monitoring the body and self-medication, and their reasons for summoning the physician influenced the way M.D.s delivered their medicine. Although they shared many of the same assumptions and materials, doctors and patients always stood on the edge of conflict, and physicians' writings frequently allude to doctor-patient tensions. Consider how Dr. Levin Smith Joynes, acting as a consultant to his colleague John Parramore, encountered an elderly man named Thomas Taylor in his home one day in Accomack County, Virginia, in 1851. Dr. Parramore thought Taylor was suffering from a bladder disorder, but he brought Joynes along to help him size up the patient's odd mental state. Joynes, for his part, found the old man to be "cheerful, collected, and quite rational." Taylor "talked connectedly & clearly about his symptoms" and, at the same time, made quite clear "his great aversion to medicine—[he] had taken little or none before: denounced the habit of physicking." This was not all Taylor had to say, either. He told the doctors about his family, about his neighbors past and present, and about how the countryside and the parish had changed over the years. "*He talked a great deal*," Joynes wrote.[1]

And Taylor continued to talk on succeeding visits, challenging the doctors, asserting himself. As much as his sickness, Taylor became a force to be reckoned with. The doctors decided that his bladder was indeed paralyzed (of his symptoms, "this pissing part is the worst of it," he told them), but Taylor remained curious and critical throughout. He approved of the sarsaparilla they had given him, but he did not like their proscription on whiskey and informed them that he intended to have his usual daily drink. He told them further that if they were going to bleed him again, to take less blood than before. As a less drastic procedure, Joynes wrote, "I proposed cupping [him] on the back of the neck." Taylor "rather objected at first, preferring that I should take blood from the arm." Everyone talked it over, "and after some argument, [he] consented" to cupping on the neck. After the procedure was finished, however, the old man "turned to John Parramore, & said in a jesting manner, 'now, sir, do you lie down here, and let us put some cups on you.' "[2]

The term "patient" scarcely describes Mr. Taylor or other afflicted people like him, and physicians frequently noted such folks refusing therapies or contesting a course of action. To some extent M.D.s encouraged this willfulness. Given the braided nature of local and orthodox practice, it is not surprising to find many physicians who preferred active, knowledgeable people able to carry out instructions, observe, and report. The hoped-for relationship, in fact, was a kind of active co-attendance with the patient and her family, and yet the physician's desire to be first among equals sparked a good deal of conflict, not least when he felt pressed to compromise his "experience." There were no hard and fast guidelines on how much compromise was too much, as Chapter 5's look at borrowed therapies shows. Indeed, many physicians, like James E. Smith in 1857, pronounced their orthodoxy even as they told how they compromised it. "I certainly would have bled and cupped him," he wrote of a man with acute gastritis, "had it not been for his *positive objections to this practice*." Dr. Andrew Kilpatrick likewise had to work around the fact that his patient was determined to use "only . . . a little medicine" regardless of ailment and "would not allow any setons to be introduced" no matter what.[3]

Matters grew touchier for a physician when he went from eliminating medicines and procedures patients disliked to endorsing ones they did. Dr. Robert Pusey, practicing in Elizabethtown, Kentucky, in the 1870s, certainly was not alone in rationalizing the fact that he gave many patients what they demanded. He bled "the Irish" because *they* thought it preventative, though in his memoirs he was somewhat apologetic about it. For people in certain kinds of pain, Pusey prescribed morphine at the patient's request. Despite his uneasiness over drug addiction, Pusey nonetheless reasoned that the patient may as well "have enough to stop the pain, and people . . . who have been taking morphine, know how much they need." Too, most physicians seem not infrequently to have agreed to patients' desires they thought ridiculous or useless, as long as there was no outright harm. In a bizarre incident, a South Carolina physician early in the century accompanied another doctor to a grave site, exhumed the body (buried two months), cut out the lungs, and burned them—all at the request of the deceased's sister, who, sick with a "complaint of her Breast," was convinced that "the Lungs of the dead fed on those of the living" and that this was the remedy for her case. The physician thought this a "strange whim" and compared it to African voodoo. But he went along with the patient's desires, telling himself that certain strong convictions were "not to be reasoned upon."[4]

So powerful was the urge to acquiesce to patients, to fit in at the bedside, that for some doctors it obtained even with slaves. Physician R. S. Bailey noted in 1856 that slaves treated tonsillitis ("which they call a 'falling down of the almonds of the ears'") by tying up their hair to keep the almonds from falling. Bailey thought this foolish, but, at the bedside, "I have generally acquiesced, not desiring to lesson their confidence in the means employed" or, doubtless, their willingness to cooperate with him. In 1846, Charles Hentz, examining several slaves at their master's request, "would *like to have pulled* a tooth for a negro woman, but she backed out," and he decided not to push the issue, nor did her master. Indeed, another doctor remarked on the frustrating reality that "the master . . . is not unfrequently impressed with the same opinion" as his slaves and therefore could be expected to pressure the doctor to modify *his* treatment in favor of the slave's wishes.[5]

Overall, then, the dynamic of forging co-attendance at the bedside required the physician to assert himself but also to go along, dissemble, and keep quiet. Each visit brought the physician into a new matrix of remedies, assumptions, and humors where he had to placate and praise. Sometimes his frustrations boiled over. Physicians resorted to getting around patients' resistance by tricking them; suddenly pulling a patient's tooth, for example, or thrusting a pill down his throat, after asking to have only a look. They deliberately mystified patients by pronouncing Latin phrases and doling out placebos. Did the treatment fail? It was the patient's fault. People medicate themselves with "Doctors Tom, Dick & Harry's pills and syrups," one Kentucky physician observed angrily in 1847; then, once their physical "system is completely ruined" by years of "folly in tampering with panaceas and nostrums," they call upon the M.D., who is blamed when he is unable to reverse years of self-abuse. What happened to patient Henry Stone and his doctor happened all the time, according to physicians. So sick was Stone with a congestive fever that he had allowed to worsen, when he arrived home one evening he had to be carried into the house. Called much too late, the physician declared in disgust that he "might as well have thrown all the medicine into the yard."[6]

Although growing from such individual instances, conflict often flared up to reveal the fault lines of southern social relations, exposing fissures of gender, class, and race that served, among other things, to raise the emotional stakes in a case. Childbirth was one such highly charged encounter. Birthing, with its fearsome risks for child and mother, insured an intense family scene. The conventional wisdom that women were "naturally" ready for childbirth clashed with equally widespread misgivings about feminine frailty, thus exposing the contradiction involved in praising women by stressing their limits. Moreover, because childbirth often drew more than the usual number of people to the bedside, and because most rural physicians did comparatively little obstetrical work, the physician stood a greater chance of being second-guessed or outguessed in full view of the neighbors. Many doctors, on edge, reacted by criticizing women as a sex. All women were by nature vulnerable and knew it, doctors told themselves and anyone who would listen, and yet they created their own childbirth problems by neglecting what health they possessed. Dr. W. P. Reese, for example, thought that "a perfectly healthy married lady is very rarely met with . . . throughout South Alabama" in the late 1840s because of women's vanity and ignorance about their bodies. The childbed was surrounded by such women. Wilson Yandell, waiting out a neighbor's "tedious labor," was at first annoyed, then angry, when the woman's friends pestered him to gossip about difficult births he had seen. They told a few "dreadful" stories of their own, including one "of an old sweet heart of mine dying" in childbirth. Yandell had to utter "threats of leaving" to prevent them from terrifying their laboring friend with their tales.[7]

Women as mothers came in for blanket criticism as well. Children were a worrisome kind of patient and childhood malady so fierce that, as one doctor put it, children frequently "get up from playing with toys and die." Physicians criticized mothers for going either too far or not far enough. A Louisiana physician in 1866 noted instructing a woman how to protect her child's convalescence, but the "foolish mother took it to the circus and it relapsed." Simon Baruch explained to a child's mother that the blister he prescribed should be left intact to create a reddening effect on the child's skin but should not be allowed to produce pain. "As I might have known," he wrote bitterly, "the mother waited until the patient complained of pain. . . . [The] blister became very intractable and contributed greatly to the fatal issue of the case." In 1851, frustration with mothers got the better of Dr. M. Rouanet, who took the unusual step of publishing a general criticism of women "killing their children" through their ignorance of certain commonsense measures, such as making sure that rooms were well ventilated and that children did not eat too much fresh fruit.[8]

Other groups singled out for condemnation were the white poor and, after the Civil War, freed people. As we have seen, physicians' lack of enthusiasm for charity care, evident in the conflicted way such care was rationalized during schooling, often hardened into outright class and racial hostility. Simon Baruch, after disagreeing with the husband of an impoverished freedwoman over the woman's fatal sickness, pronounced a well-worn "aphorism" of experienced men that fixed blame for the conflict solely in terms of class and race: "Place not too much reliance on the statements of negroes & ignorant people, but trust in preference to your own influences." Although most M.D.s had scruples against giving lesser medicines to the poor, giving less time to them was commonplace. William Holcombe, for example, exhausted after a night's work in 1855 caring for a poor white family, regretted "such sacrifices of time and comfort" and resolved in the future to give each of his "pauper" cases only "a brief visit and prescription." Holcombe's diary reveals him as caring and conscientious with neighbors he respected, but he turned a very different face toward the "ignorant, vacillating, prejudiced" white poor, "surrounded always by vulgar, meddling, pirating neighbors" for whom good medicine was "entirely above their comprehension."[9]

The supposed propensity among slaves to feign sickness went to the center of physicians' hostility and distrust with regard to black patients, and, in key ways, illuminates wider issues of conflict and co-attendance around rural southern bedsides. In particular, with regard to slaves, the issue of feigning stirred up the problematic relation between slavery and race: even after emancipation, white doctors expected that African American patients would mislead them. In a larger sense, feigning raised the issue of how physicians confronted *illness* at the bedside, as opposed to tracking disease, and thus how "experience" was shaped by conflict that extended beyond the exercise of therapeutic authority into the deeper subjectivity of being ill.

On the one hand, many physicians, like masters, viewed slave feigning ("possuming" was the popular term) as a straightforward matter of labor control, as one more form of annoying obfuscation to be expected from a class of people who wished to avoid work and manipulate authority. In this regard, authorities on medical jurisprudence considered feigning among slaves as identical to feigning among prisoners, soldiers, and criminals. On the other hand, among southern physicians, "possuming" by slaves had a racial cast, sometimes spoken of as an African "universal disposition to deception." Thus, feigning raised the vexing issue of whether a slave was doing something deliberate or was merely in the grip of her "racial" propensity. This, in turn, made problematic what a physician actually was seeing when he saw a sick slave. Indeed, many doctors approached slave patients by looking for symptoms that were *not* genuine, noting that slaves feigning seizures (considered a typical dodge), for example, would be unable to duplicate the "rigidity of muscles" and "rapidity of action" characteristic of true convulsions. It was a complicated matter, because some feigning included authentic physiological responses to "various stimulants" and other unknown "African" drugs that feigners employed. In the same vein, slaves used "flour or chalk . . . to whiten the tongue" and a coarse brush to artificially redden the skin so as to appear fever-inflamed. Thus, the physician had to suspect more than simple playacting.[10]

In fact, the more physicians considered it, feigning became a venture into the subjectivity—and potential conflict—surrounding all treatment, which, to some extent, involved imperfect trust and hidden fears. Even at a historical distance, the questions raised by feigning are deeper than mere tactical questions of power. Certainly there were individuals who faked sickness in order to assert themselves against their masters. But at least some "feigning" seems to have been a more complicated matter in which slave patients plumbed the relation between their bondage as a physical fact and the means—physical and otherwise—by which they could manipulate both body and bondage. Degrees of feigning revealed as permeable the line between well-being and illness. An individual might in fact feel ill, for instance, but exaggerate it for what he hoped would be his greater benefit; or he might not feel ill at first but act ill with such intensity as to become so. In some instances, slaves experienced, or devised, elaborate afflictions. A slave in South Carolina, over a period of time, appeared to vomit up pins along with mysterious dark lumps that could not be identified. In the judgment of the physician called in by the master, the slave had not ingested the pins but had learned to hold them somehow in his mouth, and the mysterious lumps consisted of finely knotted thread that he had swallowed for the purpose of regurgitating. If this doctor took into consideration the use of pins and threads in African conjure, he did not say so; but this was perhaps another dimension of whatever the man was doing.[11]

Was this man "truly" ill? There is no clear answer then or now. What is clear is that such instances shed much light on the way slavery made layers of conflict inextricable from caregiving. These layers, in turn, fed back into the daily social relations of slavery, roiling up the trickery, vengeance, and guilt at the heart of the most ordinary personal relationships. Health and illness became one more way to replay slavery's question of who was riding whom, with all of its heady frustrations and subtle rules. Thus one slave owner, typical of many, was disgusted by her maid feigning sickness, she thought, in order to get out of a morning's work. This servant "would *never get sick*," the mistress observed, "if not called upon until after breakfast." Though seething with a sense of being wronged, she decided to postpone the start of the workday until after breakfast. The mistress did much with this small act. She gave her servant what she wanted but, at the same time, reserved for herself the definition of true sickness. She avoided open conflict, but every such concession would be revisited in future struggles.[12]

Such twisted relationships lay beneath each slave or "Negro call" a physician received, leading him to help forge the link between slave illness and whatever else whites considered to be "Negro." The everyday scale of treatment where this link was forged—the unreflective ordinariness of it—made it far stronger than anything suggested by abstract racial theory. Thus a Florida physician wrote a note to himself about a pregnant slave woman who broke a varicose vein and fainted while working in the field that she "possumed afterwards." He noted this not because it had influenced his course of treatment for what he believed was a genuine fainting spell but because it placed this particular case and patient, for future reference, into a larger category of "Negro" behavior. Similarly, for Georgia mistress Gertrude Thomas, slavery shaped her response to her slave Daniel's fainting spell one day. Thomas suspected fakery, and, as Daniel fell to the floor, she reacted stonily: "I sat perfectly still, rather admiring his skill in effecting it so cleverly." Later, though, Thomas was chagrined to discover that "I was wrong. He was really sick as was proven." In subtle and tenacious ways, such judgments opened up the larger reality of illness' subjectivity as a spur for conflict at the bedside. The intimate and irreducible sense each person had of her own discomfort, unease, or apprehension could not be determined by any means of doctoring and so was left open to conflicts bred of suspicion and dependence.[13]

Physicians understood how such conflicts might easily spin outward from the bedside into the community, making the encounter with illness even more problematic. Again, slavery's racial logic of mistrust and subterfuge sheds light on the larger issue of who decides what defines "real" illness and how it is pronounced as such. Consider the many social and racial layers peeled back by a single "medical" word used by Dr. Wilson Yandell, who practiced near Murfreesboro, Tennessee, in the mid-1820s. Indeed, Yandell related the story to his son, a medical student, as an example of how community conflict might grow from the smallest of seeds. This particular uproar, the elder Yandell wrote, arose from "an expression I used in a letter to old capt. John Wade." Wade was the owner of a slave named Frank, whom he had sent to Yandell for treatment of "an irruption on his genetels." The doctor determined that Frank's ailment was not venereal disease but "of an *Erysipelatus* nature." Using this phrase in a letter to Wade, the doctor gave the letter to Frank and sent him home. On his way, Frank stopped to visit his wife, owned by a man named Newman, who demanded to see the letter. When "he came to the word *Erysipelatus* . . . Mr.

Newman exclaimed [']You have the foul disease you dog! Begone! For that is a latin word, & Dr. Yandell would not write latin if that [venereal disease] was not the case! So never shew your face on my place again!' " Frank hastily returned to Yandell's to ask the doctor to explain to Newman (and Frank's master as well) that the slave did not have a venereal disease. Yandell did so; the word "erysipelatus," he told the two masters, "signifies *St. Anthony's* fire . . . not the foul disease."

Frank was cleared, but the confrontation festered. Frank, his wife, and the two slave owners were members of the same Baptist church. Frank brought a charge against Newman under church disciplinary rules "for parting man & wife," and even as Yandell wrote all of this to his son, the Baptists were planning to assemble the following Sunday to hear evidence. The doctor was concerned about Frank's fate because only Baptists could testify and Yandell was a Methodist. If no Baptist knew the proper meaning of "erysipelatus," Yandell worried, "the majority might decide against my poor patient." Moreover, the incident thus pointed to a wider difficulty of such "news" spreading uncontrollably from one bedside into the community. What should have been a simple diagnosis and prescription, a word of closure from the physician, instead ignited a general conflict. Attempting to capture malady in words, like attempting to corner it with drugs, might end up spreading its influence even further. Yet physicians, trained to put what they saw into writing, could scarcely do otherwise. And in what follows, we will see physicians exploring their words for the relation between what they saw at the bedside and the kind of doctors they wished to be.[14]

WRITING ORTHODOXY AT THE BEDSIDE

It is an impressive mark of orthodoxy's reliance on texts that so many rural southern physicians continued to keep bedside notes long after school. Such notes benefited the physician by being a prompt to memory, of course, and they have been valuable to medical historians as a source of information about medicines, procedures, and clinical change. But bedside notes also are valuable for the way they reveal physicians' continuing commitment to medicine as intellectual work, resulting in a powerful continuity in the way they inscribed the social bedside and the troubling relation between disease, their medicine, and the experience of illness. Compared to the standardized and quantified medical charts that replaced them, mid-nineteenth-century notes vary considerably from doctor to doctor; and yet, overall, they occupied a consistent range of observation and writing during the entire period considered here. In their closely focused and personally inflected descriptions of body and events, bedside notes were a major textual means of performing a country orthodoxy esteemed for its courageous—indeed, "modern"—reliance on individual practitioners.

Such bedside notes are not an immediately welcoming text to read. The uncontextualized mass of observations, along with doctors' use of abbreviations and colloquial drug names, make most notes appear to be an unappealing forest of words. But with some persistence, they may be read both as a script for orthodox ideals and as a transcript of country practice. The aim is to read them against the grain of their merely practical purpose in order to glimpse how physicians forged their personal experience from the heat of sickroom events. Bedside notes were crucial in making each new, unruly bedside a doctor's own, and a doctor's vision of medicine real. Thus, even though each of the three physicians considered here kept notes in ways typical of many others, each did so from a particular place on the spectrum of orthodox style. All three employed similar therapeutic choices and a similar sense of visually witnessing a body under the assault of both disease and medicine; all three attempted in some fashion to diagnose and explain observed physical changes. But each man did so in his own signature way. As with other contexts of orthodox practice we have seen, the fact that each man's personal style enlarged rather than transgressed orthodoxy is the key to understanding how orthodoxy retained its powerful continuity on the rural, domestic scene.

The first set of notes that follow belonged to John Knox, a physician practicing in Chester County, South Carolina, who filled two bound volumes with nearly 200 of his cases in the 1840s and early 1850s. Of the three, Knox's notemaking style is the sparest and most uniform across the range of his cases, suggesting that he used his orthodox vision to smooth out the lives of others and, in doing so, muted bedside conflict, as well as patients' suffering. The second physician, Charles A. Hentz, who practiced in the Florida panhandle town of Quincy, left notes on some 150 cases to which he was called during the years between 1858 and 1863. His style of note-making includes many more particular substances and imperiled bodies than Knox's, deepening our sense of how a doctor worked through his notes to fit the potential chaos of the sickroom into a kind of "case time" that was his alone to relate. The final set of notes are those of Courtney A. Clark, who recorded about 50 cases from his practice in Jacksonville, Alabama, during the 1840s. Clark's notes share the basic style of the other two, especially Hentz's, but they also show glimpses of a physician trying to go beyond the transfixing power of a single case in order to understand how disease (and thus his work) transcended individual bedsides and lives.

Three case descriptions from John Knox's casebook:

[April 25, 1852] I visited a negro (Henry) of J. R. C; Hepatitis, & some derangement of the Left Lung. I bled him & put on a blister, & ordered a dose of B[lue] Pill at night &c. April 30th Henry is in a bad state today following Inflammation of the urethra. May 1st He has made no water since morning. I injected the penis with a solution of A. Lead & ordered B. gum and bark tea. I also gave him a dose of Copaiba. Towards evening he made water freely—Ordered Copaiba 3 times a day, to use the injection twice a day, to take salts occasionally & to live on a light diet &c. May 3 Henry is some better. May 6th Henry is better the White discharge stopped.

[October 8, 1852] Mary Dunlap was taken down with fever today. Ordered a dose of Cal[omel] & c. Oct. 9th M. D. seems a little better—Quinine—Oct. 10th M. D. has cold feet & hands this morning followed by fever. I left her Tulley's Powder—evening—M. D. is very sick. I gave her a B. Pill & afterwards Se[i]dlitz Powder—her bowels acted well—at bed time, I gave her a Tulley's Powder. Oct. 11th M. D. is cool—I gave her 5 grs. Quinine. Oct. [no date entered] M. D. has been lingering for some days—her courses has appeared which is irregular. I have ordered Cologogne & charcoal.

[January 20, 1853] I visited two little negroes at A. Dickey's. Typhus fever. Phebe is very much prostrated. Ordered B. Pill at bed time. I gave Dovers Powders. 21st The negroes seem a little better—Dovers Powders &c. 22nd The negroes appear better. I gave them Wrights Pills & ordered Dovers Powders & Brandy. 24th Phebe has been rather worse—high fever & delirium. She had delirium the first day I saw her. I put a blister on the back of her neck. She appears to be doing better. I gave 1 drop of viride & in an hour a Dovers Powders & brandy. 26th Both the negroes seem a little better. Phebe is nervous & has fever. The same treat[ment]. 27th Hannah has had a chill but she seems Pert. Phebe's better. 28th Phebe is very low, but the nerves are quiet—Hannah doing well. 29th Phebe is much the same, Hannah improving. 30th, 31st Better. Feb. 1st the little negroes appear quite relieved.

Days of caregiving pass swiftly in Knox's compact paragraphs. Their practical value aside, they raise interesting questions about how Knox inscribed over time a certain vision of patients and sickness. In particular, his style of detail and language reveals precisely how country orthodoxy was a subjective reality built from a practitioner's characteristic themes and omissions. For instance, Knox's notes are striking for their uniformity and order. The repetition of certain essentials, case after case, evens out the varied circumstances of each call, aligning all of them, so to say, at a certain preferred height and angle. His voice is calm, even remote, combining an immediate diagnosis with an economical account of the course of treatment; no one's case seems more important than anyone else's, no day seems more alarming than the next.[15]

To be sure, Knox marks certain social distinctions among his patients, but just barely—"negro (Henry)" clearly is a slave, as he is denoted as being "of" another person, a peculiar, though typical, usage that inscribed slaves as derivative and thus all the more dependent. It is doubtless indicative, too, of Mary Dunlap's low social standing that she is not given the honorific "Miss" or "Mrs.," which Knox gave most of the women in his notes. Even more striking than the minimal attention given to patients' social standing is the absence of the social bedside in Knox's notes. All of his patients seem alone. Certainly slave patients, who account for nearly one-quarter of his cases, have no social ties worth mentioning. We know the owner of the children Phebe and Hannah in the case above but nothing of their other relations. Even white families, who must have been present in their sickrooms, are barely included within Knox's angle of vision. Over time, case after case, this isolating vision highlighted only the doctor and the sick individual, making others seem superfluous when almost certainly they were not.[16]

In this way, Knox wrote himself as he doubtless hoped others would see him, as a figure of skill and action. This self-image is bolstered by the fact that he says almost nothing about the suffering and pain he must have seen. Neither illness nor his medicine seem to cause much distress for Henry, Mary Dunlap, the youngsters Phebe and Hannah, and most of his other patients, although Knox obviously laid on with a vigorous combination of orthodox and vernacular drugs. Rather, his patients seem uniformly stoic. They "do" better or worse; they are relieved, "low," or "pert." Their bodies exhibit symptoms, they respond to medicines, but they do not suffer. Although we may not expect a doctor to elaborate on suffering in every case, it is important to ask why Knox (like many others) so consistently excluded suffering from nearly all of his bedside notes, and with what consequences. Indeed, his notes suggest that suffering had to be actively omitted from the written significance of a bedside encounter. Perhaps he found that accounts of suffering detracted from his main purpose of recording how he routed disease. The silence may also suggest that suffering, like the patient's social relations, was beyond the doctor's control and so best ignored if possible. In any event, suffering did not merit either recollection or curiosity, and, in fact, too much attention to it undercut what needed to be remembered: the physician's account of his own actions as he pursued disease.[17]

Thus, Knox wrote a spareness and a stillness into his vision of doctoring, making the outcome of each encounter the main focus of his notes. Outcome, not process, is how he oriented himself to his bedside; people appear, submit to his treatment, get results, and disappear. His paragraphs suggest an ideal of quick, intelligible practice and imply that writing about it in terms of outcome was itself a means of establishing it. In this regard, it is important, too, that there are very few bodies seen whole or for very long in Knox's cases. Although he is eager to name the disease in each instance, Knox omits any account of *how* he discovered it hidden in the body. It is doubtful that Knox actually omitted physical diagnosis; he was trained at the Medical College of Georgia, a school in the forefront of new techniques and high allopathic standards. Instead, the absence of closely seen bodies in his notes suggests how a notational style might serve to insulate certain routine aspects of orthodoxy from a physician's own scrutiny. In not detailing his rote methods of physical diagnosis, that is, Knox in effect put these methods beyond re-examination and self-criticism; he did not expect his empirical methods to come up for revision.

This endgame notational style shaped the way Knox wrote about disease, as well as diagnosis. His notes jump over any consideration of disease as a process, and, by doing so, they further inscribe the tension between orthodox ideas and the practice of orthodoxy. As we have seen, physicians' understanding of disease as a protean force saturating the environment was fundamental to orthodoxy. Indeed, the point of empirical observation was to lay bare disease's many trans-formations in order to seize the right time for intervention. However, Knox's outcome-oriented approach to writing a case suggests how, in everyday practice, the notion of protean disease arose as a kind of self-fulfilling reality. That is, because he did not record the transformations of disease, Knox could not review his notes and find much except an essentially undifferentiated flux of sickness. He thus stood little chance of reconsidering disease as anything other than everywhere and protean.

This way of writing orthodoxy by outcome—common to a large number of physicians—also suggests the significance of how the orthodox vision, shaped by the personal style of each doctor, reduced the complexity of the social circumstances surrounding sickness. "Very sick," "relieved," and other simple terms Knox typically used to denote patients' experience are drawn from a way of seeing and intervening in the sickroom that he never bothers to articulate. In thus obscuring what he actually was doing with bodies, pain, and the other people at the bedside, Knox's text reins in curiosity about *illness*, about patients as people whose lives have collapsed into their ailments. Like their bodies, people's voices are largely missing from Knox's accounts, and so, too, is any sense of patients' approbation or resistance to his means, which he records imperatively: "I ordered," "I gave," "I injected." Conflict and co-attendance are not available for scrutiny in this style of note-making; people seem merely compliant and accepting of his care, regardless of age, race, or gender, from the "lingering" Mary Dunlap to the "pert" Hannah. Their feelings and desires were neither relevant nor memorable within the context of what the physician thought he needed to write: that the outcome at each bedside was the result of *his* actions.

Thus, in a strikingly consistent way, Knox fit a wide variety of patients into a narrow textual vision of what ailed people generally. He developed a kind of template for patienthood, as well as a kind of ethical baseline for being a good doctor, doubtless giving him confidence going into a case. Yet this approach also implies a certain inflexibility once he became engaged in giving care. In the rare instances where he mentions conflict with patients, whole new dimensions of his care may be glimpsed, reminding us of what he must have left out of his standard, trim accounts. In cases where we can see patients resisting Knox, even for a moment, it is clear how force lay just beneath the cool surface of his vision. Once, treating a neighbor named Nancy Eldee, Knox admitted that he "had to struggle against prejudice & superstitious notions—from the first. She expected to die, & sometimes refused to take medicine." Although he does not reveal how he got Mrs. Eldee's compliance, Knox *does* tell how he persuaded Bets, a slave woman, when she refused to comply with his plan. Bets became "boisterous" and complained about the painful blisters he had applied. When she became "obstinate and refuse[d] to answer me," Knox erased the boundary between caregiving and coercion: "I spoke roughly to her & threatened to put a blister on her breast" if she did not cooperate. "2 P.M.," his next note reads. "Bets is quiet"; a final note, a few days later: "Bets seems better."[18]

In the largest sense, then, Knox's notes permitted him to imagine himself in control of the sickroom by excluding from his text all sorts of conflict, anxiety, and pain. By not articulating how he actually exercised his authority while laying hands on his patients, Knox could simply embrace whatever authority he possessed as rightly his, as a physician and a white man. This is not to suggest he did so with malign intent, of course, or even consciously. But it is important that he adopted a notational style that gave patients no voice and deflected questions about process. He thus created a text in which key issues across a whole range of doctor-patient relations went unexamined, issues ranging from the value of empirical methods to the morality of patients' demands, their consent, and the ways they were fooled or cajoled or threatened. Nor does this notational style speak to the value of scientific discovery or the way Knox coupled orthodox and vernacular therapy. Instead, it is a text that funneled everything toward the specific outcome of each, isolated case, which is to say, toward himself and the outcome he directed.

Consider Henry's case above with these things in mind. Knox's initial diagnosis was hepatitis and a "derangement of the Left Lung." But these seem forgotten when the momentum of his notes takes hold: Knox depicts himself wading in with his medicine and determining (on what grounds? what did he see?) that the seat of Henry's affliction was his urinary tract. The shift from lung to urinary tract, with hepatitis simply vanishing, raised no issues worth recording. His medicines had exposed the culprit; prodigal disease easily fulfilled his expectations by changing form, and he responded in kind. The only pressing question was who would win, and the implication is that the physician would win only if he had a free hand with bodies and drugs. The story of Mary Dunlap, too, has the elements of a therapeutic tale that Knox and other practitioners recombined many times over: a tale of fever, first surging through the body, then countered by the doctor as his harsher measures took hold, and, then, finally giving way to measures that soothed, especially food, the surest sign that sickness had been tamed. Knox's medicines here, as elsewhere, were stunningly inclusive. Mainstream allopathic drugs abound—calomel, quinine, castor oil, blue pill, and laudanum. He also used the domestic standbys of brandy, charcoal, bark tea, and camphor, as well as substances associated with African American pharmacology: red oak bark, snakeroot, sassafras. Throughout, as he wrote it, the physician was not merely dosing; he uniquely orchestrated everything into a *course* of medicine calculated to transform disease from predator into prey. And so with Mary Dunlap, he begins with the M.D.'s heavy drugs, joining a calomel purge to quinine's controlling effect on fever; diuretics and cooling cathartics follow, summoning the bowels to their healing action. Finally, placating tonics—almost demimedicines—sooth the damaged body, wrapping up the case with the benediction of domestic remedies: "I have ordered Cologogne & charcoal."[19]

The writing of bedside after bedside in this self-affirming style goes well beyond the practical purposes of memory to suggest a deep, personal commitment to one's art. Read through, these are episodes to be admired, savored. What mattered was not what Knox saw of the body or heard from the patient but how he had bested disease. It is not the absence of modern clinical method and measures that is striking in such notes but the manifest satisfaction of transforming someone else's suffering into a personal achievement. This is what kept practitioners like Knox hard at work and feeling worthy. Learning from one's work meant inscribing one's own subjectivity as the center of a routine of evaluations and actions; it meant staking out a landscape of practice as irreducibly personal as illness itself.

CHARLES HENTZ: MAKING CASE-TIME

Charles Hentz's bedside notes bear a family resemblance to Knox's, but in key ways they cut in a markedly different path. Like Knox, Hentz wrote cases of his neighbors and their slaves who suffered from difficult but hardly exotic ailments—the fevers, pneumonia, and dysentery common to the fertile plantation district of panhandle Florida where he practiced. And like Knox, Hentz appears to have recorded certain bedsides not only because he might be in a similar fix in the future but also because of the memorably dramatic way malady tested his abilities and confirmed his performance of orthodox medicine. However, Hentz's notational style does much more than Knox's to evoke caregiving's contingencies and surprises. It is a style of greater contour and detail, capturing the shock of medicine on the body and the rush of physical signs, as well as the moral challenges, that made each bedside its own risky place to be.

It is also a style, no less than Knox's, that translated patients' struggle against malady into the *doctor's* struggle, though in a different way. Hentz's writing is structured not by outcome but by the daily or even hourly shifts in malady's signs and his corresponding response. Even on the surface, Hentz's pages look different from Knox's succession of trim paragraphs. Hentz was a scrawler; a single case sometimes spreads out over more than one page of his large ledger. He amended his entries; many bristle with marginal notes he added when rereading them. His tone is rougher and warmer, and he almost always includes the details of physical examination and the names and dosages of medicines. One result of all this is that Hentz's notes are harder to wade through than Knox's. But the effort is worth it because their transcriptlike quality yields an invaluable sense of the timing of bedside decision-making and crisis. Indeed, Hentz's notes are unified by his struggle to make from the potential chaos of each bedside an ordered "case-time" bearing the mark of his intervention.

Two cases from Hentz's medical notebook, both concerning people sick with pneumonia—one a white woman, the other a slave man—take us into Hentz's case-time and thus further into how bedside notes made orthodox and vernacular medicine inseparable. First, the case of Mrs. Goodson:

[November 16, 1860] Mrs. Jesse W. Goodson—*Pneumonia*—Nov. 16—
Mother of 12 or 15 children—taken suddenly sick on 15th with chill—had
been complaining for some days—cheeks very flushed—breathing very
quick & short, with pain in top of right shoulder—severe pain in *knee*
of same side, & in back—some in side—pain in shoulder aggravated in
breathing—pulse 132—tongue coated, rough & dry—skin moist—pulse
very soft & compressible. Respiratory sounds much muffled on rt. side—
rusty colored sputa. Large Blister over back of right side, & below
mamma—

Calomel 2 gr[ain]s—Ipec. gr. ⅓—every 3 hours—co[nfection] syr[up]
scill[ae]—every 2 hours with boneset tea—with the calomel give T[in-
ctu]r[e] Veratrum every 3 hours, beginning with 6 drops—

[November 17] Verat. had caused vomiting—Boneset also—pulse 120—
Easier—sputa still rusty—skin moist—Bowels just right—

Stop Veratr. & Boneset—continue the rest—have blister about 5 by 9
or 10 [inches] for from upper part of rt. side, to be applied tomorrow
morning—

[November 18] Better—pulse 110—perfectly easy—breathing still fast,
but not near so much so—draws long breath without pain—Sputa clear
and more easy—

[November 20] Worse—"fever rose" night of 18th—Pulse today 132
or more—breathing very fast—cheeks flushed—Bowels right—actions
[i.e., stool] bilious & not too often—no bronchial respiration—breathing
sounds muffled somewhat, but resp. murmur plain—Sputa clear, with
tough dark yellow expect[oration].

Blisters very sore—Distressed—gave 8 grs. quinine at 3 P.M.—and enema of 3 [drachms] Gum Water, with 12 drops tr. Veratr. The same doses
of quinine to be repeated every 2 hours for 2 or 3 times, or till ears buzz—
The veratr. given as above, or by mouth—the calomel & co. syr. scill—
continued—Cheeks lost flush before I left.[20]

For Hentz, it was the intense dialectic of disease and therapy—not the outcome, as for Knox—that made for a memorable bedside. Everything Hentz
wrote pivoted on his sensory engagement with the play of his drugs on the
patient's body. Mrs. Goodson's body was a kind of landscape of shifting appearances and impulses that the medicines and disease together created in a
classic allopathic search for balance. Specifically, during the first two days here,
Hentz laid on with the heavy-gauge drugs, opening up the beleaguered body in

much the same way that a firefighter opens up the roof of a building, "ventilating" it to better expose the nests of fire. His intense visualization of her body is the motif of his authority. Such detailed visualizing created the expectation—for him and doubtless for some of his patients, too—that the very act of inscribing certain signs created the potential for controlling them. Closely seen details implied closely calibrated therapy, and in this way precise notation was not simply an account of bedside work but actually part of carrying it out.

Six days into Mrs. Goodson's struggles, however, on the twenty-first, Hentz seemed no closer to ousting the foe; but then, on the twenty-third, in the midst of the orchestration of drugs, body, and timing, the case suddenly broke and a happy outcome followed:

[November 21] Was (by report of Mr. G.) under the influence of Veratr. last night—pulse was very slow—extremities very cold, sweaty &c.

Pulse 120 today—expectoration was easier—no flush to cheeks—no pain. Bowels too free—very restless & "sick." Gave 30 gtt [gutta, i.e., drops] sol[ution] of mur[iatic] morph[ine] (at 3 p.m.) & left Hydr[argyrus] c[um] creta—gr[ains] iii with ½ gr. calomel & ¼ gr. syr[up] scill[ae] co[nfection]. A large new blister on left side thorax. Tongue cleaner & moister.

[November 22] Pulse 120 & weak today on my arrival (2 o'clock p.m.). Pale—very weak—breathing much slower. Expectoration freer & easier, but more rust colored—bowels not too free—no pain.

Gave at 2 p.m. 5 grs. quinine—(the fever rises at night) with a little coffee and & 3 oz. Brandy—to be repeated every 2 hours till 15 grs. (or 1 s[cruple]) of quinine is taken—

The Brandy is to be used with judgment according to its good effect. The mercurial powders & syr. scill. co. also. A decoct[ion] of cohosh & seneka—a tablespoonful every 2 hours with the mercurial powder. Wine whey & chicken tea, &c, &c.

[November 23] Mrs. Goodson. 9th day—change for the better—she is very weak—free from pain or sickness—pulse 102—soft. Breathing easy and slower. Expectoration easier, but yet a good deal rust-colored. Bowels right—too loose last night—but has had only one action today, & that thicker. Gums very sore. Skin rather too relaxed & cool. Left her on cohosh tea—a tablespoonful every 2 or 3 hours. Brandy occasionally—syr. scill. co. when the expectoration seems to require it—quinine 4 grs. at 2, 5 & 8 o'clock unless it affects her head.

Elixir vitri[ol] if she sweats too much.

[November 24] Seems better—rests well—skin warm & pleasant—expectoration easy & not colored nor glutinous—not much cough—no pain—no flush—bowels right—mouth quite sore—pulse 110.

Left her on decoct. Seneka when cohosh is used up—tablespoonful every 3 or 4 hours—syr. scill. co. if cough requires it—a tea of asclepias root if cough gets tight &c—

Wine whey &c—[21]

The tactile (if not exactly carnal) and troubled body that Hentz here inscribes makes the abstract, screened-off bodies in John Knox's notes seem remote by comparison. Mrs. Goodson is reduced to her body, but her body is not a passive object. It is a topography of surprise, a field for the swift unfolding of malady's shocks and turns, and the doctor's somewhat breathless notes are pushed ahead by a drama that is starkly physical and urgent. All his hopes for entering into and solving this puzzle are caught up in how he writes his way forward into the mystery, day by day, using time to buy time. The patient's pulse sets the diagnostic stage each day; her breathing concerns him nearly as often, as do the temperature and changing "flush" of her skin and her "rusty" sputa. We can infer Hentz's manipulations of her body from his account of her expectorations, her deep breathing, and her blisters and enema.

Despite the orthodox tenet that a patient's environment mattered, Hentz's notational style barely gives a glimpse of it. He briefly remarks on the onset of her sickness, observing that although she was "taken" by malady the day before his intervention, she had been feeling unwell "for some days" prior to this. Although wholly inconclusive, this observation at least opens the door to what else in Mrs. Goodson's life might be relevant to her illness. So does his note that she was the "Mother of 12 or 15 children," which succinctly places her among a group of mature women whose constitutions had been tested before. Finally, there is a hint of co-attendance at the bedside. Mr. Goodson is mentioned, and either he or the patient herself is the voice behind the reports on the twentieth and twenty-first—that Mrs. Goodson's "fever rose" and that she was "sick." In noting these assessments as not his own, it is unclear whether Hentz meant to register skepticism or to mark them as memorable for some other reason, but either way, they are evidence of his dependence on others. So is the way Hentz phrased his therapeutic measures in language that mixed description with imperative. That is, while he mostly records his therapy in a record-keeping past tense, as on the twenty-first ("gave 30 gtt sol[ution] of mur[iatic] morph[ine]"), he sometimes reverts to immediate, present-tense imperatives, as on the seventeenth ("Stop Veratr[um] & Boneset—continue the rest"), which suggest conversation with others. And he sometimes alludes to his reliance on others' skill in recognizing symptoms and following through, as when, on the twenty-second, he prescribes brandy "to be used with judgment according to its good effect" and, on the twenty-third, suggests elixir of vitriol "if she sweats too much." In these small but significant ways, Hentz's notes show precisely how orthodox and vernacular medicine were woven together by the reciprocities of bedside caregiving. They reveal how much "his" bedside did *not* belong to him despite the notes that make him seem in charge.

This said, however, the larger context for Mrs. Goodson's world remains on the fringe of Hentz's writing. The main weight of his style, like Knox's more buffered approach, rests on the drama of the doctor's own measures and insights, and on the belief in the allopathic warfare between disease and medicine. At the crisis, which seems to have come between the twentieth and the twenty-first, it was Mrs. Goodson's troubled body and his own time-bound measures that the doctor most intensely wished to describe. We see him adding new mercurials on the twenty-first, even while continuing the former ones. Here Mrs. Goodson's body was most severely tried, saturated by malady and belabored by the doctor's relentless medicine. She had taken veratrum by enema "or by mouth," was given quinine "till her ears buzz," and, despite her sore blisters (she was "distressed" by them), the doctor ordered "a large new" one.[22]

The following day, the twenty-second, the watched and mastered body at last tacked toward recovery. Mrs. Goodson's breathing became "slower," her expectoration "freer & easier"; there was "no pain." Words of release and recovery. Hentz quickly reconfigured allopathic therapy once again, choosing teas over enemas, and easily stepping further into the domestic realm with prescriptions of brandy, "wine whey" (a milk and wine mixture), and the comfort of chicken tea. The thundering medicines had rolled by, the body had been thrashed and shaken. Now Hentz focused on the body's fluid telltales, stool, saliva, and sweat—signs as much his creation as malady's—and he acted on his patient's body as an object intimately his own, manipulating textures, temperatures, and substances in ways to confirm malady's departure. Not everything looked satisfactory; Mrs. Goodson was coughing yet, and her "too relaxed" skin troubled him. But he began to loosen somewhat his closely calibrated therapies, slipping into more comfortable rule-of-thumb notations ("&c, &c"), and his patient emerged from her sickness and exited from his pages.[23]

Taken together, all of these elements of Hentz's note-making style—the chronicle of drugs, symptoms, and signs, the image of a manipulated, reactive body, the obedient presence of others—impart the importance of close timing in the doctor's artful balance of acting and witnessing. What mattered in Hentz's style of bedside notes was that the doctor was able to recount a time-bound trail of exactly what he saw and did. He thus inscribed good medicine not as an outcome but as a succession of *means* made sensible by their calibration in time. Tracking these, and marking all of the seams and pivots that made for the "breaks" in a case, Hentz wrote orthodoxy not as doctrine but as something contingent and irreducibly personal. To be sure, there are silences in this otherwise forthcoming style. Nothing that Hentz writes reveals the extent to which he allowed his patients to see him mystified or improvising, for instance. Nor does he give any sense of how he specifically framed his authority in making a co-attendance with them. He does not give a clear sense of his clinical reasoning, either: *why* he chose to do one thing over another remains implicit. Nevertheless, his notes illuminate one central feat of a man of experience: he took malady's chaos and the memory of a healthy body's quiet, unremarked time and wrote them into a personal, therapeutic sense of time, case-time.

Although this style is consistent across his cases, the case of another patient with pneumonia, coming only four months after Mrs. Goodson, sheds further light on conflict, note-making, and the social bedside. Because this second patient at one point resisted Hentz's medicine, we can see more clearly how conflict and co-attendance were not opposite poles so much as a spectrum of shifting relationships. Because this patient nearly died, Hentz revealed how he let go his therapy—and then, suddenly, how he embraced success. And because this patient, Jim, was a slave, this case suggests why physicians in the throes of bedside work viewed "race" as more a social than biological condition.

From Hentz's medical diary, 1861, about four months after Mrs. Goodson's case:

[March 31] Pneumonia—Negro Jim—belonging to Misses Cash—sick since 28th—Left lung inflamed—pretty generally—crepitation more audible than bronchial respiration—rusty colored sputa—pulse 96—tongue heavily coated with dirty white fur, papillae sticking through. Bowels not at all irritated. Likely boy—18 or 20 years old—coughs pretty hard—; expectorates tolerably. Cupped freely on side—followed by large Blister.

Calomel 1½ gr[ains] with 3 [drachms] syrup scill[ae] co[nfection] every 3 hours. The syr. scill. to be given ½ way between times also.

Veratrum with the calomel—begin with 5 gtt [gutta, i.e., drops].

[April 1] The Veratr. brot. pulse down to 56 by close of Apr. 1st—but caused vomiting & great nervous disturbance—dose of 7 gtt produced the effect—

[April 2] Had to discontinue the Veratr. on the 2nd. Continue the other remedies.

[April 3] On the 3rd seemed doing better—gave him teaspoonful doses of oil—moved bowels greatly—dejections [i.e., stool] black—relieved by their passage.[24]

Here, in typical fashion, Hentz's vision takes in Jim's body. The doctor then imagines how his medicines seize it, in ways much like his treatment of Mrs. Goodson; there is the same calomel, squill syrup, and veratrum viride, with the latter once again disappointing him. Jim's initial dosages were a bit lighter—½ grain less of calomel and a drop less of the veratrum tincture. Moreover, in addition to blistering Jim (as he did Mrs. Goodson), Hentz cupped him "on the side" as well, probably reflecting what seems to be the doctor's greater concern from the outset with Jim's lung sounds ("crepitation" refers to a dry, softly crackling sound Hentz hears). Essentially, though, Hentz's pneumonia therapy for a youthful black man appears to recapitulate that for a middle-aged white woman.[25]

As important as this similarity is, however, the context of race doubtless was not absent from Hentz's calculations, and his measures suggest how M.D.s' everyday bedside work tentatively implicated theoretical notions of "race." It is possible, for instance, that Hentz's initial interest in Jim's lungs derived in part from the axiomatic view that African Americans had weak lungs. It is possible, too, that the somewhat smaller dosages of certain drugs may reflect the allopathic sense that blacks tolerated medicines less well than whites. But we cannot know for certain, and the role of racial theory remains a vexed issue. It seems clear that "race," in an expansive, theoretical sense, imparted little or no help to Hentz in his notation of timing drugs and watching the body. At the same time, bedside notes helped preserve racial theory for precisely this reason. Because "race" in the largest sense fell outside the pressures of case-time, nothing a physician did called racial theory into question. Thus, whatever notions of "African" or "white" Hentz had in his head when he visited Jim—and most likely they were the standard racist notions of most white doctors—nothing of their inchoate power would be exposed or revised by the bedside actions recorded in notes.

Much more telling, in terms of the relationship between Hentz and Jim, are the quiet but sharp ways Hentz marks Jim's social status as a slave. In this sense, as we saw earlier, to note "Negro" before a man's name, with no other qualifiers, was as much a way of denoting a slave as it was a way of describing a person of African descent. Hentz underscored this in his notes by commenting that Jim was a "likely boy." "Boy," of course, was the typical white usage diminishing adult male slaves. And "likely," a marketplace word that also carried a sense of "good" character, summed up a slave's overall health and promise (not unlike Mrs. Goodson's "12 or 15" children summed up hers)—a crisp assessment of Jim's value as a *slave* if he could be made well again. Thus, while Jim's race, seen in terms of physiology, called at most for small alterations in Hentz's basic pneumonia therapy, Jim's status as a slave framed the larger, more dynamic social context of treatment.[26]

This mingling of race and servitude must be kept in mind as we watch Hentz become fiercely engaged with this case when, on April 4, Jim's pneumonia turned into something very different from Mrs. Goodson's. Although Hentz had succeeded in engaging the disease with his drugs during four days of treatment, Jim's affliction burst this bond and broke away from the doctor's understanding and control. The way Hentz tells this story underscores how physicians strove to control malady by making case-time from chaos, by knowing when to act and when to witness. Caregiving, that is, was importantly a struggle for the control of time, and timing was inscribed at the heart of a physician's case notes.

The disturbing new element on April 4 was Jim's delirium, which, among other things, led Hentz to do what he (and other allopaths) rarely did—give in to a patient's desire for favorite foods in the midst of a course of heroic drugs:

[April 4] On the 4th pulse 80—soft—tongue creamy, bad—papillae prominent—Expectoration looks creamy, curdy, unctuous—sweat sticky—dejections very dark, gelatinous—thick—nervous system much excited—wild—delirious—quiet at times—

Put him on use of Grave's Tartar Emetic & laudanum mixt.—use flaxseed tea alone—syr. scillae co. & calomel continued—Blister to back of neck—3 × 6 [inches]—at night but little better—pulse 95—weak—Bronchial resper. very distinct—loud—over upper part of left lung—

Gave hydr[argyrus] c[um] creta 4 or 5 grs.—with 3 or 4 of calomel every 2 hours thro' night—; mixed in just enough Hive syrup to mix them—use Flaxseed tea—Drop everything else—Give Brandy if he gets crazy again—Give him Broiled young chicken & Buttermilk & water (the latter with caution—he craves it.)

[April 6] Continue the same directions for the day—at night crepitation plainly returning in left lung—pulse 88—skin moist—tongue better—some very dark gelatinous dejections—sputa white & frothy—give doses at 4 hours apart during night—

[April 7] [Hentz wrote "not so well" but crossed it out; he also wrote and partially erased "pulse quicker."] Gave 3 [drachms] oil every 5 or 6 hours till the bowels moved off very black, very thick gelatinous stools. The lung gradually improved & resp. murmur became completely [illegible]—But he got worse—these strange stools kept coming—became fetid (were odorless for long while)—pulse got faster & weaker—spells of craziness & excitement came on—his tongue became exceedingly coated—a white universal coat—[illegible] where large papillae lay under it—a curdy abundant coat. Unnatural excitement of expression, & quickness of movement when turning about in bed—

[April 8] On the 8th I prescr. wine whey—(tried Brandy but it excited him very much)—gave 20 [drops] of sp[irits] turpentine in emuls[ion]—every 3 or 4 hours—[27]

At this point, Hentz's rapid-fire, breathless notes suggest a practitioner fully engaged yet terribly puzzled at his patient's mental state, which distorted any attempt to record and interpret the usual physical signs. Underlying all of the troubling particulars was the shifting balance of conflict and co-attendance with Jim. Indeed, the case shows exactly how one was the twin of the other, in this case tilting toward open conflict because of Jim's "craziness & excitement." The crisis came during the following two days, with a shift toward recovery on the third:

[April 9] On the 9th I gave up the case as hopeless—he was very sick—breathing with gasps & laboriously—pulse 120 & weak—cold ½ way to the elbow—very much excited when I talked to him—talked about dying—got quite delirious—Left him to wine whey and Brandy—

[April 10] On the 10th he became about noon very wild & excited—it took several men to hold him—for nearly ½ an hour he struggled violently with those who held him—after this was over he spit up several mouthfuls of pure blood—and became quiet—has been quiet ever since—

[April 11] Says he is better—pulse 120—full & bounding—tongue very thickly coated on back part—very strangely so & rough—he coughs up very bloody sputa—not rust colored, but glutinous & bloody—Left lung perfectly clear—resp. murmur perfect. Has pain in lower lobe of right lung—resp. sounds very obscure & dull there—hear a sort of bubbling sound that I don't understand—Dejection passed yesterday looks better—not so black—Left him to nourishment & Brandy—left some croton oil to rub on right side, & sat[urated] sol[ution] chlor[ide] Postass. to wash his mouth with—[28]

During these three days, Jim's struggle became one against his caregivers, as well as his disease. Such conflict was alarming in any case, but it was additionally significant here because Jim was a slave resisting "those who held him." In the doctor's account, nonetheless, Jim's extremity seems to ride above his servitude, his needs and terrors for the moment the equal of any sick person's. Hentz's own mounting anxiety is clear, and under the circumstances, his note on the ninth, "left him to wine whey and Brandy," takes on an entirely different sense than it did in Mrs. Goodson's case. For her to be "left to" these medicines was the sign of her immanent recovery; for Jim, it has the character of a last rite, a closing benediction on a day where, Hentz says bluntly, "I gave up the case as hopeless."

And yet the doctor would be surprised; Jim pulled through. The crucial change occurred on the tenth; Jim "became quiet," a welcome but mysterious change for the better. Indeed, overall, Hentz's notes capture the fine line at the bedside between "expectancy" and sheer mystification in the face of illness. For the first few days, Hentz proceeded at full therapeutic gallop. But by the seventh, drugs and observation notwithstanding, Jim had crossed over into mystery, with his "strange" stools and "unnatural" excitement. Everything seemed beyond the doctor's experience, even Jim's odd "quickness of movement when turning about in bed." In the very act of writing up the entry for the seventh, in fact, Hentz appears critically unsure of his own judgment, deleting an opening assessment ("not so well"), which seems apt enough, and later, despite seeing some symptoms improve, having to conclude that "he got worse" nonetheless. When Hentz backed away from his aggressive therapy on the seventh, then, in what would have been seen as an appropriately "expectant" move by supporters of such practice (and as simple exhaustion by its opponents) his decision may be seen as arising from both of these—from nothing more or less than the unfolding drama of Jim's illness.[29]

The contingent nature of a healer's "experience," shaped by how a patient's illness swept aside measures aimed at disease, may also be behind the fact that Hentz claims no victory in Jim's case; nor did he note any new insight into pneumonia or the drugs he used. If he had any desire to advance science, it found no articulation in his bedside notes. Indeed, Hentz rings down the curtain on Jim's sickbed with the *patient's* view of things: "[he] says he is better." Hentz's notes thus imply that the most a doctor could do was welcome a happy outcome and leave the greater mystery alone, writing notes that served as the signature of *his* experience of being locked into the case-time of a single case. In this way, although case notes allowed the M.D. to give order to his bedside work (and cast him as a "modern," individualistic hero in the Romantic vein), their organization and language made it impossible to reconstruct certain other aspects of caregiving: why he abandoned one course of action for another, for instance, or why the views of the sick person should count for something or not. In his notes, each bedside encounter remained essentially a solo one, standing alone and strangely new.[30]

COURTNEY CLARK: LOOKING FOR CONNECTIONS

With these issues in mind, consider the cases of Courtney A. Clark, of Jacksonville, Alabama. More like Hentz than Knox, Clark created notes in the 1840s that captured each body in distress day by day, building a logic of case-time against unruly malady. He carefully logged the measures he took to ensnare disease, and, in doing so, again like Hentz, he wrote sometimes as an actor and sometimes as a witness, alternately directing events and standing amazed. In two main ways, though, Clark's style of writing cases extends our sense of how a doctor wrote his subjectivity into the very grain of orthodoxy. First, Clark was a physician who, more than most, made a place in his notes for the views and even the voices of patients. Although the latitude he allowed to patient voices varied from case to case, his style suggests with striking immediacy how the personal dynamics of conflict and co-attendance might dominate the physician's bedside labors and, in fact, the very definition of case-time. Second, and even more unusual, Clark's notes reveal how he tentatively revisited his interesting cases, looking for links among them. He attempted—haltingly—to see how several different cases of a given disease might yield some clue that would lead to a general understanding and treatment, thus using his notes to get past the intellectual approach to the bedside, which, as we have seen with both Knox and Hentz, typically walled off one case from another.[31]

One difficult patient whose views, as well as body, appear in Clark's notes was a Mrs. White, whose 1849 case Clark wrote under the title "*Typhoid Fever.*" Mrs. White was afflicted in late November, and in an entry for the twenty-third of that month, Clark noted:

Visited her in the night for first time. Very much excited when I entered. Commenced perspiring freely: talked incessantly in an excited manner as if partially delirious. Said she did not think there was much the matter and had desired me to visit her in the night so that the neighbours might not know of it. Pulse small, quick, 115, skin cool & covered with perspiration with feverish odour. Very slight increase in the pulsation of the temporals. Tongue furred all over the top except about a [line?] at each edge, moist, natural colour. Had three evacuations today from some Cooks pills, first one thick, the other two thinner.

Rx: aqua camph[or] [one ounce]; tinct. opii [dose illegible] every hour until she sleeps.[32]

"She said she did not think there was much the matter" is an observation that many physicians doubtless heard but relatively few acknowledged in writing. Of course, Clark's observation that Mrs. White was "partially delirious" called her judgment into question. But this does not detract from the significance of his making a place for her views, including the intriguing fact that she did not want her neighbors to see him calling. Giving his patient a voice at the outset, Clark in effect wrote a certain kind of "expectancy" that held open the chance that what the patient said might be useful at a later time. His initial drug therapy was mild and watchful, too; the camphorated water and opium tincture seem intended not to attack the typhoid, as he would have done by blazing away with purges, but rather to more obliquely "open" her body and thus to quiet her emotional restlessness as well.

During the next few days, Mrs. White's body *and* her opposition to Clark's care together shaped the physician's text. His notes thus permitted him to enter some way into her illness, as well as search for her disease.

[November 25] Pills operative twice this morning. Stools yellow natural & healthy. Was slightly delirious last night; slept but little. Arose early this morning, ordered something to eat, put on her clothes and thought she should be well without further trouble. After being up two hours lay down again, and about one became greatly alarmed, thinking she was going to die. Complains of ringing in her ears and roaring in her head: feels queer, talkative, eccentric and partially delirious. Skin moist, no heat of skin. Pulse 118, small, quick. Tongue more fur, dry on top. Mouth clammy, feels dry, frequently wants a little water to wet it. Abdomen somewhat tympanitic in the region of the transverse and descending colon. No Gurgling. Considerable hacking cough. (Blister nape of the neck; acidulated gum water per hour; ½ gr. Morphea at Bed time—foot bath.)[33]

Clark visited her twice a day for the next two days, seeing and doing much the same kind of thing. He wove Mrs. White's routine, sensations, and expressions, into the standard orthodox depiction of pulse, skin, and bowel sounds. His notes show him struggling as much to know his patient's mental state as her physical one. How and why did her emotions matter? Clark was indecisive but fascinated. In one sense, her talkativeness was a symptom of her sickness, or at least something that interfered with his treatment. "Very loquacious," Clark wrote on the twenty-sixth. "Talks so much and so fast I could scarcely get to ask her questions." At other moments, although "near delirium," the patient seemed to come close to making sense. Overall, to his frustration, she "is conscious that her mind wanders and her ideas [are] confused" while the next minute she "says there is nothing the matter with her." Clark was enough of an allopath to want to forge ahead with his medicines and turn the case around. Yet he was not able to dismiss her version of things, leaving open the possibility that he might use her illness to unlock the secret of her disease.[34]

Thus Clark wrote the crisis, when it came, not simply as disease having its way but as a story of his relationship to Mrs. White; therapy was inescapably a matter of conflict and co-attendance. Although Mrs. White's physical symptoms had worsened by November 29, Clark's account was more concerned with a rupture in their relationship:

[November 29] Awake all night; more delirious than on any previous night; talked incessantly; wanted to get up in the latter part of the night and put on her clothes; insisted that there was nothing the matter with her, and that it was wrong for her to be abed; sometimes threatened her attendants when they would not permit her to get up & sometimes begged them; said I was doing wrong to keep her in bed, and she would tell me so when I came. When I called [she was] sitting up in bed. Insists on getting up; that there is nothing the matter; is very indignant at having "her privileges taken away"; declares she will submit to it no longer; has fallen out with me and abuses me for mistreating her & taking away her privileges; declares she will not take any more medicine from me, or follow my directions; consented at last to remain in the bed a few days longer. Pulse 138, small, quick; face & forehead & arms bedewed with cold, clammy perspiration. Passes urine incontinently. Tongue not altered; other symptoms as on yesterday. The medicines and Glysters [i.e., enemas] have not operated. (Take 2 tablespoonfuls oil & repeat in 3 hours; blister to the legs.) Oil produced two copious operations, the first thick, the other thin; feet became cold; mustard poultices applied; sat up in the bed most of the day; pulse rapid & small; face bathed in perspiration; talks incessantly when anyone is in the room, and to herself when alone.[35]

For Mrs. White, it seems clear, not painful procedures or harsh medicines but her own autonomy was most at issue. Her challenge to Clark was couched in moral, not physiological, terms: it was "wrong" for her to be required to submit. In a sense, Clark responded in kind; he did not portray her resistance as merely something to be quelled. Rather, he recorded the struggle of wills, obtaining her consent "at last."

Even with her consent, however, as Clark continued to give Mrs. White a voice, his overall assessment of her words remained ambiguous. Clark thus arrived at the difficult point of acknowledging that the subjectivity of illness was the key to everything. Then, as so often happened, the patient's physical symptoms unexpectedly began to resolve. Two days after the November 29 crisis she began to sleep comfortably, her pulse quieted and slowed, her blisters "drew well." Clark *did* know what to make of these welcome physical signs, and, if this were all, he might have written the end of the case with an easy mind. But he continued to engage with his patient, and Mrs. White's volatile emotions continued to baffle him; one minute she was "crack[ing] jokes" and moving about normally and the next "still talk[ing] foolishly" in a manner Clark dubbed "quiet mania." And if this oxymoron were not troubling enough, Clark concluded his notes with a further anomaly. He thought that Mrs. White's "mental alienation," or whatever it was, should have impaired her memory of the days of sickness just passed. But, to the contrary, he was amazed to find that "she recollects almost everything that transpired during her illness," including her opposition to him.[36]

Clark's inclusion of his patient's views did not, of course, make his notes on her case any less *his* story in the end. Indeed, his story reveals personal moral and intellectual depths in his practice far beyond those revealed by the more typical accounts of bodies manipulated, drugs applied, and outcomes sealed. Though at first Clark seemed bluntly controlling, interpreting his patient's desire for autonomy as part of her illness, his doctoring involved more than this. Neither accepting nor dismissing her views, Clark wove her words into his and himself into her illness. Thus we may glimpse precisely how a country orthodoxy compensated for the fact that schooled, mainstream orthodoxy provided few means for resolving the practitioner's own disquiet in a difficult case. Although bedside notes included elements that can be seen as "objective," Clark's show how such observations ultimately fed a greater need, the need for the healer, tied to the self-reflective locus of his work, to bear witness to the subjective power of illness.

Schooled orthodoxy's shortcomings also were the context for a second impulse in Courtney Clark's note-making. This was his effort—exceptional in everyday practice, though explored in published articles by a few physicians—to grasp important medical links between his cases. That is, Clark periodically struggled within the context of his bedside notes to escape the confines of the solo case that so powerfully fascinated most physicians and shaped, as it did for Knox and Hentz, the boundaries of their vision. Even while a case was current, Clark occasionally strove to make generalizations, arrive at constants, and ponder over anomalies raised by a *collection* of similar cases. He thus attempted to integrate into his bedside work something of orthodoxy's schooled impulse to link observation to type and then move on to prognosis. And yet here, too, Clark's writing was shaped by the mis-fit between broad science and the compelling personal domain of daily work. Following Clark's rough thoughts, it is possible to take another sounding of how a practitioner's "experience" gave rise to a country orthodox style that necessarily, though uneasily, joined performance and precept. We can see him, that is, thinking an orthodox ideal into existence in the course of his everyday work.

One link among his cases that Clark struggled to establish had to do with fever's ability to travel through the countryside. How to explain fever's portability was an urgent puzzle. Most physicians until the very end of the century believed that most fevers were not contagious—not spread person to person—but arose instead from the ripening of some complex mixture of environmental conditions and personal susceptibility. Anticontagionists pointed out that, because so many people "exposed" to fever did *not* get it, contagion was a weak explanation for fever's spread. M.D.s were challenged in this view, however, by widespread popular belief to the contrary, and so the problem of fever's transmission remained a pressing one for physicians, not the least because they would have to decide whether to support or argue against families' efforts to minimize person-to-person contact.

Courtney Clark's tentative bedside speculations along these lines reveal the significance not only of how neighborhood rounds gave a physician a broader view of disease than most people's but also of how the notational style of isolating each case from others posed a conceptual limit to understanding something like contagion. As we have seen, a doctor usually considered his work finished when a patient could be "left to" some palliative means. Clark's notes, however, may be seen as a halting effort to question this practice as the proper end of things, moving instead toward a kind of ground-level epidemiology. This was at work in the care he gave to a fever-struck family named Jennings in 1844. Clark was called upon by Mr. Jennings in August for what the doctor diagnosed as typhoid fever. Jennings's household included his wife, three young sons, and two slaves—a "negro woman" and a "mulatto girl"—all of whom exhibited symptoms of fever at different levels of "danger," as Clark observed on his first visit. He recorded his bedside activities in his usual detailed way. After several days' urgent treatment, Mr. Jennings, his sons, and the two slave women pulled through; Mrs. Jennings did not.

However, instead of tying off his bedside notes when treatment stopped, Clark was moved to speculate further, breaking through the boundary of the solo case. He turned his attention to the Jennings household as a whole, pondering their self-help efforts, not simply as a help or hindrance to him, but as possibly signifying something about the nature of disease itself. Reviewing his notes, Clark realized that the fever had dogged the household for longer than he had initially thought and under circumstances far more complex. The first member of the household to be stricken, he realized, was the fourteen-year-old slave girl who he now believed had sickened more than two weeks before he was called to treat the whole household. Then, "as soon as this patient was well enough to be moved," Clark noted, "Mr. Jennings removed his whole family eight miles into another neighborhood" on the assumption that he could thereby elude a "local" fever. On reflection, Clark thought Jennings had acted wisely (and in accord with orthodox standards) by moving his still-healthy family to "an elevated and airy situation at some distance from anything like marshy land," where fever was thought to lurk. And yet, horribly, the fever confounded Jennings's maneuvers; his youngest son, seven years of age, was attacked in their new location, and, from this point on, the entire household fell into the fever's grip.[37]

Running the case back through his mind, Clark first of all questioned his own therapy but concluded that it had been properly expectant: "symptoms were treated as they arose and no attempt was made to cut short the fever" by massive heroic means. But he was troubled by the fact that Jennings's relocation failed to evade the fever, something that clearly suggested some other locus for infection, perhaps contagion. Intrigued, Clark groped his way toward challenging the orthodox view—his view—that fever was environmental. The Jennings case became part of his episodic but long-term reconsideration of typhoid fever in his notes, including the case of the strangely sane/delirious Mrs. White. Struggling intellectually against the grain of seeing each solo account as its own world, Clark reviewed the household relationships in several of his cases and then revisited the Jennings's move to the "airy" abode to seize upon a new aspect: they had taken up residence with another family there—a family that did not sicken despite the fact that the house was "a very small one having but one room and both families lived together until Jennings' wife died, a period of 21 or 22 days." Reasoning this way made contagion seem *less* likely as an explanation, as most M.D.s preferred to believe. Indeed, Clark noted with some satisfaction that even though "many of the neighbors visited and nursed the sick family, not a single individual either of the visitors or the other family had any symptoms of the disease."[38]

With this self-affirming observation, Clark's struggle to generalize about typhoid fades away. Seen from the heights of the history of pathology, of course, his ruminations do not amount to much. Indeed, if his diagnosis was correct, he was heading in a wrong direction; typhoid may quite easily be transmitted from person to person. But seen as ground-level texts of practice, Clark's notes reveal much about case notes and intellectual process in country orthodoxy, in particular why pulling general truths from the parade of cases was difficult conceptual work. In one sense, the individual people and places at the heart of a doctor's notes—their homes and personalities—lent a powerful continuity to the dominant way of thinking about cases one by one. Again and again, despite his efforts to generalize, Clark based his medical reasoning squarely on the familiarity of known people—on "the case of Nancy Nabors" and those of "Richard Weever, Mrs. Vandiver, Miss Fanny Green, Leonidas Grant." Though inspiring him to seek the wider view, Clark's collected notes also pulled him back to locality, neighbors, and what he still called "our Typhoid Fever." And yet, at the same time, his writing suggests how note-making might reveal a counterpoint to the dominant, local way of thinking. Episodic though they were, Clark's ruminations sparked a kind of proto-epidemiology that went beyond personality. When he jotted down who else was at the bedside with him, it was not just to keep a list of witnesses or whom to thank. It also was because they might be implicated in fever's spread. And so for brief stretches in his notes, Clark transformed his neighbors into something more abstract: carriers of affliction, vectors of disease.[39]

It is striking and even poignant to see physicians like Knox, Hentz, and Clark laboring away over their notes in the homes of their neighbors. In a sense, their notes were the most markedly orthodox aspect of their daily routine, and, in a way, the most "modern," in the sense of twentieth-century medical values. The very conviction that written observations gave a man valuable insights into his doctoring—and, perhaps, a purchase on new knowledge—embodied the physician's faith in the conceptual superiority and ultimate effectiveness of his medicine, even when a case dragged on. And yet, like all texts, bedside notes extended beyond any single set of intentions, gathering up contradictions. Most important, as all three physicians here reveal, notes did not simply record schooled habits but reified the practitioner's subjective grasp on his work, especially his need to control the body and the social bedside. They reveal his uneasy sense that he, too, was a kind of domestic healer after all, and that his everyday work was immersed in the suppositions, remedies, and desires of both his patients and wily disease. And so, even as the physician was compelled to acknowledge orthodoxy as rooted in his community, he strove nevertheless to write himself at the center of events. To that extent, he effaced the lives of others, drawing his vision downward into the troubled body, focusing it on the familiarity of his own therapies, and inscribing a control over events he never quite possessed.

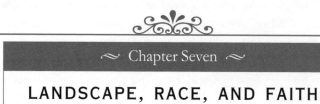

~ Chapter Seven ~

LANDSCAPE, RACE, AND FAITH

Because so much of what physicians wrote about concerned the drama of individual sickrooms and the complexity of other people's bodies and lives, it is striking to see M.D.s stepping back from the bedside to speak as critics and advisers with an overview. Yet many ordinary physicians did just that, projecting their experience onto the larger backdrop of society and nature. For many doctors, it seems, speaking broadly about health provided some intellectual and emotional respite from the sickroom's demands. Moreover, a wide-angled view followed logically from their conviction that individual practice encapsulated science in the most direct, inclusive sense. These physicians felt obligated to represent themselves as belonging to their southern place, to speak out for its physical and moral soundness, actual or desired. Writing as social observers but also (they hoped) as trusted advisers, physicians thus imagined a powerful but troubled extension of their country orthodoxy into far-reaching realms of southerners' well-being.

In one sense, by writing broadly, physicians experimented with what would become the modern voice of professional authority. And yet the means—the texts—available to them to speak in this all-encompassing fashion did at least as much to bolster the individual, parochial texture of traditional rural practice. In fact, as we will see, much of the appeal of becoming public spokesmen for shared values was the sense of belonging it conveyed. Physicians could think of themselves as preserving social continuity, as well as the continuity of their individual patients' lives in the face of malady's threatened chaos.

This chapter considers three contexts for physicians writing their medicine large. In the first, the physician acted as a social ethnographer and critic by writing one of the canonical texts of orthodox medicine, an essay form called the "medical topography." Here he viewed a community (usually his own) as a complex social and natural environment for health and sickness. He criticized shortcomings and advocated improvements. In the second, physicians struggled with the social significance of race and slavery. Here, too, physicians aimed to be broadly "topographic," taking what they had observed about race—what made for a "Negro case," how black patients compared to white, how black disease might differ—and giving it a stable, interpretive shape within the structure of slavery. Finally, many practitioners reflected on the unpredictability and contingency of their work by giving it a transcendent meaning in terms of Christian faith. For most religious physicians in the South, this meant an evangelical Protestantism, a faith premised on lifting individuals out of the prison-house of body and time but not out of their devotion to neighbors, work, and locale. Remaining largely constant in form during the mid-nineteenth century, each of these three contexts preserved abiding expectations and beliefs central to the practice of everyday medicine, even as orthodoxy stood on the edge of change in other ways.

LANDSCAPES OF KNOWLEDGE

Physicians could not have hit upon a better term than "topography" for the texts in which they undertook to describe the natural, social, and medical worlds that supported, stymied, or in any case surrounded their daily work. Essays with titles like "On the Topography, Climate, and Diseases of Washington, Texas" and "On the Medical Topography of Bowling Green and its Vicinity" aimed to characterize a southern place in terms of its achieved healthiness and its potential for improving it. Although sickrooms are not absent from topographies, their significance is shrunken; they are merely thresholds on an intellectually higher ground. Most topographers began with a sketch of the literal, geographical topography of a place or community, an overview of its population, and often a sketch of its history. These descriptions shaded into the author's interpretation of how local habits either furthered or impaired general health. In all, the hundreds of medical topographies produced in this era, on both sides of the Civil War, are an immense reservoir of the intellectual energy local practitioners found in their work. In stepping away from the everyday parade of cases, topographers reconfigured the particulars of their work into an image of themselves as the Good Doctor: a socially conscious man whose clear-eyed advice was matched by his loyalty to the southern place he loved.[1]

Most topographers came to their task with a kind of almanacker's energy, mixing the inquires of scientist, journalist, and folklorist. The topographer himself inevitably was topographed along with everything else, and the personal style of these texts reveal as much about the subjectivity of their physician authors as they do the landscapes they looked upon. Not just the neighborhood's demography and mortality but its flora and fauna, annual rainfall, diet, medicinal plants, game birds, livestock, farming practices, and commercial interests came under review—along with attention to local fevers and the spectrum of healers. Topographers found inspiration in the local and discovered science along the road. For instance, H. V. Wooten wrote his 1850 topography of Lowndesboro, Alabama, after it struck him that in choosing the route for his rounds, a route shaped like "an irregular cone," he had unconsciously traced a larger geographic reality of his region that naturally "divided into three sections—the Flats, the Prairies, and the Ridge," each with its own risks and remedies for disease. He encouraged his readers to look for correspondences between their own rounds and geography. C. E. Lavender offered a similar discovery about his rounds near Selma, Alabama, in 1849, which turned out to be nothing less than "a perfect laboratory of miasm" affording fresh study each day as he rode past undrained swamps and huge thickets of brush and trees uprooted by planters. Such practical science was the apotheosis of solo practice. There was no greater rebuke of orthodoxy's critics, and no better demonstration of the essential intellectual democracy of all orthodox M.D.s, as Robert Little wrote in 1842, than to show through topographies how the "greatness" of medical men was "not in the glare of their theories . . . or in the hardihood of their assumptions, but in their profound and judicious observation."[2]

Everything topographers saw was framed by the weather, water, elevations, and air of the South. Risk and disease were introduced—and held at bay for a moment—by a naturalist's inclusive vision, one that included a sense of beauty. In Virginia, for instance, the Shenandoah River is "a bold, dashing stream that comes thundering along over its rugged bed with such a fearful rapidity as to make the surrounding hills vocal with its pastoral music." In another writer's view, the sand hills of South Carolina, seductive in their beauty, were a mixed paradise: "the rank and luxuriant vegetation is full of flowers of the richest kind, making the hot air heavy with a perfume as stifling as the incense of a sacrifice, yet is loaded, even in daylight, with noxious exhalations, and myriads of flies and mosquitoes." Rounding through the countryside opened such visions to the practitioner with a topographer's eye, with science shading into lyricism and a booster's happy prose. As one physician wrote of South Carolina in 1851, "there are few spots on earth where the wants and comforts of many can be more bountifully supplied. . . . [M]isery and crime are almost strangers to the land."[3]

The heart of a medical topography was its view of southern people in their social, as well as natural, habitat. Thinking of themselves as natural scientists, topographers nonetheless spoke most clearly as ethnographers, elaborating on social themes alluded to in their daybooks or bedside notes. They wrote of their neighbors from a certain critical, generalizing distance not permitted by the bedside, and their characterizations of social life mingled sharp criticism with a local man's devotion to place. One frequent topic was the prevailing taste in medicines and habits of self-medication. Topographers generally agreed that southerners loved their medicines to a fault, and people's rampant self-drugging confirmed that the stiffest opposition to physicians' "expectancy" was among ordinary people, not rival doctors. J. B. Suddarth, for instance, thought that self-medication among all classes of people, including slaves, in Simpson County, Kentucky, in 1856 was "very considerable," mostly because people had no trouble finding one healer among many who would give them what they wanted. In Madison County, Alabama, according to John Young Bassett, on top of every dose of calomel, self-prescribed, people took three doses of quinine and a fair amount of castor oil. The thirty doctors in the county, he added pointedly, were busy adding to this overconsumption.[4]

In prizing moderation and breadth of knowledge, and in attempting to reform popular habits, the topographer embraced a vision of hoped-for modernity based on medical science. And yet it was a sharply bounded vision, arising from *within* the community under critique, in which the objective voice of the M.D. observer mingled with the subjectivity of a man who had a personal stake in how things turned out. Thus, although authors often portrayed their fellow southerners as isolated, credulous people in need of enlightenment, they also testified to progressive trends slowly taking shape. One such trend, to some extent countering the rage for self-drugging, was that people expected to have more choice in who doctored them. Gilbert Tennent, sketching Abbeville District, South Carolina, in 1829, reported that "30 or 40 years back . . . people had to rely on the resources of nature, or their own simple remedies." Many in Abbeville District had called upon a legendary "urinomaniac," who diagnosed only from urine, "conveyed to him in bottles, without [his] ever seeing the patient." Although admittedly impressed that "people [had] flocked . . . from all parts of the country" to this "extraordinary man," Tennent nonetheless believed that people were now better off and knew it. John Young Bassett, too, in his acerbic way, thought healers slowly were improving in quality throughout his Alabama county in the 1840s, largely because physicians were systematically schooled. Bassett recalled a low point twenty years earlier when most M.D.s in the region were dilettantish "young Virginians of good families . . . whose out-fit in life generally consisted of a pretty fair education, a genteel suit of clothes, a good horse and a mulatto servant; and whose object in life . . . was like that of our young preachers, to marry." If their communities still lagged in some ways, at least topographers were able to report that the momentum of history was on the side of improvement.[5]

Still, most topographers found much to worry them in taking the broad view. Many detected an underlying want of collective purpose sapping their community's betterment. The persistence of unhealthy farming practices was a common concern. From the 1830s onward, most physicians decried as a source of fever the stagnant mounds of rotting vegetation left over from land clearing, and by the 1850s, many M.D.s joined those warning of the misuse of fertilizers and reckless modes of cultivation that resulted in ruined soil. Intelligent management of water also was lacking in many locales, and topographies combined fact-finding and homily in recommending careful study and a public-minded spirit in all aspects of farming. Dr. John F. Posey, for example, reminded his rural Georgia neighbors in 1858 that their exploitation of nature masked their dependence on it, especially on the supply and management of water. The crucial balance, which physicians urged upon their farmer neighbors, was to collect enough water for their needs but not so much that it stood in brackish pools breeding fever. Posey, like other topographers, recommended that physicians act collectively in the name of public health, even if their communities did not, monitoring water supplies and admonishing neighbors.[6]

However, Posey and other authors seldom articulated a clear program that would realize their recommendations for reform. Rather, they tended to drift from their reformist purposes into detailed accounts of local customs and language that ended up simply informing or appreciating. For instance, Posey spent some time carefully recording the local language for watered areas: "bay-gulls" was the term for the small stream-valleys draining the region; "tie-tie" the term for berries that grew in healthy well-watered areas. The local water was tasty, he observed, but highly mineralized, imparting a "yellowish hue" to washed clothes, and he puzzled briefly over whether there might be an implication for health in this. Indeed, most topographers reveled in details of this kind. S. C. Farrar's topography of the area around Jackson, Mississippi, in 1849, for instance, was shaped by his closely seen accounts of weather, water, and agriculture, as informed and devoted as any thoughtful farmer's. The month of May, he wrote, "was unpropitious to the planter, and unpleasant to all, from the frequent rains." November, though, stayed above freezing, and "tomatoes, beans, and other tender vegetables retained their verdure, and on the last day, green peas were gathered."[7]

Thus, though struggling toward a definition of broad reform, topographers remained wedded to local details, a feature of published topographies that only gained force by the 1850s and persisted well after the Civil War. Whether or not they possessed the insight they thought they did—and published topographies varied from the well argued to the weirdly idiosyncratic—physicians wrote in a way that uneasily combined an attraction to a vision of change with an ambition to belong to the communities they critiqued. Engaging with the large issues discussed in the profession nationally, topographers nonetheless wrote as local men who wished to be admired by their neighbors.

Similarly mixing the voices of moralist and scientist, authors further implored southern communities to control social disorder, as well as disease. In the medical topographer's vision, a community that did not embrace the midcentury moral ideal of self-improvement and local pride could not be healthy. Efforts to clean up stagnant ponds thus had to be linked to making new roads, attracting trade, and appealing to a "better class" of people. So, in a way both republican and Whiggish, physicians applauded civic virtue and commercial opportunity. Dr. James A. Briggs, for example, in 1851 praised the progressive citizens of Warren County, formerly fever-ridden and "known by the memorable name as the Grave Yard of Kentucky," who had acted to clean up various health hazards and attract new settlers. Mississippi physician S. C. Farrar similarly praised his neighbors for overcoming political inertia to adopt a cistern plan that would insure a reliable supply of clean water by having "one or more of these [cisterns] . . . made an essential piece of property to every improved lot." "Improvement" was the byword, the promise of a South filled with communities known for their well-drained fields and good air.[8]

At their most expansive, topographers embraced a kind of aesthetic vision of harmonious social order in rural neighborhoods, where science was in service of beauty and people took pleasure in the attractiveness of their communities. Such authors spoke as caring if critical stewards. "The town is not more dirty than villages usually are," one physician wrote hopefully of Cahaba, Alabama, in 1855. Indeed, his town had grown quite "attractive," although "it has not the neat swept appearance which would be desirable, and it is only moderately supplied with shade trees." Looking about their neighborhoods, physicians hoped to be able to say what John Harden said in 1845 of Liberty County, Georgia, when he praised in general the "habits of the people. The black population is better fed and clothed now than formerly, and the habitations of both white and black are greatly improved. . . . The system of practice [of medicine], both domestic and professional, has been greatly altered for the better. Less drastic and poisonous medicines are now employed, and indeed the heroic treatment . . . has been exchanged for the milder and more rational method of *assisting Nature.*"[9]

Nonetheless, this ideal proved difficult to realize. Distilling expansive social ideals from solo practice, speaking as both outsiders and insiders, physicians came up against the limits of the topographical form, as well as those imposed by the many interests and irrationalities undercutting public health in southern communities. Many M.D.s responded aggressively, writing direct challenges to those who resisted reform and, by implication, orthodox medicine. With varying degrees of spleen or sorrow, more topographies than might be expected deplored in detail foolish or atavistic habits that undercut both health and citizenship. Frederick Becton ticked off a list of his fellow citizens' bad habits in 1832, including the fact that "we in Rutherford County generally eat as if for a wager against time, swallowing our food mashed, but not masticated," sending it to the stomach "floating in strong hot coffee," certain to end in a chronic—indeed, epidemic—dyspepsia impervious to medicines. Moreover, people bathed themselves and changed their clothes too infrequently, and Becton was equally critical of those individuals who did not wear enough clothes at all, interestingly pairing "the almost entire nudity of some of the fashionable belles, and the little negroes." Worst of all was drunkenness, which topographies underscored as the single greatest impairment of healthy living in the South. A Mississippi doctor in 1856 condemned the ubiquitous "doggery," or drinking place, usually no more than "a small cabin" found "at almost every cross road." He fervently praised temperance societies, with their "language of love, and hope and consolation," which he thought would do more against drunkenness than any of his medicines.[10]

There is a sense in much of this writing of physicians projecting the frustrations of their daily practice onto a people exposed as corrupt, yielding a portrait of isolated, ignorant southern communities familiar from other mid-nineteenth-century sources. But doctors seem peculiarly caught between the cool critique of a social witness and the desperation of a man embroiled in a moral drama. Thus the descriptions of sparkling rivers in the opening pages of a topography might well empty out into a flood of harsh social critique at the end. Time and again, rural southern neighborhoods were portrayed as peopled with folks lacking the social coherence that good health required. Washington, Texas, in 1856, J. J. Heard concluded, still bore the ill effects of its haphazard founding years earlier by a group of "transient persons . . . , consisting of disbanded soldiers, adventurers from the states of Europe, flock[ing] in rapidly." A certain flawed recklessness pervaded the social life of such places, and even when they despaired of changing it, physicians seem driven to report it. R. T.

Gibbes portrayed DeSoto Parish, Louisiana, in 1850 as twisted by tensions between French, Spanish, and U.S. citizens, resulting in a social pathology manifested by vicious economic competition and heavy drinking. Moreover, the widespread "sumptuous living" by the newly rich was the cause of more ill health among the "better" people than the "malarious exhalations" of the swamps they neglected to clear. Thus many topographers peered over into the greatest abyss of all, the perhaps bottomless one where generations of bad habits served a decadence beyond the reach of medicine.[11]

Few had imaginations more richly bleak than Alabaman John Young Bassett, and yet he was not unique in what he concluded in 1849 about southerners' self-destructive ways. Called to a site in his town, Huntsville, Alabama, where a workman had uncovered a skeleton with a shattered skull, Bassett had a kind of epiphany of the history of southern settlement. The broken skull was an old one, he concluded, probably belonging to an early settler who had met a violent end at the hands of a fellow Huntsvillian. Speaking as a man moved both by moral outrage and by intellectual discovery, Bassett reflected on southerners' resort to violence as doing double damage to the health of their communities. Violence became a kind of tradition that made worse the already terrible intractability of disease and the abuse of self-medication. But beyond this, social violence impaired efforts to imagine any other way of living, erasing a recorded history that might have served public health. "Such a race leave but short records of their diseases," Bassett wrote of the forebear settlers, mixing images of repair and slaughter. "Where bloodshed is always epidemic and every man his own surgeon, the few that recover feel grateful to none, and hang no 'votive tablet' on the natural columns of their forests" to mark their grief or lessons learned; indeed, "it would puzzle Hippocrates himself to collate the cases" from such a community's past. And yet, Bassett grimly concluded, there was one legacy over all: "these early squatters have . . . made their mark" in the way their descendants had learned to cherish their ignorant and murderous ways.[12]

Speaking from such a topographical overlook, whether from hope or despair, physicians strove to translate their bedside insights into an objectifying vision in which their orthodoxy became a kind of social science. Through their efforts, we, too, can see some of the ill health consequences of southern communities' prized "independence" and understand how certain debilitating habits cut across the entire South. But physicians' topographical vision was even more essentially a moral one, arising from everyday work recast as social commentary. It was a vision in which the doctor manifested his experience as the spokesman for his community's best instincts and worse fears. And it was a vision of social reform that had less to do with mobilizing political forces for change than with how well he used insights from his practice to foster the moral continuity of his community.

SLAVERY AND RACE

As we have seen, everyday practice brought white physicians into frequent contact with the bodies, needs, and self-care of black patients. As a result, some physicians became curious about the wider meaning of African American health and probed deeper into questions of race and slavery. In fact, more broadly than most other social contexts in the slave South, medical practice opened up a view of African American experience to those whites who cared to look. To be sure, it was a distorted view, and most did not look very deeply. Even those physicians who were curious became entangled in a practice-oriented vision that both diffused and circumscribed their broader imagination of African American health. Nonetheless, their texts are the ones that best sum up what we have so far seen of M.D.s' view of slavery and race.

Physicians' broad consideration of African American health often took a "topographical" form into which authors poured both empirical data and unexamined racial notions, reading orthodoxy at large from the standpoint of their personal experience. As we will see, and as physicians' education and bedside work already have suggested, this perspective led M.D.s to three main, overlapping assumptions about African American sickness. First, the visible structures of slavery as a social institution took precedence over more amorphous speculations about the biological nature of race. Second, physicians pushed for reforms aimed at benefiting slave health but in ways aimed at strengthening slavery. Third, the vexing question of the nature and extent of "Negro disease" remained interesting but largely unsettled—talked about but yielding no clear course of medical action.

Before looking at how physicians approached such matters, however, it is important to put their topographical view of race and slavery into its intellectual context within orthodox medicine. For one thing, given that everyday practice was the source of most physicians' curiosity about African Americans, it is important to appreciate the contrast between this quotidian curiosity and the comparative silence about both race and slavery in medical school. It is a contrast that emphasizes how doctors' interest in black health grew from the practical problems of work-a-day medicine. Too, despite their distortions and uncertainties, working M.D.s were more reflective than most other whites who engaged in caregiving for and with African Americans. Certainly physicians moved beyond the minimal health talk of most masters, and their relative volu-bility contrasts, too, with the striking near silence on slavery and race in the many books of popular health advice in southern circulation. Popular authors A. G. Goodlett, Samuel Jennings, and others, addressing themselves specifically to a southern audience, wrote hundreds of pages on prevention, symptoms, disease, and drugs but managed to mention slaves only a few times, and then only in passing. These authors may have believed racial differences were either inconsequential or so well known as to be taken for granted, or they may have feared treading on the prerogatives of masters. Whatever the combination of motives, however, popular advisers were mute in comparison to those physi-cians who addressed the topographical shape of race and slavery.[13]

Finally, most physicians' emphasis on the practical and the everyday should not, of course, imply that no M.D.s were interested in speculative racial theory. Certain southern physicians took the lead in a national discussion of race, men like Mobile, Alabama, M.D. Josiah Nott, for example, and Mississippi's Samuel A. Cartwright (about whom more later). Nott is particularly well known as an influential contributor to white racial thought during the century; he was an aggressive opponent of clergy and others who argued that God had made no racial distinctions at Creation. Nott argued combatively that whites and blacks always had been separate and must remain so. And yet if some doctors found interest in his biotheology, it is significant that few of them incorporated such ruminations into their topographical writings about African Americans.[14]

Thus we return to what obviously did carry explanatory weight for most physicians: a practitioner's "experience" and the insights extrapolated from everyday encounters between the races within the strictures of slavery. Recall some of the ways the physician's eye and texts shaped these encounters: he spe-cially highlighted and to some extent segregated his black patients (as "Negro Jack" or "the woman Lucy") in his personal record-keeping; he singled out hues of "colored" skin for particular diagnostic attention; he borrowed freely from African American pharmacology but dismissed black interpretations of disease; he actively sought black patients, charged the same fees for slave and free, and in other ways shaped his livelihood to the power relations of slavery—for example, tailoring his treatment to the monetary cap set by the master.

When physicians stepped back from these immediate routines to take stock of what they observed about African American patients generally, they tended to favor three approaches to sizing up black sickness that grew from and bol-stered the main assumptions about black health noted earlier. The first of these approaches viewed slavery as a kind of epidemiological terrain. Here physicians tallied numbers of slaves in a given region, noted slaves' collective susceptibility to disease, and commented on patterns of health, weather, and diet. A second, and more frequent, approach attempted to size up particular settings for slaves' health, mostly in terms of plantation life, and to make recommendations to masters. Finally, physicians discussed the extent to which "Negro disease" was distinctive.

Consider, first, physicians' sense of African American health as something with epidemiological significance, which is to say, as adding to doctors' understanding of widespread patterns of sickness in the South. Most physicians proceeded along topographical lines in reasoning that "place"—an area's water, climate, geography, and health habits—was far more important than abstract or inherent qualities of "race." The mixture of natural and social conditions, not raw biology, comprised the salient medical world. Some physician observers, for instance, were interested in the sheer numbers of slaves in their region and so tallied numbers, broke them down by county and geographic zones, and attempted to use these numbers to help them discover the "incidence" of sickness and mortality. Indeed, medical authors quantified no other social group in this fashion—not even women, whose collective health problems also interested many doctors.

Such quantification at times implied that blacks were an aggregate "other," but more often the effect was to include the black population in the local social scene, albeit as part of a white landscape. To this end, some physicians, like J. B. Suddarth, writing in 1856 from Simpson County, Kentucky, took a historical interest in an area's slaves, integrating African Americans (and slavery) into his largely positive view of what made his region unique. Thus, as a point of interest, he traced some of his county's slaves as descending from Virginia Africans, others from the Carolinas. Before this, he discovered, they "were of distinct tribes, principally of Upper and Lower Guinea." All of these peoples and their scattered origins, along with white settlers, now were in synchrony in Simpson County. The slaves, no less than whites, "through admixture . . . have now become one peculiar class bearing the physical impress of our climate and social habits among them."[15]

Broad-based, environmental considerations of this kind were related to the longtime white interest in how to assess black "acclimation" to local climate and diseases, a subject still unresolved at midcentury after more than 200 years of white medical thought, with each new generation of doctors in effect reinventing observations of black susceptibility or immunity to disease. A few elite physicians, Josiah Nott for one, maintained that African Americans were capable of acclimating to fevers of all kinds. More mainstream, however, was the view that, in most regions, blacks, like whites, never became acclimated to *endemic* fevers (evidenced by the fact that these fevers never completely disappeared), though blacks probably possessed greater resistance than whites to most *epidemic* fevers. It was a vexed question, however, and one clearly of economic interest to slave owners. So many variables applied, and physicians wished to be the ones the white community relied upon to sort and organize them: up-country versus low-country fevers; fevers that varied by region versus fevers that varied by season; long-term resident slaves versus new arrivals.

Although the big picture grew cloudy in the medical literature, tied as it was to the irreducible particularity of scores of local topographies, the tireless topographer E. D. Fenner spoke for midcentury conventional wisdom when he wrote that *some* kind of acclimation must take place among *all* southern creatures ("even the dogs, turkeys, and chickens") because otherwise every immigrant population would have been wiped out by disease long ago. Moreover, most physicians seemed to agree that "race" in some absolute sense did not deserve to be privileged in the assessment of acclimation. Thomas Affleck's view typically gave the nod to place over race. Even when whites and blacks differed in their susceptibility to fever, Affleck argued, the different environmental circumstances of each race probably explained the variation. And nothing shaped environmental differences like slavery. In fact, Affleck concluded that the races were "equally liable, under the same circumstances of food, exposure, etc.," to fever. That is, absent the conditions imposed by slavery, blacks and whites stood an equal chance with disease.[16]

Thinking along these aggregate, epidemiological lines, physician authors struggled throughout midcentury to define certain basic characteristics of slave health that would fill out the little they had learned in school or recorded at the bedside: infant mortality was much more prevalent among blacks than whites—two to one in many instances—although the former had greater longevity once childhood was survived; blacks were less susceptible to intermittent fever (malaria); blacks were more susceptible to respiratory diseases and to diseases associated with cold weather; blacks had more dental disease; black women were "naturally" more adept at "easy" childbirth, although this advantage frequently was undercut by strenuous field work, which put pregnancies at risk. Again, although such generalizations sometimes took on a collective "racial" cast, most doctors seem to have used them as broad guidelines for treatment with little interest in the gloss of theory. Because local observations carried equal weight throughout the profession, a doctor's challenge was to sort through the flood of empirical findings for the ones that best fit his situation rather than to speculate on biology.

The observations of one sharp-eyed medical topographer, William L. Mc-

Caa, in 1822, writing as a student on nervous diseases among slaves in South Carolina, suggest the way race and slavery were wrapped up together in orthodox generalizations. McCaa simply accepted the necessity of slavery, but he produced a reading of black health that credited African Americans with tendencies similar to whites'. For instance, McCaa observed that slaves did not suffer from nervous diseases resulting from "disappointments in love, [or] in ambitious pursuits." Not race but the social dynamics of slavery explained this difference from whites: in terms of love, no ties of marriage prevented a enslaved man from moving on to another woman as "soon as . . . affection dies," so there was no need for a sickly despondence. Similarly, because slave life and labor demanded no personal ambition, in McCaa's estimation, slaves did not become mentally disturbed over whether they possessed enough of it. At the same time, by thus channeling blacks' health into their status as slaves, McCaa saw African Americans sharing certain other, more basic, traits with whites. So he concluded by asking, "What . . . can excite ambition in the slave" if not love or work? His answer, startlingly, was freedom. In his observation of slaves in his region, "nought that I know of save a glimmering spark of hope for that liberty of which they are now deprived" inspired slave ambition. "It is true that this aspiring hope has cost some of them their lives, but so far as I know, it has not stolen from them any [of] their reason."[17]

Writing in the 1820s, McCaa was not as guarded about mentioning black freedom as physicians even a decade later would be. But his emphasis on the social conditions of slavery was typical of the reasoning that would continue throughout midcentury. This same emphasis gave rise to proposals for the reform of slavery, proposals that in no way countered masters' power, of course, but, by the same token, did not lock African Americans into a static realm of biology either. Here, as elsewhere, physicians treated slavery and black health as something malleable, overriding certain essentialist questions about "race" and begging others.[18]

Frequently, for instance, authors appealed for improvements in slaves' health by appealing to the slave owner's self-interest. Thus Thomas Affleck in 1850 informed himself on slave diet by visiting the best-run plantations in his region and publicizing them as models of good slave management. He described in detail the amounts and preparation of pork and cornmeal per hand, per dinner, and how it was delivered still hot to each worker in "a small tin bucket, with a cover" by way of "an old man and cart." Although he observed a need for greater variety in slave diet, the doctor concluded that such meals, like slaves' sixteen-by-twenty-foot houses and their woolen clothing in winter, were "generally quite good" on the best plantations and recommended that all slave owners adopt these as a standard. Similarly, H. W. Moore thought the slaves of his region of South Carolina in the mid-1850s were "generally well fed" by partaking three times a day of pork, meal, and sometimes chicken. He noted, moreover, that "the negro . . . is something of an Epicure" and relished raising his own garden, a true health benefit for masters wise enough to allow it. He also praised a "native" bed devised by slaves from "common Spanish Moss and cornshock," declaring it "an admirable mattress" worthy of adoption throughout the region.[19]

Sometimes, however, physicians spoke critically, using rounds-gathered facts to build a case for change. Despite the risk of being the bearer of unwelcome information, C. H. Jordan wrote of his practice in 1832, "I always . . . reveal the situation of the negroes as nearly as I can to the master." Slave housing, more than diet or overwork, came in for the greatest criticism among medical topographers of slavery. A Virginia physician in 1859 observed of his region, "The farmers do not, in a general way, give sufficient attention to the subject of proper ventilation . . . in their buildings erected for the occupancy of their negroes—often crowding too many in a small, ill ventilated room. . . . All negro cabins should have at least two windows, fronting each other." Another doctor advocated changing local slave-owning practice so as to give each slave family its own quarters. "Privacy gives self-respect, and the latter always tends to moral elevation," which he urged as the key to health for blacks, as well as whites.[20]

Overall, whether couched in terms of praise for "good" plantation practice, or in more critical terms, physicians' focus on bettering specific conditions of African American life led them to make no more than remedial suggestions for reform. Nothing they said touched the essentially arbitrary nature of each master's power over the bodies and living conditions of slaves. More tellingly, doctors' implicit definition of what was "medical" excluded certain subjects from the conversation. For instance, their uniform silence in published writings on whippings, imprisonment, and sexual and other abuses of slaves is striking. It was a silence that in effect put these aspects of slavery, as commonplace as matters of food and housing, completely outside the topography of slave health. A few writers contented themselves with recommending "kindness" in a general way. H. W. Moore in 1856 was exceptional in mentioning that "much might be said against the almost universal prostitution that prevails among the Blacks," although by this he meant extramarital sexual unions between slaves rather than sexual abuse of slaves by masters. In any event, he beat a hasty literary retreat, noting that his topography "has already extended beyond our intended limit and we must lay our pen aside."[21]

Thus, the selective, remedial quality of doctors' proposed reforms arose from and fed back into the profoundly local boundaries of their topographical advice. Caught up in the satisfactions of describing their own surroundings, and trained to focus on work at hand even as they attempted to speak broadly, very few ordinary physicians developed a view of the slave system as a whole. Rather, their local vision bolstered the resolute individualism that infused all aspects of country orthodoxy. Taking pride in speaking with equal authority, whether from prime cotton country or backcountry, M.D.s writing on race further enshrined the conceptual limitations of their determinedly personal vision of doctoring. Topographies on race, therefore, not only deferred to local standards of "management" determined by masters, they also made it intellectually acceptable for the physician to conflate the health of individual slaves under his purview with the health of "Negroes" at large. Thus, while most physicians avoided embracing the most oppressive, virulent potential of racist theory, their particular angle of vision permitted certain "ordinary" abuses to live on unexamined, making their writing one more text shoring up whites' belief in the rightness of their power.[22]

Growing directly from their interest in both epidemiology and the social conditions of slavery, physicians' interest in the relative distinctiveness of African American disease reached a peak in antebellum medical writing. Discussions of distinctive "Negro diseases," like discussions of slaves' labor and living conditions, also privileged individual practice, folding the details of a practitioner's "experience" into unexamined notions of race in a way physicians never quite sorted out. In the name of pathology, they wove racially inflected rationalizations of slavery into their close clinical descriptions, simultaneously weaving their own subjective sense of the tie between sickness and bondage.

The central orthodox consensus on "Negro disease," hammered out in medical journals essay by essay, supported the view (which many masters accepted on their own authority) that sickness among blacks and whites differed in terms of degree rather than kind. This view supposed that there were certain slave afflictions worth naming—"Negro consumption," for example—which might be more or less exotic in certain settings. But these afflictions never were wholly alien to whites. This consensus pointed in two different directions. On the one hand, the supposed similarity between the races supported bringing black and white patients together under a single plan of care. Slaves were portrayed as a people well within the southern domain of sickness and therapy: purges, tonics, and surgery had similar effects; vaccination against smallpox "took" regardless of the racial source of the vaccine; lungs yielded similar sounds, black bodies exhibited familiar responses, the heart beat in everyone. On the other hand, when physicians wrote expansively, which is to say speculatively, about black disease, many alluded to a sense of black difference in a way that furthered white uneasiness over possible unknown risks to health lurking in a racial "other."

Thus, although mid-nineteenth-century medical journals contain a fair number of essays on this or that "Negro disease," authors tended to beg the question of how to define, much less measure, racial difference. Instead, most practitioners contented themselves with describing the action they took, deepening their bedside notes rather than delving into vexed questions of theory that might seem fatalistic or prove to be divisive. In this context, the black diseases most often written about were those that followed from the general susceptibilities noted earlier, conceptualized as variations (more or less virulent) on white afflictions. Among these diseases were relatively intractable cases of trismus nascentium (infant tetanus) and "marasmus," a term used to indicate infant "wasting away" from causes unknown. M.D.s also observed blacks being afflicted more acutely by certain diseases (especially fevers) that took on a "typhoid" state, which seemed to mean an alarming general debility of the vital signs. Many physicians referred to "Negro consumption" in this way but, again, tended to be satisfied with asserting the name and letting it suffice for pathology.[23]

This way of thinking about disease is evident even in the discussion of a sickness at the exotic end of the spectrum, most notably cachexia africana or "dirt-eating." Though widely referred to as a "Negro disease," and assumed to have an "African" origin, in fact most M.D. writers did not draw as deep a racial line as might be supposed. Cachexia africana was observed in some poor whites as well, and white physicians noted many similarities. Although the image of cachexic slaves, with their "invincible craving for earthy substances" leading them to devise "cunning plans" for deceiving whites, added to the white stereotype of deceptive black patients, the mainstream view by working rural doctors was that this disease nonetheless deserved broad attention as a "poor people's" environmental and social affliction.[24]

The individual, practice-based nature of orthodox generalizations about African American disease—its perceived similarity to white sickness and the priority given to the concrete details of slavery over the murky question of race—may be summed up with a look at physician Samuel A. Cartwright and his critics. Cartwright merits such a look not only because he published widely on slave disease but also because he has been, mistakenly, singled out as representative of a view that black disease was essentially racial. Cartwright, who practiced in Natchez, Mississippi, and in New Orleans, in the 1840s and 1850s, was in indefatigable writer on a wide range of medical reforms, including the need for more southern medical schools and the desirability of compiling accurate statistics on regional disease. He also was an outspoken defender of slavery and of the southern physician as uniquely qualified to treat slaves. However, he has become best known for identifying (and giving innovative names to) supposed slave diseases such as "drapetomania," the disease which caused slaves to run away, and "dysæsthesia æthiopis," a disease "called by overseers 'rascality'." Here his influence has been misread in two ways. First, despite the dogmatic gloss imparted by the names he gave to his "diseases," Cartwright, like most physicians, emphasized the conditions of slavery, not biological race, as the key to the afflictions. Moreover, when he did focus on certain racial characteristics of blacks, Cartwright clearly strayed from the orthodox mainstream, as his many critics reveal.[25]

Inventing diseases such as drapetomania seems, at first look, to imply a degraded, "racial" explanation for slaves' behavior. But, in fact, the maladjustments of slavery, not racial determinism, were behind Cartwright's essentially remedial vision. For example, he explained running away and "Negro rascality," which included feigning, as rooted in conditions of slave management which intelligent masters could change. Indeed, Cartwright discussed diseases like "rascality" as problems mostly for the master (that is, slaves appeared not to suffer, except morally by not doing their duty) for which the solution lay in the shrewd, but also caring, manipulation of slaves' environment. Although Cartwright believed that certain behaviors and aptitudes made up a composite slave character, this character, too, was something essentially moral which could be modified by the master's reliance on his own moral stewardship, as well as by medicine. To this extent, Cartwright's views, though more expansive and theoretically phrased than those of most physicians, fit into the general topographic sense of blacks as part of a manipulable white social landscape. If there was a Cartwrightian emphasis, it was psychological, not physiological; his impetus was to medicalize social relations in order to "cure" social ills. "Negroes are very jealous and suspicious," he wrote, typically. "Hence, if they are slighted or imposed on in any way, or over-tasked, or do not get what they call their rights, they are apt to fall into a morbid state of mind. . . . It is bad government to let them remain in this sulky, dissatisfied mood, without inquiring into its causes, and removing them." The physician's role, in Cartwright's view, was to advise a master to think not of the whip but of changing his management; to think of "bad" slaves as being sick but quite open to "cure."[26]

In one aspect of his work, however, Cartwright did highlight race, claiming to find, in the course of doing anatomical dissections, certain specific, physiological characteristics of blacks meriting scientific curiosity. Here, revealingly, his views came under fire by peers who believed he was stepping over the empirical line into unsubstantiated speculation. He was criticized, first, for putting forward ambiguous physiological evidence with no clear therapeutic value. Although his various claims—that African Americans' brain size, blood color, eyeballs, and sub-epidermal tissue all differed from whites'—resonate ominously with the racist biology prevalent a half-century later, Cartwright had almost nothing to say about the medical implications of his assertions. More than this, though, it was Cartwright's aggressive certainty—and the fact that few if any fellow physicians could corroborate his observations—which seemed to call forth his critics. Even an editor who published Cartwright on such topics, E. D. Fenner, took open exception to Cartwright's aberrant racial speculations. Cartwright's assertion of race-specific physiology, Fenner wrote bluntly by way of introducing one of Cartwright's essays in 1850, "will be somewhat startling to those physicians who have been familiar with negroes all their lives, in health and sickness, and even in the *dissecting-room*, without having observed these things." Indeed, Fenner, widely respected for his own medical topographies, noted that he had rejected an earlier version of one of Cartwright's articles, and indicated he might well have rejected this one, too, had it come from "a writer of less experience and exalted reputation." Though paying respect to "experience," Fenner nonetheless made it clear that Cartwright's work lay far outside what most experienced men were reporting from the field. Fenner made it clear, too, that he was troubled not only by Cartwright's careless use of clinical evidence (and by his forays into theology, as well as speculative biology) but also by the likelihood that the man's extreme views on race would be mistaken as the mainstream of southern orthodoxy. Fenner was concerned that non-southerners in the growing slavery debate ("the greatest question of the day in this country") would think that all southern physicians were as extreme as Dr. Cartwright.[27]

Other physicians concurred, finding Cartwright's racial physiology unsubstantiated and his innovative slave diseases misconceived and even dangerous. H. V. Wooten, of Alabama, for instance, took Cartwright to task for slighting the observations of blacks made by many other medical topographers who had seen nothing of the distinctive blood or tissue that Cartwright claimed to find. Moreover, Wooten sharply criticized Cartwright for simply asserting the existence of "negro dysentery" when the question of a separate black disease was exactly the issue under debate. This critique, which essentially faulted Cartwright for his lack of respect for others' experience, was joined to another that scored him for medicalizing behavior better understood as bad behavior. Rascality was rascality, not illness, his critics argued, and to say otherwise was to invite an epidemic of dissembling and resistance by slaves who would claim they were ill. As Louisiana practitioner James T. Smith pointed out, medicalizing "rascality" opened the door to "a very numerous class of diseases hitherto never dreamed of as being anything but vices; for if a strong desire to do what is wrong be a disease, the violation of any one of the ten commandments will furnish us with a new one."[28]

Understanding that Cartwright himself placed more emphasis on slavery than race in his notorious diagnoses of slave "diseases," and understanding, too, that when he strayed into racial speculation he was taken to task by his empirical-minded peers, emphasizes how most midcentury physicians looked to slavery and not biology in their commentary on African American sickness. It was an emphasis consistent with the demands of daily practice and with the way race had been marginalized by physicians' schooling. At the same time, however, it is evident that physicians' conflation of race and slavery kept alive the possibility for an expansive biological racism. Their deep immersion in the social structure of slavery, like that of most other whites, merely forestalled physicians' focus on race, a focus that would obtain with terrible effect at the end of the century after the structure of slavery had fallen away.

In the meantime, during the midcentury decades, most physicians centered their attention on the piecemeal reform of slavery, speaking as the most widely experienced, comprehensive advisers on such matters as slave diet, housing, and preventive health care. Such reform not only buttressed the white social order generally, it also more firmly rooted the country style of orthodoxy in the local context of each man's practice, where the continuity of personal experience shaped the most significant observations, remedies, and homilies orthodox medicine had to offer.

FAITH: KNOWING WHAT "PASSETH UNDERSTANDING"

Christian ways of knowing shaped a further intellectual context for nineteenth-century physicians' attempts to assert the breadth and inclusiveness of their work. Although not taking as specific a textual form as physicians' writing on the environment and on slavery, writing on religious faith nonetheless provided a similar way for doctors to see themselves as they wished to be seen: as belonging to their community yet speaking as leaders of it—as moral, as well as practical, men.

Expressions of personal faith, appearing throughout published, as well as private, writing, typically followed the channels cut by evangelical Protestant Christianity. Such expressions spoke directly to physicians' deep concern for how to reconcile the fluid phenomenology of practice with the promise of orthodox ideals. The language of faith also gave doctors an inclusive way to acknowledge, in their struggle against disease, the mysteries of illness. How expressions of faith performed this work is the focus here, beginning with a brief reminder of religion's power to refract all knowledge in this era. This is followed by a look at particular tensions marking physicians and their faith, and, finally, at how these tensions often were resolved.

Two broad features of a quotidian, "practical" Christianity alive in southern communities are key to understanding religious faith's importance in physicians' work. The first is the pervasive (and comparatively homogeneous) way in which Christian references and purposes shaped a lively intellectual culture everywhere in nineteenth-century America. Christianity supplied an adaptable, widespread heuristic unrivaled in its power to bring the thorny ways of the world to happy synthesis. Not only self-criticism and moral instruction but also social and political commentary flourished in Christian terms.

The second, more specific, and somewhat countervailing feature of Christian thought as it configured a country orthodoxy was the long-term tension between established religion and the materialist implications of positivist, empirical science. To be sure, there were ways for scientifically minded nineteenth-century Americans to alleviate this tension. Accepting natural theology's deduction that a wondrous creation implied a wonderful Creator, for instance, allowed a person to both praise God and collect specimens—in fact, to praise God *by* collecting specimens. Even so, conflict between the worlds of sense and faith sometimes was stirred to life by contentious, materialist physicians in the tradition of South Carolina's Thomas Cooper. "Man consists of a body . . . and certain phenomena connected with it," Cooper wrote with typical bluntness in 1824. Everything ultimately was material; the body, and the mind along with it, "decomposed" upon death, into an assortment of elements ("carbon, ozote, hydrogen, oxygen, phosphorous, and lime; and perhaps another substance or two"). Nowhere in this, Cooper was pleased to emphasize, was there evidence of a soul. Although most doctors by midcentury were not so confrontational, the materialist view continued to have some resonance in orthodox circles. Even by the 1880s, when many Christian physicians, more confident in their therapeutic promise, softened the edges of controversy by criticizing both religion and science for excesses, the sense of an essential conflict between science and religion persisted as an intellectual challenge to the many physicians who aspired to faith.[29]

Understanding the place of religious belief in the work of mid-nineteenth-century southern physicians, then, means understanding how the tension between faith and materialism, along with a pervasive natural theology, regularly appeared in physicians' commentary on their practice. One specific context for this tension was physicians' encounters with clergy on rounds. A community's ministers and its physicians both came daily into the lives of sick neighbors already in the grip of perplexing dualities: worldly striving and eternal reward, spirit and carnality, ambition and virtue. All of these were open questions for many sick people, through which an ambitious professional might launch his own specialized quest for answers. So it was not an inconsequential matter for a doctor coming into the sickroom to squeeze uncomfortably past a minister of God also making his way to the bedside. Medical and clerical literature throughout the century was shot through with one profession giving advice to—and criticizing—the other. Ministers may be found giving lectures on belief and character to medical students in 1880 much as they did in 1820, although M.D.s did not do much speaking at religious convocations until the 1880s. Each urged the other to think beyond narrow professional goals. A hymn may sometimes do more than a drug in the sickroom, a minister typically admonished his medical audience. The physician "who systematically excludes the minister from his sick room or admits him only as the ghostly precursor of the undertaker . . . is ignorant of some of the deepest facts of human nature, and unfit to practice his noble profession."[30]

Doctors sparring with clergy uncovered a deeper issue, the fear that medical work uniquely bred a personal Godlessness that threatened a practitioner's own soul. Bedside failures, as well as preoccupation with bodies and drugs, took a toll on the will to believe in something transcendent. The aged clerical adviser of Lunsford Yandell, who had earlier considered becoming a clergyman himself, pleaded in 1839 with the younger man to choose the enduring truths of Scripture over the limited ones of physiology. Yes, the old clergyman allowed, medicine had a "propensity" for intellectual excitement. However, "God will not be mocked with impunity. . . . [You] may be right to indulge this native propensity, within its legitimate bounds. But the danger is, in giving [it] too much rein." The highly charged, oddly impersonal physical intimacies of diagnosis and the sometimes harshness of treatment distanced the doctor emotionally from his patients. But worse, in a way, was the fact that the daily demands of solo medical work isolated a doctor from his community generally.[31]

An atmosphere of materialism and alienation from Christian brotherhood thus swirled around the physician. His interests and his livelihood presented simple but nonetheless fundamental challenges to religious life; for instance, doctors faced "the formidable difficulty [of] . . . their frequent want of the Sabbath." Physicians worried the issue of their attendance at church, some remorsefully, others combatively defensive, all testifying to how the claims of faith raised a doctor's doubts about belonging to his community. South Carolina physician Samuel Leland in the 1850s frequently noted in his diary when his medical duties interfered with his practice of religion, explaining to himself, repeatedly, how he had intended to read his Bible but was interrupted by an urgent call and "before I could go there and back the Sabbath was gone." John A. Robinson, often so busy on Sundays in 1871 that he "cannot possibly get to church," took this as a warning "that my practice is growing too extensive." Other doctors, at first regretting their separation from others, ended up embracing it. Arkansas physician Frank James reacted angrily to importunities from his Baptist neighbors that he attend church. "The Baptists seem to have everything their own way in this community," he raged in his diary. "Their narrow-minded, blood-thirsty creed just suits the ignorance of the people." Such conflict was about a man's character, of course, but also about the terms of his acceptance into his community. At least some physicians found these tensions reviving old fears from medical school, fears about becoming hardened to what Joseph LeConte described as the huge gap between the "awful responsibilities" of doctoring and most men's moral readiness for it. Another physician worried that "*Science* may not foster irreligion, but the *medical life* might," seeing signs in himself of the "calloused feelings" that resulted from long practice. Professing one's faith and attending church with neighbors were guards against a cold materialism that led many a doctor to see a medical emergency—for instance, an injured, bleeding neighbor—not as a moment of transfiguring human need but only as impersonal Nature "diverting the course of a little red fluid."[32]

Disturbed by the all-too-public instances of the mis-fit between medical practice and religious belief, devout physicians strove to make real a faith that would set their everyday work aglow against a backdrop of Christian meaning. They embraced the idea that doctoring itself was a kind of social ministry and therefore a form of worship. Its benefits were not measured by hours spent in church but by hours spent with patients. In this view, medicine was less a natural science than it was humanitarian labor, and as such, it was an especially apt form of an "active" Christianity prized by Jesus, "the great Master Physician." Some nonevangelical physicians also embraced this notion in terms of a natural theology. Charles Caldwell, for instance, hardly an evangelical Christian, nonetheless defended "natural religion" as fully Christian in the "best" sense, maintaining that through their version of natural theology physicians had realized how to love the world exactly in proportion to its wonders. The most profound calls to faith, Caldwell proposed, were not the "faint and feeble" metaphors of the Bible (God riding a whirlwind, for example) but the actual marvels of the natural world ("a universe consisting of millions of orbs"). Caldwell, a combative man, doubtless knew that he was raising the hackles of ministers everywhere. Nonetheless, there is an authentic intensity in the way he anchored his insights firmly to the bedside by arguing that medical work, deeply bound up with the mysteries of suffering and healing, was a kind of microcosm of Christian devotion. Lest he be misunderstood, Caldwell spelled it out: "[M]y meaning is . . . that a physician is much more *religiously*, as well as *usefully* employed, in the chamber of disease . . . than in a place of public worship."[33]

Though in part self-serving, even self-deluding, there was yet a greater depth to doctors' sense of this bond between self, work, and redemption. The physician is seen as a man of spiritual fortitude because he deliberately rejected the world-weariness he might easily have chosen. A Tennessee doctor in 1830 thus drew great strength from the thought that the unique challenges of a medical career provided the best proof that "man was designed [by God] to be an active rather than passive being." A truly Christian doctor, in the words of William Holcombe in 1855, is one who "*works* and *works* and *works*." And a youthful J. Marion Sims wrote to his wife words that expressed the hoped-for unity of healing and faith when he rejoiced at the close of a successful case, "Oh! what a glorious thing it is to feel . . . that you are a blessed instrument in the hands of God."[34]

Closely tied to the sense of medical work as ministry was the conviction that practice vouchsafed for a Christian doctor a privileged witnessing of God's powerful mysteries. Bearing witness—in a Christian sense—brought unified meaning to the physician's difficult balance of action and witnessing in the sickroom. Witnessing God's glory embraced—and for some doctors exalted—the tedious routines of their work: waiting and observing, probing and recording; it unified these into a kind of devotional metatext that only a healer could inscribe. Thus, the onslaught of challenges to a physician's knowledge might, by faith, be turned into a resource, with a doctor understanding how he might truly "learn your profession by [living] a Christian life." So it was that many physicians, fearing that medical work would deplete what one doctor called his "conscience toward God," found renewed energy and purpose in the doctor's privilege of bearing witness to transfigured Nature, a kind of apotheosis of all of their social and physical observations. Here was a Nature neither cold nor savage but one combining a Romantic sense of natural beauty with a practical natural theology celebrating God's handiwork everywhere and nearby. In his notebook, John Lindsley answered his own question, "Why nature is worthy of man's study" by the simple declaration, "It is God's idea." Medical students, hearing such views from their mentors, reaffirmed them in their M.D. theses. "I believe the Great Supreme Being has implanted in our soil and climate medicinal plants well adopted to cure our diseases," wrote Kentucky student James

Sterrett in 1821. Thomas Hardin argued that in "modern Chemistry nothing is better sustained by proof than the sublime fact that in the hands of the Creator . . . the most trifling means are made adequate to the most wonderful results."[35]

Even the body itself rose above the material world. Religious doctors cherished the human body for how wonderfully suited it was to human needs, thereby placing the vulnerabilities of particular bodies onto a larger, more serene stage. In considering mother's milk, for instance, a young doctor concluded that its adaption to "the infantile organs of digestion" was proof of "the wise and benevolent order of Providence." Samuel Dickson, certainly no evangelical, nonetheless told his students in the 1850s that "I find a Supreme Being absolutely necessary," and he taught them that no matter how many sick bodies they were to see to never forget that the body ultimately resisted empirical reduction, was "fearfully and wonderfully made." For Thomas Powell, in 1860, study of the body revealed an even grander vision of medicine's promise. As a true science, Powell admitted, medicine was "comparatively sleeping." Nonetheless, medicine's growing knowledge of the body implicated the physician in the most meaningful of all events when, at Judgment Day, the resurrected body— "refined, glorified, and beautiful"—rose above all Nature. "We know of no material thing which will live beyond these awful scenes of dying nature," he wrote, "but this human body." Knowledge of the immortal body, as well as bedside caring for bodies, thus fed into a faith in divine justice at the end of days. Under the canopy of Nature and Nature's God, this vision became a kind of exalted witnessing in which medical practice was more than merely contingent on the pressure to act.[36]

Though seeking certainty, the language of belief was not rigid, and its very flexibility was both a strength and a weakness in the midst of doctors' work. Religious discourse was strikingly adaptable, its weight and meaning suddenly shifting from one register to another. Thus, for some physicians, religious belief was a comparatively remote backdrop for other, more immediate acquirements. As Thomas S. Powell expressed it, religion was mostly important because "only religion . . . can center in a man all the graces and finish him for the walks of life." Belief was first of all a great stabilizer of social relations. "You should always respect religion," Powell thought, "whether you believe in its truths or not, because, true or false . . . it is calculated to improve and ennoble society." For other doctors, though, it was precisely the concrete, epigrammatic power of religious truths that mattered, turned over and over like amulets or relied upon like familiar drugs. Thus a doctor might sum up his successful efforts for the day with the terse but satisfying observation that both the healer and the sick were, once again, "spared for some wise purpose." Jeptha McKinney repeated to his wife what he typically told critically ill patients: "God is with us all, under whose Protection I hope we may always remain."[37]

However awkwardly truth and truism mingled in these religious epigrams of practice, they provided doctors with their most expansive language for sympathy and concern for patients' suffering. Nothing in their schooling, or in their other topographies of meaning, came close to the sheer moral reach of religious words. " 'The cold, clear atmosphere of reason' may do for natural science," as one adviser warned in 1876, "but it will utterly fail where human nature is involved." Sympathy grounded in faith was fundamental to a doctor's ministrations, much like "the mother's kiss is often the sweetest balm for her children's hurts." Though vast, faith thus circled back to address—though not to interrogate—the deeply personal frame of solo practice. Despite the drugs and skills you bring to your work, one clergyman reminded physicians, in reality "you only bring yourself. . . . But you bring all of yourself—your integrity, your honor, your sympathy, your strength of heart, your courage, and your hope."[38]

Thus religious understanding may be seen as a key way—for many doctors, the central way—in which the local, personal context of physicians' work importantly shaped the overall meaning of their country orthodoxy. By belonging to patients, as well as doctors, faith became a major avenue by which vernacular meaning flooded into orthodox thought—diluting it, some physicians would say, or revitalizing it, in the view of many others. Certainly, the common language of faith undercut physicians' ability to alone control the definition of their "experience" and their professional realm. A Tennessee patient in 1838 took charge of his case when he directed his physician, who had become "baffled [in] his skill," to "pray the Lord to divert [your] mind to some article of [your] medicine] to afford relief." And yet faith allowed both patients and their doctors to accept worldly limits to therapy, to acknowledge failure, and to rely, as one sick man said, on "the will of God 'who pitieth us even as a Father pitieth his children.' " Patients thus tied their personal physicians, and the whole process of their relief and recovery, directly to God and his mercy. In this way, a North Carolina woman, like countless other patients, perceived her recovery as arising from "God's blessing on the means used by our kind Dr."[39]

Many physicians thus were strengthened in their daily work by a household's faith that renovated their own. Doing all that he could for his young patient, a Louisiana physician in 1865 concluded his labors by praying with the family. Together they implored God to let the boy recover; but even if his death were to come tonight (they prayed) "may [he] be a blessing to the family, in showing to them the power, the mercy, and the blessings of a Heavenly Master." Less evangelistically, but no less intensely, Lunsford Yandell was moved in 1824 to make some notes on what he called "the continuance of hope in Consumption" after visiting an old woman whom he believed to be dying but who nevertheless impressed him with her optimism and good cheer. Yandell paused to reflect upon what he perceived as a compelling mixture of faith and "fancy." His patient was staring at the very face of death, her body at its limits. "Her muscular energies are completely exhausted," Yandell wrote. "She has wasted away to a skeleton." And yet, ignoring the looming evidence of her mortality, she saw instead the continuity of life, talking to him about what she would do when she was freed from her illness. For her, Yandell marveled, "the torch of hope is still alive & appears to burn brighter & brighter as the prospects of success fade away," carrying her past the bonds of her sick body. Her faith counterpointed the doctor's slow relinquishment of treatment, showing him, he thought, how to let her go.[40]

A person's deathbed thus brought the power of faith to its sharpest focus as the occasion for witnessing and completion in evangelical Christian faith. Many physicians took the time to tell deathbed stories precisely for this reason. Lunsford Yandell's physician father admonished him to be receptive to the "solemn impression" of deathbeds, recalling his own youthful consternation when called "to the bedside of the dying before acquiring that familiarity with deathbed scenes which our profession necessarily intails [sic]." Death refreshed faith; deathbeds afforded not only hope but instruction. A South Carolina woman's grieving account of her mother's death nevertheless praised her deathbed as "truly an edifying scene." Another woman similarly related her friend's death as an event that "was my privilege to see." William Martin, though mourning his son's passing, wrote with pride of how the dying young man had calmly divided up his belongings among friends who were present, "talked much about the glorious prospects . . . [and] conversed with the utmost composure." Telling this story gave the father strength to believe that "my lovely son, 'is not dead but sleepeth.'" A friend told Eweretta Middleton about a young woman's deathbed where she asked people to pray with her, "took leave of all around her separately & with the greatest affection" and said as she died, "Oh how happy I feel."[41]

Such stories are remarkable for many reasons, not the least for how frequently doctors told them; their form and intensity changed little over the century. Physicians related them in much the same way as patients, including them even in medical journal articles. There were a few differences in detail; physicians seem to give more attention to bodies, for instance, describing how the dying person's "body was tossed painfully" or how "the last struggles were writhing the frame of [the] patient." But for the most part, the physician, like the patient, strove to turn death from the wordless horror of loss into a story of Christian triumph. Emerging from the drugs and the blood was the wisdom of recognizing earthly limits. Work hard for your dying patients, James Milligan urged his young physician son, treat them "carefully & kindly . . . and leave the event with God." An Alabama doctor acted the ideal when, after a frenzy of cupping and stimulating a dying young woman, he stepped back from the bed, saying to her, "Go to heaven, sweet sister." Thus the work of doctoring crossed into another realm. Young J. M. Richardson, after a night of fierce struggle to save a sick man, believed, at the moment of death, "the chariot of the Lord came, and his [patient's] spirit took its flight for eternal worlds, on the pinions of faith it soared."[42]

At the heart of these stories of release from worldly ties and bedside labors was the final convergence of spent bodies and spiritual peace. Dr. Samuel Leland's diary account of the death of a young man named Jacob combines these themes in a striking way, not least because Jacob was Leland's slave:

> We know not what a day may bring forth. Yesterday I recorded that my boy Jacob came home from the Rail road, sick. To day he is a corpse, and his soul is in Eternity. Poor fellow he had but short notice. . . . When I saw him he was speechless, and dying. The poor fellow though struggling for breath, when I exhorted him to turn his dying thoughts to the Savior, and request[ed] him, if he understood me, to squeeze my hand, he made every effort to do so. He was what the world would call a valuable negro. . . . But at this time, if I only knew that all was well with his soul, I would cheerfully resign his body. He was a Faithfull & honest servant, and I thought much of him.[43]

Leland's image of the two men holding hands at the moment of death is a powerful image of Christian faith crossing the gulf between slave and master. Even so, there is a striking turn of phrase that reveals how deep the gulf remained: Leland, hoping that Jacob was bound for heaven, says he would "cheerfully resign" Jacob's body if he could only be sure of the man's salvation. Before God, as before the law, Jacob's body was his owner's to release. Yet even this unconscious claim to mastery has ironic power, metaphorically uniting slave and master even as it divided them.

In all these ways, it was at once profoundly instructive and consoling—and, above all, shared with other Christians—to take the long view that in medical crisis, as in everything else, "at best the journey of human life is a journey of afflictions and trials" that "passeth understanding." No language better than the language of faith strengthened the continuity of meaning in everyday practice across the midcentury decades. From this perspective, an older Tennessee physician, looking back on his career, realized that while he had learned much about the particulars of biology and practical prevention of epidemic disease over the years, it was still best *seen* through the language of Scripture as " 'the pestilence that walketh in darkness, and wasteth at noonday.' "[44]

In a sense, this impulse to frame sickness with the larger truths of human life was the aim of all three expressions of expansive orthodoxy considered here. And yet, notwithstanding the energy that many physicians put into such writing, their vision was overmatched by deeply entrenched problems acknowledged but unsolved: southern social life continued to be fractured by isolation and disease; poisonous racial assumptions remained hidden in the remedies for slavery's ills; religious faith renewed hope but did not recast social vision. Nevertheless, despite these limits—indeed, because of them—each way of speaking broadly from his experience gave the physician a claim on orthodoxy's social worth. Each suggested that orthodox medicine's peculiar engagement with southern society and culture would clarify much broader prospects. Each allowed a practitioner the opportunity to inscribe the image of the Good Doctor on his practice, writing for himself an inclusive, stable meaning from the tenuous position of being both actor and witness. Immersed in the daily relations of his neighbors and slaves, friends and antagonists, the M.D. was able by these means to reach toward the wider fraternity of physicians, and then toward his community, for help and consolation. He was able to balance, for a space, all that might yet be discovered about the natural world, disease, and illness with the few things he knew for certain. By making these broad, social meanings from their work, physicians made their personal "experience" in medicine essentially, irreducibly moral.

For all of its potential, however, it was a troubling route to take into the heart of medical practice if one took it seriously. Many physicians, for instance, failed to take it very far into self-knowledge, or into the subjectivity of their patients, with the latter perhaps doctors' greatest failing as they struggled to believe in their own importance. It was a failure of imagination, among other things, and it helped to shape a more self-centered, inward-looking text to be explored in the final chapter. Not faith alone, and certainly not science, but plot-bound, personal stories of practice held the key—or, better, keys—to the troubled experience of being a doctor.

Chapter Eight

WITNESSING

In multiple ways—in school, at the bedside, at their most professionally expansive—physicians aspired to an overarching orthodoxy while invariably casting it in terms of self, locale, and everyday work. In all of these places and forms of practice, because physicians were such insistent writers of their work, they continually reinscribed the objectivity of someone else's sickness within the plane of their own subjective "experience." The case narrative was the physician's most sophisticated way of doing this. It brought together the essentials: a doctor's personal story of something gone wrong, peoples' debility and need, and his efforts to set things right. These elements acquired explanatory power in the way narratives joined observant science to a practitioner's self-disclosure, and, therefore, they were the most subtle instance of the homological relation of medical text and work. That is, narratives took their shape from the rhythm of practice and then validated practice by reproducing it as a text widely used by other doctors as both practical lesson and moral example. A close look at depth and variety of narratives serves to conclude this study, as these stories most fully capture the work-bound imagination of orthodoxy underlying physicians' allegiance to their personal style of practice.

Examples taken from practitioners' case narratives appear throughout this study, as illustrations of disease and therapy, as lessons learned and proof acquired. Prototypes of these stories took shape, as we have seen, in lectures, daybook notes, case histories, and physicians' correspondence. Narratives were published as stand-alone items in medical journals, but they also appear in the midst of larger essays on pathology or topography. Compared to other ways of writing medicine, narratives not only were more ubiquitous but also persisted longest over time. As important, they linked easily to other forms of personal storytelling in a century awash with novels, travel accounts, and personal memoirs. Borrowing from these, in fact, physicians' stories gathered up the cultural possibilities and wishes captured by medical work and lay them out to view. While narratives feature the doctor as active and initiating—indeed, in most cases, he is the center of it all—they also reveal him, ultimately, as a witness to all that he could not change.

This chapter explores the pivotal character of case narratives, first, by looking at them briefly for likenesses of theme and form, tying these to what we know about physicians' concern for their identity, their knowledge, and the moral scrim through which they saw their work. Then it looks closely at four doctors and the case narratives they chose to tell once upon a time. The aim is to conclude this study of the everyday practice of medicine in the South by airing its central themes—what country orthodoxy owed to the vernacular, the subjectivity of practical "experience," the physician's desire to be both distinct from his community and a moral force in it—not by way of a general synthesis but by entering more fully into physicians' own interpretive work; by telling stories about the storytellers.

CASE NARRATIVES: ORTHODOXY'S STORIES

It is not just that case narratives informed and entertained, though they did both. The more important point is that no orthodox text was more professionally authoritative throughout the mid-nineteenth century than the case narrative. Indeed, narratives drawn from an individual's practice were the featured genre of medicine's literature, and, as such, they came to represent physicians' peculiarly conflicted relationship with an ideal modernity that was itself in flux. The significance of narratives' central place in medical epistemology is illuminated by the contrast with what replaced them. By the early twentieth century, the intellectual authority of bedside narratives gave way to formal reports on research carried out in laboratories and generated by protocols created to control variables and systematically compare outcomes. Although case stories still flourished in personal correspondence and conversation, the professional demotion of the published case narrative meant that the orthodox writing that carried the intellectual weight of the new medicine became increasingly impersonal and divorced from daily caregiving. This new medicine, touted in terms of self-evident progress, valued certain things most rural doctors found difficult to acquire or accept: access to a laboratory, the instrumental abstraction of the body, and the muting of everyone's personal voice. But this particular view of progress drew upon only one stream of modernity at midcentury. Another was the stream that made personal writing so compelling generally in the mid-nineteenth century, a sense of the transcendent individual and the romantic adventure of character. Much about physicians' stories allowed them to belong fully to this equally "modern," subjective realm of imagination and self.[1]

The texture of personal experience—in particular, the case as part of the drama of the *physician's* life—was the essence of a narrative's medical meaning, as well as its larger meaning. In narratives, the individual practitioner was the active figure at the center of events, initiating and transcribing them: "March 16th, 1833, [I] was called before sunrise to visit a negro woman." "I took from her twelve ounces of blood." "I waited about fifteen minutes, when she had a severe convulsion." "I unloosed the bandage from her arm." The genre was willfully local and prized continuity. Narratives did not aim to transform the meaning of daily practice, nor even to standardize it; their consistent purpose was to represent its truths as belonging to the individual practitioner. At the same time, because stories invited the physician to wander curiously through the routines of his doctoring, narratives sometimes turned up new and unsettling meaning in the work he thought he knew well. As a result, through the free flow of case narratives, orthodoxy itself rode atop a sea of incidents, of "episodes," framed by plots and characters that compelled like those in history or fiction. Thus, doctors admired narratives as "interesting," a word carrying its full charge of both intellectual merit and entertainment, no matter that a great many stories had no particular lesson to teach, and certainly no scientific breakthrough to announce. Their interest was in how they made a conceptual world from the dramatic power of autobiography at the heart of every clinical tale.[2]

One kind of "interesting" story that appeared frequently in physicians' writing, published and unpublished, one that underscores the unabashed personal voice of narratives, was the call for help. This tale from practice was a kind of shout in the woods of everyday work, where the author told about a puzzling case in hopes of finding a reader who had resolved something similar. Consider Dr. Henry A. Ramsay's attendance on Ben, a slave living on a plantation near Raysville, Georgia—a young, strong man who one day came down with a chill serious enough to alarm his owner. Ramsay wrote about how he examined Ben physically in the usual way, noting his muscular body and generally strong constitution. Ben's abdomen was disturbingly unyielding to the touch, however; Ben said that he had been suffering pain from a blow he had received. Ramsay drew off a gallon of Ben's urine, gave him opium and calomel for inflammation, prescribed a warm bath, and left the plantation thinking matters well in hand. Returning the following day, the doctor was shocked to discover that Ben had died during the night. In his brief account, Ramsay wondered whether a diseased spleen (his tentative diagnosis of Ben's abdominal pain) might somehow be implicated. But the doctor did not speculate further on the cause of death or in any way develop his diagnosis. His purpose in writing was simply to call for help, hoping aloud that someone had the experience he could make use of next time: "Are such cases common? Could such a case have been remedied?"[3]

A related kind of "interesting" case that moved many physicians to write involved unusually stressful calls and, especially, times of failure. Like the call for help, the story of a runaway episode often had no specific advice or finding to relate. The sense of things being terribly out of control was the reason enough to write. Infused with personal drama of a trial by fire, such narratives rehearsed stories of doctors as embattled heroes. F. A. Bates's 1849 account of the scarlet fever that swept through his community was a story of general disaster but told in terms of *his* personal trial. He wrote of examining the distressed bodies of his patients and told of how he arrived at his therapy of "light" diet and mucilaginous drinks. He told of the rapid pulses of the victims, the "alarming diarrhea," and wrote, in summary of his overmatched experience, "Every effort was made to arrest this condition, but without avail. The hot air bath, frictions, enemata of tr. Opii, sinapisms, calomel and opium all failed." Similarly, the title of J. M. Hamilton's case story posed the agonized question, "How Long Shall We Wait" to crush the skull of an undeliverable fetus in order to save the life of the woman in labor. But nowhere in his essay did he answer—or even ask—this practical question. Instead, he simply told about his harrowing experience with a craniotomy he performed one day at a neighbor's.[4]

The autobiographical texture of such narratives and their emotional resonance are as tangible in case stories that have neither mystery nor disaster to relate but speak instead of the sheer strangeness of life opened to the physician's view. A doctor is summoned and finds something weird or amazing. Strangeness itself was a reality of medical work that needed telling. The doctor saw things not dreamed of in many philosophies, so he told stories of wonders: of a woman sickened by the "exhalations" of her husband's body; of a black woman whose skin was turning white; of a child born to a dead woman at her wake; of a man suffering a gunshot wound in 1840, with the bullet not recovered until his death twenty years later, when it was found in the chambers of his heart; of an unfortunate man who tried to cure his piles (as he said he read somewhere) by inserting a greased half-pint whiskey flask into his rectum.[5]

Most of these stories weave together distress, humor, and empirical observation, just as they were found in practice. Thus there also is an unmistakable moral edge to most of them, an opportunity for a doctor to witness and also judge the spectrum of human nature, which, inevitably, led him to test the moral quality of his own subjectivity. When Dr. Samuel Leland failed to arrive in time to assist a woman in childbirth, instead of *not* writing about it, he wrote a case story of the woman delivering her child alone; his main point: her courage was "some pumpkins!" and a moral inspiration to all. Like many other physicians, Charles Hentz praised patients for their willingness to undergo painful therapies, to be faithful observers, and to otherwise cooperate with him, just as he wrote stories to criticize "possuming" slaves and "shiftless" poor whites. And many wrote narratives as they pushed for reforms: the need for trained midwives, for example, or the importance of rethinking therapies that seemed not to be working.[6]

In all of these types of narratives, from calls for help to moral tales, the common thread was that the work of the physician as bedside witness was not complete until he became a storyteller. The autobiographical work-story thus became a kind of public testimony to the M.D.'s role as a trusted figure in the community. Moreover, even if there was nothing new to report, the story imagined the doctor's bond with brother practitioners separated by time and distance. Every narrative created an intellectual bridge between doctors' empiricism— their drive to collect and objectify—and their desire for moral esteem. Each one had the potential to make a practitioner's life and work consonant with the "modern" mid-nineteenth-century Romantic fascination with emotional life and the individual's struggle to find his identity. Seen in terms of the narrower, cooler twentieth-century professionalism that would replace them, however, stories that featured everyday work rather than the new, generalizable innovations of clinic and lab did not contribute to reform. In fact, individual stories held this new professionalism at bay.

Despite their roughness and apparent jumbled variety, most case stories were comprised of two narrative elements: patients' bodies and their biographies. As in doctors' bedside notes, certain aspects of the body and its corresponding products—blood, stool, and organs such as the tongue and skin—took on a significance that case narratives further underscored by developing them into stories with plot and context. Physicians wrote eagerly of their encounter with the body's signs and symptoms as a journey taken or a mystery solved. The body became a constant source of the familiar and the new. Patients' biographies are less clearly seen in narratives, mostly those aspects immediately transformed by injury or illness. But in writing a case, most physicians pulled scattered observations of a patient's family and habits into a sense of plot and characterization, a sense of *predicament*. Most—though not all—cases revolved around individual patients, usually identified in terms of race, sex, and sometimes family relationship (wife, son), though seldom by age, much as they were in bedside notes. And yet the crafted case story reveals interesting differences. Naming the patient in published narratives, for instance, exposed a tension between a physician's desire to be persuasive (nothing persuaded like authenticity) and his desire to be discreet. Empiricism's ethic of full disclosure conflicted with the dictates of modesty. Most doctors settled on the now-familiar convention of using a person's initial ("Mrs. A."), a device that clearly signaled sex and class and that sometimes took a graphic form reminiscent of fiction ("Mrs. F******* of Natchez"), almost enticing the reader to guess the patient's identity.[7]

However they were combined in a narrative, body and biography pushed the physician to tell about illness, as well as disease. Narratives opened easily to the subjective drama of lives altered by accident and suffering. The shattering biographical truth of illness was that it appeared out of the blue to physically strike a person down. The plot of case after case is that malady lay hidden in the folds of daily life in the South. As Hannah, a slave, was "lifting a heavy piece of timber, she felt something give way in the lower part of the abdomen." "Mrs. L****, . . . whilst stretching out a hank of cotton yarn, suddenly felt pain" in her arm, and now the "limb is painful and almost useless." Narratives are thickly populated with people like the Alabama merchant "sitting on a chair . . . his features greatly contracted, his countenance anxious," the young Virginian "scarcely able to walk about his chamber," and the woman Dr. J. S. Dyer recalled in 1852 only as "the misshaped patient." Transformed, too, was the physician's life. The steady flow of narratives tell a story of personal surprise and struggle that for a great many doctors never became too familiar to tell.[8]

Opening onto the life of the sick person, many narratives allowed family and friends to come forward, just as they did at the bedside. Here, too, the personal texture of people, place, and emotion afforded by the narrative's autobiographical form inscribed the individual doctor's sense of his social relationships as indispensable to medical fact. Many stories feature harmonious visits and grateful patients, doors swinging open, care embraced. But physicians also recorded their difficulties as outsiders seeking entry into people's homes and their trust. Frequently, his *not* belonging is what the doctor described. "When I walked into the room she looked on me with an eye of distrust," W. A. Shands reported of one new patient. Like Shands, many narrators were not at all reluctant to tell about their own relative powerlessness at the bedside. So William P. Hort related in 1847 his inability to follow a certain procedure because "the prejudices of the family . . . were very strong, and they would not tolerate it." Another practitioner urged the husband of a woman in labor to send for a consulting physician, but "the case being one of emergency, he declined calling in any other help" because it would take too much time. Though provoking great anxiety in the doctor, the husband's wish prevailed.[9]

Telling of such encounters bound the physician's sense of his work even more tightly to its local context, and thus to the immediate moral underpinnings of doctoring. Narratives underscored the central fact that medical care was made piecemeal by both physicians and others, and that no matter how much a doctor wanted his story to be about his competence, he told a tale of working in full public view, in need of others. Many physicians, like H. V. Wooten of Alabama in 1850, recounted cases in which they never spoke to the patient at all, gathering information from family, neighbors, and, in this case, even the patient's landlady. At other times, patients' own words break into the story with particular power. A white woman giving birth screams, "O Doctor, my womb is split, and I shall die!" Mary Ann, a slave, suffering in her labor, tells the doctor, "I want you to cut me open, and take out this little devil in my belly . . . for I am determined not to die." Such times were unforgettable moments in a physician's day, and in narratives built on autobiography, these personal moments became inextricable from his professionalism.[10]

Slaves appeared often in M.D.s' narratives; so often, in fact, that their presence in white medical storytelling was the greatest single social difference between southern physicians' narratives and those of M.D.s elsewhere in the United States. A physician in New York or Philadelphia might tell of an immigrant patient and urban surroundings, but so might a doctor in New Orleans or Baltimore; slaves' ubiquity in narratives was a constant reminder of southern distinctiveness. Slaves were portrayed in an importantly different way from most southern white patients, a way that reinforced how slavery made a slave's sickness refer to something other than her own well-being—to her owner's interest, for example, or his ability to pay, or his sentiment. Although the bodies of slaves appear in ways comparable to whites' bodies, slave patients almost always seem alone in physicians' narratives. Typically, even slaves who are given names and voices (as poor white urban hospital patients almost never are) have no friends or family around; white doctor and black patient are a lonely couple unlike any other in physicians' tales. Courtney J. Clark, for example, the observant writer of case notes, narrated in 1850 the case of an eighteen-year-old slave patient, Charles, in a way that shows how physicians' stories helped make African American social life irrelevant to whites. Clark portrays Charles in a lively way, which makes the young man engaging and sympathetic: the doctor knows Charles's medical past ("he has always been a very healthy boy"), reports Charles's self-assessments ("he felt better"), and gives his readers a vibrant, colloquial body ("his pulse was thumping away"). But no one else enters into this encounter. The doctor's thinking is not mediated in any way by family and friends, as it was in nearly all of the stories he told of white patients.[11]

While it cannot be known for certain whether Charles's friends and family were in fact nearby, it is certain that the collective effect of many similarly solitary slave patients in narratives meant that even though their bodies were closely seen, their biographies were scarcely at issue. Thus, the lives of slave patients, as inscribed by M.D.s, were comparatively atomized and physical, making it an easier matter for a physician to objectify and dominate them. In a striking way, then, the case story made explicit the disturbing reality that the doctor was not the *slave's* physician at all. He was called by the master and inscribed the slave's life as nested within the life of her owner. Others had no place in the plot. And so, in white physicians' narratives, African Americans were simpler patients who could never be as "interesting" as most white patients. Their illness did not compel the physician to achieve the precarious balance he established with white patients, between manipulating their bodies and acknowledging the context of their lives. He did not, through his story, invest his own life in theirs.[12]

Given this difference, however, the broad characteristics of all case narratives—slave and free—grew from, and reconfirmed, the consensus among physicians that an individual doctor's practice had unique explanatory power in medicine. Available to practitioners in various locales across a spectrum of experience, narratives were sown back into practice by physicians writing, reading, and using them as guides in the dreary-dramatic course of their daily work. This homological relation of text and work thus meant that the physician continually inscribed what he owed to the vernacular, as well as the professional, world. The narratives of the four physicians that follow suggest how the expression of this country orthodoxy was woven from both professional ideals and social context, plan and contingency. Indeed, narratives were compelling precisely because they were both inclusive and open-ended. They unified personal practice and abstract principle like no other device at an M.D.'s command by linking science to self-portrayal and making personal experience the main conduit for medical understanding. Telling such stories doubtless strengthened the resolve of many practitioners by infusing their work with intellectual purpose and a Romantic emotional power shared by other physicians. Simultaneously, though, because narratives reinvested a practitioner fully in the "usual" way of good practice—his personal way—they made orthodoxy indistinguishable from a man's sense of self-esteem and thus made change in orthodoxy all the more difficult to effect.

DR. PATTESON: TECHNIQUE AND TRANSCENDENCE

Consider, first, the cases of Kentucky physician A. A. Patteson, published in the *Transylvania Medical Journal* in 1850, which he assembled in order to argue for a certain way of treating cancer. All of the thirteen cases date from between 1847 and 1849. Although Patteson is not always clear just how he came to be at a given bedside, he seems to have met most of the patients in his own rural practice. And yet the prominent surgeon Benjamin Dudley makes an appearance in one instance, so it seems possible that Patteson may have kept a tie to his alma mater, the Transylvania school. This association would help explain Patteson's school-inflected effort to draw a general recommendation from his array of cases.[13]

This recommendation was that Patteson's fellow physicians be less surgical and more "expectant" in cases of cancer. And yet, as will be seen, Patteson's style of recounting his cases in strikingly different ways, which in turn suggested the different ways a bedside practitioner might engage with his patients, undercut his effort to draw a uniform recommendation from them. Most significantly, he became transfixed by the drama of one particular case, an instance of extreme suffering and the courage of religious faith, which pushed his call for expectancy into the background. This tension between Patteson's generalizing purpose and his fascination with a compelling individual tale need not be read simply as his failure to discover the modern clinical tactics of bedside emotional detachment. Rather, it is a story of the strikingly mixed meanings—intellectual, technical, moral—that a thoughtful physician encountered when he decided to narrate his work. It is Patteson's *choice* of conflicting meanings that matters; as he attempted to channel his cancer cases in a direction that would further the treatment of disease, he simultaneously chose to linger over a story of raw illness.

Each of Patteson's thirteen cases (ten of which were fatal) comprises a single patient; twelve white males and one black female. Not framing all of his cases by stating his argument for expectant surgery at the outset, he begins conversationally, as if in the presence of the reader, by expressing the modest hope that his cases will prove "of sufficient interest, and worthy of note." Then he simply launches into a description of his first case. We may highlight Patteson's thesis even though he did not. At the close of his essay he asks, a little defensively, "why this funereal array [of cases]?" The answer—his thesis—is twofold. First, he makes his argument for privileging expectancy over immediate surgery; in cancer cases, he believes he has shown, "surgery is disarmed of its skill" and only blunts the doctor's efforts to study the disease. He then argues that if cancer cannot be cured by the "purely local means" of surgery, then it must be seen as rooted in some "vice of constitution," that is, some hidden bodily fault that can be discovered only by careful expectancy. In all, doctors must risk failure, and see their failures as lessons; they must observe every bedside from a certain distance and with a level curiosity.[14]

This impulse foreshadows the twentieth century's "objective" mode of collecting and comparing cases. And yet Patteson's narrative style, deeply implicated in the particularity of each case, and in their strikingly different moral and emotional textures, utterly overrides this impulse. For instance, he clearly knew (and cared) more about some of his cases than he did others, and his writing accentuates this unevenness. One case takes up nearly one-third of the entire essay. At the other end of the spectrum is a case that reads, in its entirety, "A boy aet. 17, from Missouri, with Fungoid tumor of left superior maxilla"; it was a case tallied but one without a story. Like other authors, Patteson saw no reason to explain or excuse the marked variation in the length and detail of his stories. Indeed, the variation was one of the truths of everyday practice, and his essay was all the more lifelike and convincing because it inscribed it: a doctor saw some patients at length, others hardly at all; some patients stayed and talked, others left quickly; sometimes he attended, other times he consulted. In telling some stories at much greater length than others, then, Patteson drew upon the familiar continuity of this aspect of physicians' personal experience.[15]

At the same time, however, even though the succession of dramatically different stories might have convinced some readers that Patteson was right about expectancy, his essay pointed toward a different unifying center: the combined case narratives are a story about the doctor himself. They are held together by Patteson's autobiographical impulse to bear witness to what he has seen. Larger than the audience of fellow M.D.s was the surrounding community who feared cancer and surgery, and perhaps expectancy as well. Patteson's narrative style reached toward everyone's hope that suffering might be transformed into a significance far greater than the timing of surgery.

The longest of Patteson's cases speaks directly to this hope, a story that includes the usual clinical details but does not stop there; it is the story of Mr. K., but it is the doctor's story, too. Mr. K. was a man about sixty years old who came under Patteson's care when already grievously afflicted with cancer, and, in the physician's eyes, beyond recovery. Patteson's physical description is typically unsparing, even a little grotesque. Mr. K.'s cancer was in and around his eyes and sinuses. The tumor "sprouted" below his right eye, "rising up so as to obstruct the vision. . . . [B]oth nostrils were then filled by the morbid mass," which extended out of sight into the skull.

And yet it was not Mr. K.'s body but his character that most impressed Patteson. Mr. K. was remarkably composed and informative. "The patient expressed his opinion, confidently," the doctor noted with approval, and did not object to the painful physical examination. But it was Mr. K.'s deep religious certainty that most moved Patteson, and this faith was the heart of the story the doctor chose to tell. Mr. K.'s courage, even when "the last ray of hope" had vanished, and his calmness as "he awaited [the] result with the firm and cheering faith of a Christian" joined medical failure and moral lesson into a single, powerful outcome. The man's struggle went far beyond medicine; Patteson writes nearly a full page on Mr. K's waning days, which includes only one item of therapeutic significance (chloroform failed to check Mr. K.'s spasms). The main story to be told was not about disease or therapy but about witnessing courage and unshakable faith.[16]

Patteson thus does not spare his readers the horror of Mr. K.'s illness; indeed it *must* be told. Mr. K.'s tumor, some weeks after Patteson first saw him, had grown to such a size as to prompt seizures. It was not a struggle between equals; Patteson leaves no doubt that malady would win. But his readers must *see* the contest as he saw it, step by step. There is a sense that Patteson wished to contribute to both medicine and Christian faith by way of an unblinking portrayal of malady's ravaging physical work. In the grip of a spasm, Mr. K.'s "mouth [was] so drawn to the left, that the patient could only breathe by thrusting his finger between the lips and pulling with all his strength in the opposite direction. The disease gradually extended to the muscles of the neck and throat, and his attendants saw him often fall back upon his couch, literally asphyxiated." He lost his ability to speak or cough, enduring convulsions of his facial muscles, "which were so powerful as to shatter several of his large and finely preserved teeth." In all of this, Patteson's failure was complete. "Everything was tried that experience could suggest," he writes, but to no avail.

There were few realities of practice more familiar or more in need of saying than the point when a patient stood alone against the onslaught. Woven into the story of Mr. K.'s Christian fortitude is a tale of the doctor forced to step back and witness. At the end of the narrative, all Patteson can do is invite his readers to do the same. "Imagine a man weighing 220 pounds; of immense muscular development and not very fleshy; possessed of perfect consciousness, except when senseless from the immediate effect of a paroxysm—imagine such a man struggling with the desperate energy of despair against death from suffocation, and a faint conception may be formed of what this unfortunate gentleman endured through seven days and nights of ceaseless agony." The physician's narrative became a kind of deathbed homily, infused with images of the body and pain transformed, and the futility of medicine became a triumph of a different sort. In telling his story this way, Patteson glanced toward his medical brothers, perhaps hoping for a nod of fraternal recognition and sympathy. He went on to argue for expectancy. Yet the story of Mr. K. remains a story for everyone, told by the doctor as Everyman, a tale joining faith to the incontrovertible facts of sickness just as he had witnessed it. The patient was a powerful man. He was conscious, too, during the week it took for him to die. Imagine it.

DR. DOWLER: SCIENTIST AND COMMUNITY

A single, brief case narrative by Dr. Bennet Dowler of Louisiana in 1854 also concerns imagination and bearing witness, but in a different way. It suggests how a single case might linger in a practitioner's memory, mingling the moral and the contingent, to give him a sense of belonging to his community. Dowler's brief tale, about a drunken youth afflicted with intestinal worms, at first seems flat, then puzzling, and, finally, points to how a case might stretch far beyond the bedside moment in what it allowed the physician to witness and to say. Dowler's case appears as a separate article in a journal that he edited. The solitary nature of this tale is part of its appeal; it invites readers to look for a unique meaning. Also intriguing is that Dowler has nothing therapeutic to recommend and describes no diagnostic procedure. It reads as if Dowler had stepped out onto a lighted stage to show a small gem picked up in the course of his work.[17]

Strikingly, the events of the case took place twenty-six years earlier. Although Dowler says nothing about his intentions in telling his belated tale, regular readers of his articles in the mid-1850s would have been familiar with his forceful writing style and broad, ebullient interests. His rural practice had supported polymathic ambitions and made him an eager advocate for orthodox medicine as the bastion of science. The story of the worms is something else again, but not completely unrelated to Dowler's intellectual energy. He fearlessly entered into the vexing professional matters of his time, advocating reform in medical education and promoting the American Medical Association's attempt to shape a truly national profession. At the same time, he believed in the importance of a southern medical education for southern doctors, arguing in a way intended to turn southern characteristics—and stereotypes—to southern advantage. He maintained, for instance, that even though many outsiders thought the hot southern climate debilitating, the sunny South had the potential for the greatness historically found in hot-climate empires: "Warm southern climates mean men need to work less hard to achieve subsistence," he pointed out, and thus they have "more leisure for mental cultivation." He concerned himself, too, with the debate over the unity of the races, siding with those who believed that the Bible showed that the races were one. He rejected Louis Agassiz, Josiah Nott, and other dual creationists with the warning that "he who will not accept the Mosaic history, abandons the last plank, and must sink in hopeless uncertainty." Scripture, not man's feeble science, was the surest guide to mankind's progress through the dimly lit eons: "Will the remote past ever reveal to science the origin of the universe? The vibrating pendulum of eternity seems to answer—*Ever*? Never! Ever? Never!"[18]

Yet, within its worldly compass, science was man's greatest achievement. Dowler was irrepressibly curious about the natural world, proud that medicine led all of science into realms where empirical methods were busily dismantling ignorance. He was enthusiastic about meteorology, for instance, not only for its value in helping people understand their environment but also because its reliance on observation and record-keeping was proof that science "is becoming more *terrene*, and less celestial—less astrological." His empirical appetite was enormous, especially with regard to the study of animals, and he dissected everything from rats to alligators. After studying the mosquito, he wrote with typical enthusiasm that the tiny insect "is an encyclopaedia of anatomy, microscopy, physiology, and natural history," proof that "a thorough knowledge of a single species will serve as a key to the whole animal kingdom." His absorbing curiosities drew him into research both on and off his rounds. Picture Dowler keeping careful track of his body temperature with his new thermometer. He informed his readers in 1855 of how he went about it in his bedroom in the morning: "Jan. 19th, 6 A.M.—Room 54 ½ [degrees]; the left hand in bed, 100 [degrees]; arose, dressed partially, in 25 m[inutes], 90½ [degrees]; applied water at 53 [degrees] to the forehead, face, and opposite hand at intervals, sitting in a room at 62½ [degrees], the back towards the fire." And so he followed himself thermometrically through the day. Or consider how his treatment of sick slaves led him to argue that slavery was the salvation of Africans, giving them health and well-being through food, shelter, and Christianity. He concluded one essay with an avid image of "uncivilized" Africa, an image of catastrophic death and a weird mixture of places and times: "Pile up the pyramid of Negro Skulls *statistically* wasted in Africa, in the West Indies, and everywhere beyond the limits of the slave-holding States, and lo! the Bunker Hill Monument, and the Egyptian Cheops will be lost in its overshadowing shade. Mount upon this *golgothan* pyramid—and from its apex survey the vast *Acledama* around its base, which expands illimitably, save a single oasis [that is, the slave South] that rises to view."[19]

This was a man of enthusiasms, then, with a bent for didacticism and unwitting self-disclosure. Medical work put him at the center of many compelling issues and entitled him to be heard, he thought, in many arenas. And so it was that Dowler believed all physicians owed it to themselves and their fraternity to think big, to read beyond professional texts and, among other things, not to dwell on "tedious histories of cases *ad infinitum*." Yet the story of the worms is a case history. How did it square with Dowler's grand aims? In one sense, it might be seen as simply inconsistent. It is written in a more subdued voice than Dowler usually adopted; perhaps the doctor merely lapsed into the comfortable case narrative form. And yet it seems more likely that Dowler knew what he was doing and that the worms narrative may be read as of a piece with his passionate sense that physicians should use the bedside to look beyond it. The tale's simplicity nearly conceals what it most interestingly suggests—that physicians tell stories because they cannot do otherwise; stories seek them out.[20]

The worms narrative concerns the thirteen-year-old son of "Mr. B. and his lady, persons of good moral character" who related the events to Dowler about four months after their occurrence. The son "had been in bad health for a long time, and had undergone several courses of treatment under different physicians without relief. His disease appeared obscure—its seat uncertain." This changed dramatically, however, during a house-raising for the B. family when, during the course of doing their neighborly duty, the men in the party got themselves and young B. drunk. Made violently sick by the alcohol, the boy subsequently passed twenty or more intestinal worms, and in the days and weeks afterward, he gained weight and energy. Having succinctly related these events, Dowler turns from the B.s to describe the worms in close detail, for more than half of the space of this one-and-one-half-page essay. He then switches back to the house-raising scene by concluding: "Whiskey, for once, seems to have acted beneficially, having doubtlessly, in this case, proved detrimental to this nest of worms. The boy recovered his health rapidly after the discharge of these worms.—He removed, not long afterward, with his parents to the West. About seven years later I met with him in New Orleans, (in 1836,) in good health, pursuing his trade, in the saddlery establishment of Mr. John Hoey, on Tchoupitoulas street."[21]

A happy ending, it seems; but the story suggests more. Dowler was not the attending physician in the case, if there was one, and he did not personally witness the house-and-hell-raising affair that resulted in young B.'s fortuitous purging. Nor did he have any scientific point to make. To be sure, there is the lengthy description of the worms couched in the baroque language of the era's naturalism: the worms' "longitudinal band," "annulated articulations with acute margins," and "parenchymatous columns" are described with care. And yet Dowler readily confesses, as if he thought he might be asked, that he has never looked at the worms microscopically and so disclaims any truly new scientific knowledge of the creatures.[22]

The key to the story is the way in which it became Dowler's to tell. Some days after the expulsion of the worms, "they were delivered to me by the parents, inclosed in a phial of whiskey." The worms, he adds, are "still in my possession." Two simple acts, the boy's drinking and the parents' presentation of the worms, frame a moral story of a physician's work and self. It is not a story born of bedside heroics or calls for help; indeed, it is a story depending on a certain distance from sickroom preoccupations. The physician, his eye falling on a jar of worms he has kept over the years, is moved to tell a tale he alone is fitted to tell. It is a story about whiskey in people's lives, as a catalyst for misadventure, as accidental medicine, and as the final preservative of the boy's burden, the worms. It is a tale of irony resolving into a moral lesson; whiskey, that bane of community life, "for once" furthered something good. It is also a tale about past and present (the worms have been on the shelf a long time). It is thus about change but also about an even more remarkable continuity. At the heart of it is a story of the doctor as someone who can say something about how things turned out—something conclusive about such otherwise transient episodes. He knows about crisis but also about hope. He knows what happened to young B: the boy grew up, became a saddler at Mr. Hoey's establishment, here in New Orleans (I saw him).

Having the worms in a jar on his shelf, then, Dowler possessed the story, and in knowing the "final" outcome he claimed for himself the patient he never treated. He could do this because he was the community's man of science, the man people brought their worms to. People thought he might find a use for such artifacts, and he did. The physician's identity was inscribed by his knowing what to do with things expelled and preserved, relics and symbols. In Dowler's tale, doctoring becomes almost a pure tale of belonging to a community, the physician as witness to himself and to once upon a time among the people he served.

In both Dowler's and Patteson's narratives we can see how physicians pursued autobiographical means to plumb the deeper meaning of their "experience," thus inscribing the close bond between medical knowledge and self-knowledge. Dr. Patteson, intent on making a general argument about cancer and expectancy, nonetheless was swept up in the story of one man's illness. Dr. Dowler departed from his usual objectifying, reformist advice to reflect on what happened when he found himself in the aftermath of a medical event instead of in the midst of it, an event he discovered reverberating through his life for more than two decades.

The case narrative form thus tied the meaning of medicine to a grammar of personal satisfaction, ordering the cases and the chaos by way of the physician's subjectivity. Narratives kept orthodoxy in the known orbit of a man's personal, moral experience. At the same time, telling stories joined him to others riding the same stream of Romantic individualism shaping the sense of the modern embraced by country orthodoxy. Even so, such expression had its limits. The tale told by Dr. Lunsford Yandell, of Murfreesboro, Tennessee, in 1836, reveals how the narrative form might conceal or suppress. Although Yandell spoke as personally as any physician-storyteller, his narrative of cases of dysentery was much less self-revealing than it seems. In fact, his published narrative actually eclipsed a deeper personal meaning, restraining a fuller autobiographical tale by presenting him in the image of a certain kind of professional man.[23]

Yandell's article is titled "Cases of Dysentery, with Remarks," and by "remarks" he meant a pointed criticism of the standard therapy for dysentery. Yandell introduces his subject by saying that his own bedside failures had led him to doubt the accepted therapy. His tone is modest if somewhat foreboding. He had been reviewing his cases and now believes that there is a new form of dysentery abroad, one of "a very different character . . . , especially when it attacks children." In the face of failure, "a conscientious man will ask himself, why?" With this as an opening, Yandell brought forward nine of his cases in order to reflect on the standard therapy, one that employed "calomel and ipecac., in small doses. With . . . hot and stimulating applications externally." Heat was the key to the approved therapy, including hot compresses and warm drinks. Building toward his criticism, Yandell became more personal, recalling for his readers the especially sharp "feelings of mortification" he felt when two of his first dysentery patients died, adding, "I have experienced the same feelings since in a more intense degree." The attentive reader might ask what the doctor meant by this, and although Yandell did not reveal it, there was a reason: Case 7 was his son Willie, recorded only as "W. Y. a boy aet. 6 years, of robust frame" who sickened and died with a suddenness unusual even in dysentery and in the teeth of the standard "heat" therapy. Case 8 was Yandell's wife, Susan, and Case 9 a young female friend of the family, both of whom recovered, but only after the approved therapy had failed them, too.[24]

By silently including his family among his cases, Yandell secretly reshaped a tragedy that had changed his life. He rewrote the excruciating collapse of his family's happiness into a measured call for general therapeutic reform, obliquely airing his sorrow by muting its most disturbing resonances. This deeper significance of his narrative may have remained hidden, save for the existence of letters Yandell wrote daily to his wife's parents as he struggled to save his son's life. These letters show how his published narrative conceals, as well as reveals, and that as he strove to portray himself as a conscientious professional man he omitted much else from the purview of the Good Doctor. The effect was to close off certain avenues of work and autobiography, faith and family, and, perhaps most significantly, to efface the terrible contingency that could reduce to a shambles even the most devoted bedside care.

Transforming his son into "W. Y.," Yandell wrote his case narrative in standard body-and-biography fashion, stressing the boy's physical symptoms and the course of his rapid decline and fall. First there was a "slight" fever, on June 9, and Yandell, writing as if he were merely W. Y.'s physician, says he induced vomiting as a preventive measure and "that evening [he] appeared well." On June 11, however, the boy had "a bad night," vomiting to exhaustion. His limbs were cold despite the application of flannels soaked in hot spirits. "Thirst moderate," the doctor wrote in clipped, bedside-note style. "And drinks toast and slippery elm water, but asks for ice." Staying with the traditional therapy, Yandell did not give the boy ice but continued with the warm drinks and compresses. The subsequent course of events, which takes just under one page to relate, races to a terrible finish: "Great tossing . . . restlessness increasing. At 12 [midnight], becomes delirious. At half past 8 in the morning, dead." To the doctor, the boy's sickness seemed "extraordinary," beyond dysentery even, as if the patient had fallen "into the collapse of cholera," where medicines made not the slightest difference.[25]

Moving on to the next two cases, Yandell had a different tale to tell. "The mother of this little boy" (his wife Susan) and "Miss C." (their friend Matilda Cantrell) began showing symptoms just after Willie's death. But this time, shaken by the failure of the standard therapy, Yandell abandoned it at the pleading of his thirsty wife for water and ice. It was an "experiment," Yandell explains as he relates giving her ice and an "effervescing" drink of soda water. Amazingly, "after eating the first lump of ice [she] felt refreshed" and slept well. "The relief afforded by the change of treatment was instantaneous." He treated Miss C. in a similar way, and she, too, recovered rapidly. The hidden heart of Yandell's family story may be heard at this point in his published essay, beating just beneath his casebook style: he wonders, perhaps anticipating a question from an attentive reader, whether ice and the soda drink might also have helped "the little boy" in Case 7. While this "cannot now be determined . . . , it is impossible to repress a feeling of regret that the experiment was not made."[26]

Paternal grief, repressed into a professional's "regret" in his essay, bursts with full force from Yandell's daily letters—amounting to a kind of diary—which he wrote to his wife's parents during Willie's illness. The first letter, on June 12, was written "under the most painful oppression." Willie was "in the most imminent danger. . . . His death, in less than 24 hours, would not surprise me! . . . O Lord! have mercy on us." Yandell's next letter, the following morning, proclaims the loss even as it occurs: "Our dear little Wilson is still alive, but to all appearance, in the article of death! The trial to us is, indeed awful. Our hearts were bound up in the lovely boy." Then, in a postscript, "It is all over. Even while writing the lines within, he began to gasp for his last breath. He died at half past 8 in the morning—being 5 years, 11 months & one day old . . . I am unfit to add more—"[27]

However, in the two weeks following Willie's death, as he cared for his sick wife and their friend, Yandell wrote a great deal more, daily letters that rode three powerful themes effaced from his professional narrative. Two of these— themes of religious faith and family feeling—are the very substance of his letters. A third, more oblique, theme concerned the mundane work of doctoring as emotionally depressing and above all treacherous, a sense quite at odds with the brisk, problem-solving style of the published narrative. As we have seen, a great many physicians did not altogether omit such themes from their professional writing, especially allusions to religious faith. Thus the disparity between Yandell's letters and his cooler published narrative suggests how hard he must have worked to mute such expression, from guilt, as well as grief. Choosing a language that drew a sharp line between his experience as a physician and his emotions as a husband and father, Yandell held at bay the life-swallowing enormity of illness. At the same time, in rewriting his family catastrophe into a critique of orthodox therapy, Yandell shed light on the meaning of both.

In his family letters, both religion and family feeling gave Yandell a powerful language that reached out for an explanation large enough to match his loss. With Willie dying in the next room, Yandell wrote to invoke "the comforts of that hope which looks beyond the grave. . . . Thank God! if we may not hold the beloved one with us, we may go to where he will shortly rest." And yet, in the hours after Willie's death, Yandell was not consoled by his religion. Indeed, he feared that "having been so luke-warm a Christian," his own lack of faith might have "caused this blow to fall upon our lovely child." He knew he should not "murmur" against the will of God, but he felt "grief and shame" nonetheless that God may have taken Willie as chastisement. Here he folded his religious doubts into his longing for family to comfort him, urging his in-laws to immediately make the two-day journey north to Murfreesboro to join him. "Time, I know, is the remedy, but how slow!" he wrote. "How much we need your society to comfort us." The parents became part of his therapy, just as he had become part of his household's pervasive illness. "Susan, as may be supposed, is low spirited," he wrote eight days after Willie's death. "How consolatory to her it would be . . . to have the society of her mother." Two days later, as if his word were not enough, he wrote that Susan herself "bids me to urge you . . . to commence your journey without delay. . . . Impatience, you know, is almost inseparable from the sickbed."[28]

The contrast between these expressions and the published narrative suggests that even as the autobiographical case narrative furthered a kind of medical understanding that privileged—even celebrated—the personal context of a doctor's work, it was crafted to exclude other ways of self-awareness. For all of its personal framing, the published article nonetheless placed a limited, clinical vision of the boy's sickness at the center of the doctor's intellectual and emotional horizon; Yandell laid Willie to rest by bringing "W. Y." to life. The implications of this go beyond Yandell's personal saga to suggest the way narratives circumscribed a physician's identity more generally. Shying away in his article from the deeper, emotional reaches of illness—and in this way demonstrating the power of professional writing to limit in this specific way what counted as true medical knowledge—Yandell in effect devised a way to distance himself from similar loss and sorrow he had witnessed many times in the homes of other frightened and grieving families. To the extent that he may be seen as stepping away from the fullness of his own religious and family feelings, then, he removed himself from his local community, trading its emotional solace for the consolation of a comparatively remote professionalism.

Perhaps most intriguing of all the contrasts between his published narrative and his letters, however, is the way Yandell's narrative diminished a pervasive reality of everyday caregiving, which his letters exposed: the way in which bedside events could outstrip not only the physician's knowledge but also his energy and morale, deceiving him into a fatal misstep. As we have seen, many practitioners freely admitted their puzzlement and failure in their published writing. But Yandell's letters, contrasted with his narrative, suggest a dimension of this experience that crafted narratives did not explore directly: the treacherous contingency at the heart of all that the physician tried to do with the bodies and needs of sick people. Orthodox therapy, that is, ultimately depended on the physician as opportunist, alive to the possibilities of the vernacular setting in every new encounter with illness. Giving care in the midst of happenstance and error was as essential to the doctor's identity as knowing the action of a drug or the location of a vein. Thus it was as important to avoid being stupefied by detail as it was to be careful in interpreting it, so that the saving insight might be recognized and seized.

In his article, Yandell portrayed himself at work in a way so essential to narratives that its artifice went unrecognized. He inscribed himself as the professional in full stride, not always knowing the answer but always in charge of the process: he "determined" actions; he "instructed" his patients; he "ordered" things to be done. But who was carrying out these directions? From his letters, it is clear that Yandell was doing most of the tiring work himself, certainly after his wife also became sick. He once notes consulting a medical colleague (who does not appear in the essay), and he may have had a slave assistant, though none is mentioned. Thus Yandell, like most rural doctors fully engaged in the care of a "dangerous" case, worked through all phases of caregiving, sleeping only when his patients slept, and giving in, as they did, to the rhythms of their illness.

The nature and course of the disease, too, are cast in a much more problematic light in Yandell's letters. In the published narrative, dysentery is a cleanly identified foe, epidemic in scope and consistent through all nine cases. But in his letters, Yandell was struck by the oddness of the affliction, which "seems almost confined to my family." Moreover, his need for advice and help, freely expressed in his letters, and his willingness to adopt therapies suggested by his patient— such as the water and ice—contrast sharply with the comparatively passive patients of his article. In sum, the cool physician of the published narratives is revealed as a man wholly swayed by the feelings and suggestions of his patients. The letters clearly show that the physician's most powerful bond with his patients was the mystery and subjectivity of illness rather than, as the essay would have it, his orchestrated attack on disease. Illness oppressed everyone. "We are, indeed, in great darkness," Yandell wrote on June 21. "And, like dying men, catch at straws to keep our hearts from utterly sinking." After more than ten days of catching at straws, the doctor craved release. "I want occupation," he wrote. "Books do not interest me, as formerly. . . . Thus depressed, I do not afford that salutary excitement which flows from a bright countenance & cheerful manner."[29]

Yandell's letters, drafts of letters, and bedside notes, lying among the medicines and instruments on the bedside table, became part of the clutter that washed back and forth between despair and hope. Their very roughness, the scratched-out sentences and altered ideas, is a transcript of his struggle to anticipate and control the contingencies of giving care. Here, finally, Yandell's letters reveal something central about his therapy that he let slip through the looser weave of his published narrative. In the latter, Yandell's discovery of the soda-and-ice treatment is the moment of revelation; this therapy was his shining ally in the last two cases, and indeed its discovery prompted him to write the article. Recall that when his wife's symptoms had reached "an alarming height," the first piece of ice gave her "instantaneous" relief. In the letters, however, the ice-and-soda drink has no such fanfare; he notes merely that it made Susan "much more comfortable." This therapy followed others, and it seemed likely that others would follow it. Rewriting events into a narrative, though, called for turning points and climaxes; what had been only dimly seen or inadvertently discovered was inscribed in the narrative as an insight boldly seized.

But was the ice and soda an accidental find? Like so many physicians, Yandell did not explain, in his essay, what led him to try a particular therapy. Yet among Yandell's letters are a few notes from Willie's last days suggesting that the provenance of this new therapy lay in the implacable contingency of events, insights, and timing that seethed around every bedside—and just below the surface of every narrative. As he wrote his daily letters, Yandell also recorded some of his son's last words and moments. "I'm sick so often," Willie said at one point, and, prefiguring Yandell's own judgment that the boy's affliction was more cruel than ordinary dysentery, "I expect I'll have smallpox next and then cholera—and that is worse than any, isn't it Pa?" Yandell told of how he carried Willie to the window to watch a parade of militiamen and of how "his last effort to rally was on Sunday, in the afternoon when he heard his puppy bark. My darling boy Wilson." Most terribly in retrospect, Willie said, "Pa couldn't I have a little ice?" But the physician, staying with the orthodox therapy, said no, even though Willie allowed it could be "a piece so small that you could hardly see it." The moment for therapeutic discovery came and went. Yandell's published narrative drops only the barest hint of its passage: "[He] drinks . . . slippery elm water but asks for ice." Later, his wife asked for ice, too. Thinking it over, watching Susan recover, and then writing his essay, Yandell buried the terrible misstep he had taken by not listening to his son.[30]

Reading the letters across the grain of the published narrative, then, we can see that even during the years that it flourished as an authoritative text, the physician's autobiographical case story diminished certain ordinary yet far-reaching aspects of the everyday practice from which it grew: the drudgery, the guilt, the wavering sense of Providence, the accidents. Yandell's writing suggests how and why physicians let these things fall out of their stories. The more fully autobiographical a doctor became in his narratives, the more he called attention to the chaos that surrounded all caregiving. An overly detailed account of practice allowed contingency to define not only medical science but also the substance of professionalism, and even one's own moral striving toward better health, better understanding, and better care for one's community. It revealed even the active, hopeful doctor to be, after all, no more than a witness. In the face of this, finding the right words for opportunities missed or chances not taken was too daunting a task. And so physicians like Yandell came to limit the personal disclosure at the heart of their medical tales. These limiting measures would grow and toughen by the end of the century, as physicians began to see that a new kind of professional authority—impersonal, objectifying—would be enhanced by further loosening the tie between work and self.

DR. BASSETT: THE ECLIPSE OF THE PROFESSIONAL

Even at the height of their professional influence, as all three of the foregoing stories suggest, case narratives had a more problematic relation to the identity of orthodox practitioners than it might at first seem, given physicians' eager traffic in stories throughout the century. With their moments of drama and respite, and with their portrayal of medicine's social engagement, case narratives supplied reasons for orthodox ways while hinting at truths beyond reasoning. At the same time, however, case narratives were so personal and elastic that they sometimes led a practitioner (Dr. Yandell was one) to arrive at the abyss of illness and face the depths of what he could *not* do or say. Either way, though, whether they resolved conflicts or stirred them up, narratives remained so commonplace that doctors accepted their influence without much scrutiny, thus obscuring the intellectual consequences of relying on a literary form that imagined the meaning of individual practice in terms akin to the emotional power of fictional tales.

The main consequence was that the texture of an individual's practice continued to be the touchstone for everything admirable in orthodox medicine, tempering any change that challenged the sway of personal experience. In this sense, narratives were among the central achievements of orthodoxy, though they were scarcely acknowledged as such. Instead, end-of-the-century elite reformers effaced the power of personal stories by portraying orthodoxy as riding a tide of preeminently impersonal laboratory-based science and institutional care sweeping all before it. In doing this, reformers not only pruned back the complex, locally rooted history of all medical care, they also facilitated the transfer of a doctor's allegiance from his daily work in a community to the new bastions of professional power in hospitals, laboratories, and schools. By the turn of the century, in fact, professional leaders were giving accounts of their immediate forebears that portrayed them simply as willing players in the rise of the new, objectifying medicine, largely by erasing the physician's deep— and deeply conflicted—personal ties to his local community and to vernacular caregiving.[31]

The significance of this transformation of country orthodoxy—and the importance of narratives generally—may be seen in the way one mid-nineteenth-century southern practitioner's case narratives vanished from his story as it came to be written by one of the foremost leaders of change at the end of the century. The practitioner in this instance was John Young Bassett, born in 1805, graduating with his M.D. from Washington Medical College, Baltimore, in 1828, and, after spending some months in the Paris clinics, returning to wife, family, and practice in Huntsville, Alabama, where he worked until his death from consumption in 1851. His memorializer was Sir William Osler, professor of internal medicine at Johns Hopkins University, the very seat of modern medicine, where he and his colleagues did more than any other group of M.D.s in the early twentieth century to reconfigure orthodoxy in the ways that became axiomatic to its authority: as rooted in institutions, founded on systematic basic science, and embodying a broad public interest that entitled M.D.s to exclusive license in the provision of medical care. A look, first, at Osler's story of Bassett and then at Bassett's story of his own struggles reveals the extent to which Osler rewrote his subject to facilitate a re-imagination of modernity. He did this in a way that reveals how the case narrative, as the fundamental imprint of a mid-century practice mentality, was the device that reformers like Osler were eager to overcome.[32]

One of the ways William Osler sought to remake orthodoxy, which was part of his larger effort to reform medical education, was to be a public spokesman for its values and its history. In lectures to students, and in essays and sketches published in medical journals and elsewhere, Osler tirelessly described the habits of intellectual and moral character that made for a good doctor, including an interest in the medical past. One piece of Osler's historical writing that became a classic in American medical education, and indeed in American medical history, is his 1896 essay "An Alabama Student," a staple of medical student reading well into the twentieth century. "An Alabama Student" was not, strictly speaking, about a medical student, but about an established (and "forgotten") physician a half century earlier—John Young Bassett—who continued to teach himself about disease and his profession despite the huge difficulties of doing so in the antebellum South.[33]

The essay, feeding a vision of an immediate medical past struggling to become what Osler wanted it to be, inspired many other physicians as well. In 1906, Osler wrote to one of Bassett's daughters, who had given him letters from her father, "I do not think that anything I have written is so frequently referred to by my correspondents as the sketch of your good father. It seems to have appealed to a great many people." Osler elsewhere described his discovery of Bassett, whose medical topographical writing he came across by chance, as an immediate and pleasurable shock of recognition. Bassett's topographical eye revealed him as nothing less than "a 'kindred to the great of old'" who seemed almost godlike in his "'likeness to the wise.'" In short, Osler seized upon Bassett as he might an ancient kinsman; as a relic and a prophet, one deserving honor because his life wonderfully incorporated the qualities of focused inquiry and sound judgment that were the harbingers of the new medicine now being realized.[34]

If anything, Osler's fascination with Bassett was enhanced by the southern context of Bassett's practice, which Osler, of course, would have seen in the context of the 1890s: a South staggered by the social tensions following from the Civil War, emancipation, the failure of Reconstruction, and hard economic times. Indeed, there is more than a hint in Osler that the southern cast to Bassett's struggles against isolation and ignorance was especially significant; there was no isolation like southern isolation. It is not that Osler misses Bassett's mistakes or portrays him as a saint without a temperament. But Bassett's redemption from obscurity was essential to Osler's writing; his story was "the story of a man of whom you have never heard, whose name is not written on the scroll of fame, but of one who heard the call and forsook all and followed the ideal." Men like Bassett, "these 'mystics' and 'chosen' are often not happy men," Osler admitted. But they were "restless spirits who . . . had ambition without opportunities" and proved that ambition was enough. The significance of Osler's Bassett was that he was motivated solely by an avid curiosity and an inductive intelligence that pointed him toward a certain vision of the modern. The "humble" lives of such men, if clearly seen, "may be a solace" to young twentieth-century physicians stepping into a very different world of practice that promised everything Bassett did not have: effective therapies, institutional authority, and the broad intellectual landscape of modern science.[35]

Yet Osler's view, for all of his liberal reading of Bassett's published topographies, strikingly ignores the *means* by which Bassett told about his practice, that is, by way of case narratives. Twenty cases roll by in Bassett's twenty-six-page 1849 topographical essay, for instance, but none is remarked upon by Osler. Bassett spoke through case stories drawn directly from the depth and texture of community life and his edgy, sometimes cynical, view of its medical politics. But Osler, eager to record Bassett's "discoveries," and himself still too close to the storytelling mode to be fully aware of it, comes close to making him Everyman and Huntsville Everyplace. Charmed by Bassett's eye for "modern" science, Osler overlooks Bassett's voice as a man of his town and his times.

In fact, the driving force behind Bassett's stories, especially those in his 1849 topography of Huntsville, is his desire to expose a vicious and venal community that has thwarted good medicine. Although Bassett was not without empirical curiosity, his narratives are mostly fueled by accounts of people's foolishness and corruption, against which Bassett portrays himself standing alone. Irony is Bassett's métier; he writes as a practitioner whose skills are far from exhausted but whose forbearance in the face of popular disrespect has about run out. His town's founders, whom he deflates as "squatters," set the moral tone for everything that followed: "They had the piratical appetite for gain natural to the English race . . . and they readily acquired the Indian taste for blood." Social life by 1849 was not much better, at least when it came to citizens making rational judgments about their health. Bassett's case narratives are a moral indictment of reckless, self-destructive behavior—sick people staying out in the night air, self-medicating to the point of suicide, refusing to help neighbors—and the lingering taste for violence. In one story, two quarreling caregivers agree on only one thing—the patient must be bled—and they compete to see who should have the grisly pleasure of doing it. Many of Bassett's cases similarly seem to have no other purpose than to expose Huntsville as a place where the practice of good medicine is impossible. Though straining toward some implicit idea of good medicine, the narratives are powerful not for their vision of reform (as Osler would have it) but for their portrayal of a man completely preoccupied with the discontents of his local practice.[36]

Other doctors, too, are fully implicated in Bassett's picture of willful ignorance and self-interest. His critique of alternate healers—chiefly Thomsonians—is not surprising, except that the wealthy are among the malfeasant; Thomsonians are "generally discontented and indolent mechanics, unemployed overseers, with a few illiterate preachers, and many respectable planters . . . in the habit of thinking for themselves in politics and religion" and thus in medicine, too. But M.D.s, too, are portrayed as corrupting good medicine. They defy expectancy and resort to the knife too early. Surgery in Bassett's tales emerges as a kind of local sport in which most M.D.s participated. In one such case, doctors arrive at the scene of a man wounded by a gunshot. As they debate the wisdom of surgery, the crowd around the victim urges them to the knife, pushing the doctors to "cut it out" without delay. Another such narrative opens with a sense of rushed, case-book immediacy: "A row at the 'Bell' [inn]—a man stabbed—Dr. O. called in." There never is a chance for a serious, professional operation; Dr. O., "praised like a new preacher" by the bystanders, responds by wading into his crowd-pleasing role with lancet and saw. The "wound was too deep for him," Bassett observes, but Dr. O. kept at it, "probed away and said nothing," until at last, "the doctor reeking with blood pronounced the wound mortal!"[37]

In short, Bassett was relentless in portraying local "care" as doctors merely pandering to a popular thirst for the high drama of big doses, sharp knives, and blood. Indeed, his 1849 essay originally included a conclusion so harsh that the journal's editor deleted it. The bitter summing up, as he explained to Bassett, coming after so much criticism already in the bone and sinew of the essay itself, seemed "calculated to be very injurious to yourself . . . [and] *no matter how true*, would be very offensive to your fellow citizens." He counseled Bassett, "It would be useless to make enemies & vain to attempt to castigate a haughty & independent community into better manners, morals, or intellectual culture." This, of course, is exactly what Bassett was using his cases to do. He grasped a fundamental aspect of being a physician—the particular knowledge of sickness as a moral register—and used it as a weapon against a community whose ignorance swamped the better instincts of the fraternity of M.D.s. Nor did he exclude himself from the general demoralization of medical practice, writing bitterly of his own "folly" in going against " 'the throned opinions of the world.' "[38]

Bassett's ripe stories, which are at times more yearning and conflicted than he might have admitted, suggest that local practice left unfulfilled two wants of a doctor in search of the crucial link between work, knowledge, and profession. In wishing to supply these wants, Bassett was not wishing for an entirely new medicine, as Osler implied, as much as he wished to find satisfaction in the kind he knew how to practice. The first want was not being able to practice "expectantly" as a man of science ought. Nearly every story about his community's ignorance concerns the evil that followed from physicians jumping into a case with drawn scalpels because they feared rivals and popular pressure. In Bassett's view, traditional "heroic" practice was wrong not because of its large doses or toxic medicines (he clearly used both) but because it was *hasty*, unreflective medicine. In this context, country orthodoxy was revealed—quite accurately—as springing from the popular impulses many M.D.s loved to scorn but in fact embraced. Tied closely to the frustration at not being able to control the timing of his work was Bassett's sense of being an outsider in his community more generally, despite his efforts to belong. In Bassett's tales, the physician attempting to deliver medicine based on serious study and professional esteem, was invariably viewed with suspicion or outright contempt by his fellow citizens.

Seen this way, Bassett's self-image as a solitary man singlehandedly keeping alive the ideals of good medicine may seem on the surface to be something like William Osler's image of him. Yet Osler's Alabama Student is a "mystic," whereas it is clear that Bassett was avidly, even desperately, attempting to inscribe how to belong to the community and embrace the country orthodoxy he needed but despaired of. Abstracting Bassett from his cases, Osler made him a simple prelude for Osler's own time, holding him up as an "even-balanced soul who 'saw life steadily and saw it whole.'" By returning Bassett to the heated world of his cases, it is possible to see that even though broad reform mattered to him, he was constantly drawn into (or *jumped* into) the compelling local setting for his large ambition: the power over bodies and the means of altering them, the fit between orthodox and community values, and the making of trust in a social world that belied it.[39]

Bassett's struggle with his community—a struggle over who should define the essentially moral meaning of a doctor's "experience"—is perhaps best seen in Bassett's narratives by looking at the longest case story among them, one which engaged with the Christian context of practice. Osler refers to this narrative but skirts the religious meaning that Bassett made central to it. Indeed, imagery drawn from the Bible colors Bassett's language throughout the essay in a way Osler either ignores or misses entirely. This may be because Osler himself lived in a professional world that remained openly, if uneasily, attached to Christian values and allusions. Indeed, "The Alabama Student" begins with an gently ambivalent allusion to "the Gospel," which, Osler observes, teaches that the spirit of self-sacrifice required of a healer is the same spirit "responsible for Christianity as it is—or rather, perhaps, as it was." He thus quickly historicizes Scripture into "ideals," placing Christianity at just the remove where it gives off a soft, inspirational light but no more.[40]

Christian belief, in its pervasive social influence, as well as its inspirational light, emerges as far more problematic for Bassett in his long case story of a slave woman and her difficult childbirth. This tale is more than twice the length of any other narrative because Bassett uses it to leap into the fierce, unresolved, and widespread debate over whether physicians were morally right to use the new anesthesia to numb the pains of childbearing women. The central question, much debated with clergymen and in the orthodox profession at large, was whether the biblical description of women as bound to give birth "in sorrow" was a proscription on anything that would lessen a woman's pain in labor. Osler only briefly mentions Bassett's taking up this issue (he omits, too, that the patient was a slave), describing it as "a very clever discussion," as if the matter were merely a quaint episode. He portrays Bassett as above the debate and obliquely criticizes midcentury clergymen who forced physicians to "logic-chop" theology at the bedside.[41]

In fact, Bassett was eager to logic-chop theology, aggressively asserting his view of the Bible, women, and physiology. He clearly welcomed the opportunity to argue the anesthesia issue as a matter of both scientific learning and community leadership. Bassett maintained, first, that the new anesthetics were not essentially different from the old ones—opium and whiskey—still much in use, and not only by M.D.s. Thus he suggests (and this *is* a clever dig at ministers) that in intruding upon doctors' turf, clergymen were in fact meddling with folkways. And when it came down to whether the people or their ministers knew more about what people needed, Bassett was delighted in this instance to show that he sided with the people. Even more striking, though, Bassett waded into the scriptural debate with gusto, parsing Hebrew text for the meaning of "pain" and "sorrow," quoting biblical commentary, and expounding on what Solomon, David, and even God most likely meant. He concluded with a more secular view of the matter, arguing that everyone would be better off if they embraced biblical values but historicized biblical events ("when Moses recorded that in sorrow Eve should bear her children, it had no reference to chloroform"). And yet, at the same time, he kept scriptural references alive in his own language, describing, for instance, his arguments for the importance of labor pain as "add[ing] my testimony to David's." In short, Osler notwithstanding, the religious context was anything but "clever" play for Bassett, who, in entering into the language and logic of this debate, reveals with particular clarity how important it was for him to be heard in his community and to belong to it. Although he took the view that medicine was best left to physicians, he did so by acknowledging the larger truth that the issues of God and pain, women and sin, were the moral center of childbirth and fittingly a matter for everyone's concern.[42]

Bassett's acid tongue doubtless worked against his being embraced by many Christians and accepted into his community as he wished, but it is not unusual for someone longing to be loved to be harsh with those who do not see his desire. Religious belief inscribed the widest circle of belonging in southern communities, and in worrying religion in his narratives Bassett showed how much his own personal ambivalence in matters of faith cost him as a both neighbor and doctor. "Dying men will have their pills and parsons," he wrote wryly of the link between medicine and faith. But when he himself was dying of consumption in 1851 he was not so aphoristic. In letters to friends, Bassett wrote another case story—his own—of approaching death, its relation to medicine and to his lack of faith. Now that he himself was seriously ill, he said with a dose of self-mockery, he saw how true it was that death was not to be resisted; yet it still had to be placed *in life*, his life.[43]

Troubled by a debilitating cough, losing weight rapidly, Bassett knew he was looking askance at a diagnosis he would have been quick to make in another. Indeed, he realized that he "intentionally stood off" from his symptoms, as he wrote to a colleague. But diagnosis would out; naming malady was a social affair after all: "[M]y friends began to say Consumption—well says I, Consumption then." In New Orleans, he asked E. D. Fenner to examine him, and Fenner "tapped me slightly on the breast and listened there a few moments, then looked me in the face with the same deep expression that my wife had when she said Consumption & and said *Consumption*." Not a colleague, but Bassett's wife, Isaphoena, became his doctor after he admitted his illness to himself. Bassett declared himself a tolerable patient, not least because he did what all patients do, which was to pick and choose which therapies suited him, never mind the advice from experienced healers. "[M]y wife took charge of the case aided by numerous voluntary sisters of Charity, with their *Liverwort* & *Tan* and *Cod Liver Oil* which was kindly received but not taken."[44]

And yet the shortcomings of medicine, which he knew all too well, did not trouble him in the final months of his life as much as the puzzles of faith. Talking about religion with his friends—mostly about his lack of belief—was more important than what was happening with his body, which he believed he understood. "I am aware I am not a christian," he wrote to his old friend George Wood in April 1851, "however much I may have for a long time past desired to be. Indeed sir if I possessed the faith which you have this day declared, nothing could add to, or take from, my happiness. Why do I not then?" Bassett could not answer his question; he could only point out, good empiricist, all of the reasons he *should* possess faith—reasons tied to his yearning to belong, to be inside a fellowship. "I am living in a religious community, my wife is a truly religious woman, my pastor is pious and learned, a most refined gentleman and my personal friend. I keep no irreligious company, am not afraid of the opinion of any man, and desire to be religious. I do not understand why I am not religious any more than I do why others are."[45]

Still, Bassett continued to strive for faith, though the irony of his seeking a deathbed conversion did not elude him. He worked at it as he had worked at discovering the course of a disease in a patient. But, as he told Wood some weeks later, "My own efforts are as fruitless as those of my friends. I lack belief." He turned instead to what he knew best as a doctor, which was death. "I have no moral or rather intellectual dread of Death," he wrote. "The raw head & bloody bones distroyer [*sic*] of the nursery has long since vanished from my imagination. I regard Him as the door to immortality. . . . I have times out of memory personified him as he came toward me over the hills. . . . I do not care whether he comes today or tomorrow—or next week. I know he will not break his word." In the meantime, Bassett lay back to witness the rounds of other people coming and going from his bedside. He knew his family and "some few friends" would miss him, and he them. "Yet I am cheerful & on the whole have reason to be. Most of my fellow citizens sympathize with me, my professional brotherhood have kindly divided my practice in a certain inheritance among themselves, my wife, children, & servants are particularly kind in small matters, receive me respectfully when I approach & look after me sorrowfully as I pass, as though I were sort of a respectable ghost—out of sight, out of mind—as soon as I vanish my orders are forgotten, at least neglected, & this makes me laugh."[46]

When death came, medicine moved on. Doctoring was a transient thing, taking its cue, finally, from the turn of events it only minimally shaped. Telling case stories was the surest way for the physician to imagine anew the constant transition in medicine from acting to witnessing and back again to action. In this way, mid-nineteenth-century doctors acknowledged the reality that practice was made from countless moments of engagement and release. Shuttling between the two was possible, even exciting; but it was troubling nonetheless, because it made the professional man a transient, too. Writing himself at the center of every narrative countered this impermanence. The story a practitioner most desired to tell was one that put him into the light, at center stage, his experience illuminating the prospect of all medicine.

In thus merging stories of self with the substance of orthodoxy, physicians played out their version of mid-nineteenth-century moral purpose and individual style, writing themselves into the era's Romantic imagination of modernity. In this sense, few scenes in mid-nineteenth-century American life were as compelling as those that told of the struggle against malady. The century's man of action and sensibility was at home here if anywhere, a place where personal character engaged with events urgent and material: stopping the blood, getting the baby out, doing something for the pain. More, doctors and Americans at large knew the sickroom as a cultural stage of another kind as well, a place of exhausted options, of everything going silent, and hoped-for salvation. Thus, ordinary physicians at work—and writing their work—shed light on these two great planes of cultural experience in the nineteenth century, ambition and release. Telling stories, they wrote and rewrote this tale about themselves many times over, whether in frustration and conflict, or in amazement, or with the satisfaction at having diverted malady from making another conquest. Doing their orthodox work, they discovered (and sometimes embraced) that the essential meaning of their medicine arose not from precept or technique but from how they were able to tell the story of their lives.

THE CIVIL WAR AND THE PERSISTENCE OF THE COUNTRY ORTHODOX STYLE

In this study, the mid-nineteenth century has been weighted toward the years before the Civil War. And yet, as noted at the outset, this should not imply that the essentials of everyday rural medicine changed sharply after the war. Although the conflict altered the lives of many individual practitioners, most ordinary physicians in the 1870s and 1880s held on to the central expectations and practices at the heart of antebellum country orthodoxy. Indeed, the persistence of the country orthodox style of practice through the Civil War is testimony to the depth of its antebellum influence and thus a good way to sum up its significance in a southern setting.

Older assessments of the Civil War's effect on medicine tended to highlight certain wartime innovations—in surgical or sanitary techniques, for example—which went on to influence turn-of-the-century advances in medical care. The current view of the war's consequences is broader and far more mixed, especially for the South, calling into question the once axiomatic link between war and "progress." Two related themes have emerged. The first is that mass casualties and a shockingly wide variation in doctors' skills impressed at least some physicians with the inadequacies of their standard therapies, especially the use of the mainstream, "stimulating" drugs like calomel and alcohol. Even so, most war-bound physicians did not radically innovate with their medicines. Instead, as John Harley Warner has suggested, wartime therapeutics may be seen as bringing antebellum orthodox therapy to its "fullest fruition." The second theme concerns the small but important number of physicians and nurses who emerged from the war to campaign for public hygiene, education reform, and the development of sophisticated, multipurpose hospitals. No simple route to progress, the reforms were hard-fought. And, as Charles Rosenberg has argued, in terms of hospitals, the war's specific effect was "substantial but elusive," less a source of wholly new ideas than an impetus to antebellum reforms such as "expectant" care, ventilation, and orderly record-keeping.[1]

Despite this new sense of complexity, medical historians have not paid much attention to the war's impact on everyday illness and medical care in southern communities (or northern ones, for that matter), nor does Reconstruction history yet have much of a medical dimension. Instead, the consequences of the war, despite their mixed nature, still have reference to the eventual "modern" changes in institutional organization and biological sciences after 1880. By taking a ground-level view of local practice, however, we can appreciate the significance of how the war did *not* alter ordinary M.D.s' expectations for what constituted a desirable practice. For the most part, in fact, the war reconfirmed southern physicians' sense of the primacy of personal experience and the ideal of medicine as a moral endeavor in a local community setting.

Although reliable figures are few, clearly hundreds, perhaps thousands, of southern physicians were killed in the war and thousands more had their careers disrupted, left the South, or quit medicine altogether. Thus, for many individual practitioners and patients, perhaps especially for emancipated African Americans, the war drastically altered the immediate social relations of health care like it altered so much else. At the same time, however, the dislocations of war worked to bolster the larger culture of antebellum rural practice as a powerful ideal, one suggested by the stories of three southern doctors going to war.

Many physicians doubtless had Dr. David Winn's unhappy experience of the war as distorting doctor-patient relationships. And yet Winn, practicing in Americus, Georgia, clung all the more tightly to his prewar domestic practice as his postwar goal. Citizens praised Winn when he volunteered to accompany the local boys to war in April 1861, and a month later, the doctor wrote with pride to his wife, Frances, that the soldiers "cannot get along without me." By October, however, everything had changed. The long march from Georgia to Virginia sickened many of the men, and supplies ran short. Along with battle casualties, this completely overwhelmed Winn's doctoring and soured his relationship with the Americus troops, who daily pressured him for special favors and leaves of absence. To Winn's disgust, several soldiers even wrote home to complain of his care. As he wrote to Frances, "My position is a wretched one. . . . These complaints are so infernally ungrateful that I am trying to get out of our company into one where I know and care for no one." And yet the ideal of community practice continued to sustain the doctor. Throughout his troubles, Winn managed to detach the hometown "wretches" he saw every day from his image of folks back home in Americus. Indeed, by going to war, he told Frances, he now saw that he had poorly served his hometown patients and "I have neglected the happiness of myself and family." The war was an aberration to be endured; genuine practice "must wait until I return home."[2]

Young Lafayette Strait, practicing in Chester District, South Carolina, with a fresh M.D. in the spring of 1861, had a more positive experience in Confederate service but was no less inspired by antebellum ideals of domestic practice than David Winn. When war broke out, Strait sought the advice of two physician uncles, both of whom had proceeded cautiously. One, W. W. Mobley, believing "my honour is at stake," reluctantly attached himself to the army, but only after extracting a promise from his neighbors that "if I return I shall always have this practice so long as I will attend to it." Strait was eager to join up, however, and by the early summer of 1861 was serving in Virginia as an assistant surgeon with the rank of captain in the Palmetto Sharp Shooters. He had survived illness and a battlefield wound in the spring and felt that he was well-liked and respected by the men in his unit. He wrote spirited letters home, relating to his mother, for instance, a pugnacious "Rx" for war made up from equal parts ammunition, weary marches, shelling, and Sharpsburg and Manassas—to be administered "ad lib," as needed. And yet, in the midst of his excitement and up until his death from dysentery in the fall of 1863, Strait kept the ideal of his hometown practice at the center of his work. He yearned to find himself back in Chester District with his patients, "if the war should ever close." Everything he learned about his profession had reference to his return home. By treating military experience as a kind of clinic, he wrote, he would burnish the esteem in which he was held back home. "I will not only be better prepared to practice my profession," he wrote of his war experience, "but the people will have more confidence in me."[3]

Dr. Samuel Maverick Van Wyck nurtured similar hopes, although, in the first days after leaving home and practice in Huntsville, Alabama, in the spring of 1861, all he could write about was his worry that he had abandoned his patients—and that his rivals would seek to supplant him. He asked his wife to pass along to individual patients his recommendations for which local physician would best replace him on a temporary basis. "Dr. Wall told me he would attend to Laura," Van Wyck wrote five months after leaving home. "Also to my anatomical specimens, tell him to get them out of my office. I have a decoction of morphine on my office shelf worth $1.50 or $2.00—sell it to Cooper or Rison."[4]

At the same time, Van Wyck was alert to learning medical lessons in the newness of army service. He was attached to Nathan Bedford Forrest's cavalry regiment in late 1861, writing of his first battle that "shot & shell fell thick and fast around me, and strange to say I was more collected and calm than when I used to pray in church." The medical needs of wounded and sick men filled his days, but Van Wyck, too, remained focused on practice after the war. Although he sometimes was disgusted that "every man think[s] he is the only sick one on the hill," looking ahead to peaceful times, he believed his army work "one of the finest positions to learn practical medicine that I know of." War work did not replace domestic practice so much as highlight the personal character of its best practitioners. All else, no matter how riveting, would pass.[5]

So Van Wyck was pleased to hear from his wife of two former patients at home who "enquired after you, as indeed everybody does, and spoke in exalted terms of you. Mrs. Jolly says she thinks it a blessing to the poor soldiers to get such a man as you with them." In October 1861, about a month before he was killed in action along the Ohio River in Kentucky, Van Wyck wrote to his wife one evening from his tent, his writing desk two stacked boxes of whiskey, promising her that his army service "will answer forever and brake that restlessness of mine." He could scarcely wait to return home and to his practice, but in the meantime war would serve as his school: "I am deeply interested in my pursuit of knowledge & experience."[6]

This faith in personal experience as the heart of doctoring, and reliance on the character of inquisitive, local practitioners, continued to define medical institutions, as well as individuals, after the war. Most notably, medical schools remained valued institutions on the urban and professional landscape. Despite great difficulties, three of the five major southern schools—Nashville, Louisville, and Louisiana—managed to remain open during most of the war. The other two, Georgia and South Carolina, shut down but were back in operation within a year after the end of the conflict. To be sure, schools tersely acknowledged the general devastation in their first postwar announcements. The Medical College of Georgia, for example, mentioned the "disastrous effects of our conflict" on "this good old institution," and MCSSC took note of how the "exhaustive war . . . broke up communications . . . and suspended the daily and weekly journals." But most schools did not dwell on the destruction. They continued to embrace the conviction that southern schools were particularly apt for the study of distinctive southern disease and that southern physicians were more than ever morally bound to tend to their communities. If anything, the antebellum sense of regionally specific medicine was given new strength by each school's postwar pride in its corner of the South. The Georgia school, for example, boasted in the mid-1870s that its chief accomplishment was to have produced "more than 1,200 graduates" serving Georgians, and in 1871 the

University of Louisiana school noted with pride that more than half of its antebellum graduates had represented the state in the Confederacy.[7]

Changes in the curriculum after the war were slow to take place and even by the mid-1870s occurred only within a larger continuity of courses and pedagogy. Reliance on lectures remained unquestioned. Traditional subject areas persisted, lecturers continued to speak in a personal voice, and individual "experience" remained the center of good learning; a few schools offered courses in "military surgery" in 1866 but dropped them within a year or two. With schools retaining the four-month, two-term requirement for graduation, the growth of the antebellum "shadow" curriculum was, if anything, furthered by the war. Uprooted or in transit, many talented men ended up in cities like Charleston and New Orleans and were given adjunct faculty status (called "supplementary" or "extraordinary" faculty), offering a variety of courses on the margins of the traditional five or six core subject areas. In part because of the presence of such teachers, hospital wards slowly became organized around specialties, and by the 1870s the well-known development of the hospital into a general care institution was fitfully under way. Yet, amid these shifts, the emphasis on the mentor-student relationship remained the heart of schools' definition of a good education. Indeed, some teachers noted that the war had made young men more receptive to their mentors, because during the conflict "they had to work for their support [and] knew the value of time." As for mentors, one school observed, postwar hardships and shortages were making "students anew of [the] teachers" and so bound them even more closely to their pupils.[8]

In the decade after the war, then, professional leaders in medical education agreed that one certainty at least might be drawn from "the gigantic mass of suffering" that was the war: the ideal of moral practitioners "who performed their arduous duties so manfully." A lecture by Dr. David W. Yandell to the incoming class of students at the University of Louisville in 1869 captured the way in which the vision of personal, moral experience remained a constant in orthodox education even after the war. To be sure, Yandell lauded certain practical innovations brought to orthodox notice by the war: the use of anesthesia, the importance of sanitation and accurate statistics; he predicted the future value of the stethoscope and the oral thermometer to ordinary, rural practice. And yet his image of the good doctor was not a technical wizard but an ordinary man with the wisdom to see that the war had confirmed "expectant" practice and individual "experience" as the essence of orthodox healing. "[E]arnest, energetic, zealously laboring for the advancement of medicine," the southern practitioner in a postwar world drew on the continuity of an orthodoxy "not less elevated in moral tone" for all of the trials of war and the uncertainties of the future. Once again, it all came down to individual experience. When patients ask, "what shall I take?" Yandell wanted the kind of physician who could answer in utter confidence, "take [my] good advice."[9]

The view that an individual's experience defined good doctoring continued to shape bedside care, as well as education. The war had done nothing to change the expectation that postwar practice would remain in the context of local communities, distinctive southern diseases, and the moral role of the physician as caregiver. Of course, many physicians were at loose ends immediately after the war, struggling for economic survival. Robert Battey, for instance, practicing near Rome, Georgia, in 1865, had become so unaccustomed to seeing cash that when he received "an old fashioned 5$ gold piece" one day, he "was so elated with my luck that I . . . actually played with the toy like a child with a new tin trumpet." Frank Ramsay, practicing in Memphis, Tennessee, after the war was touched when he received a letter from thirty former patients in Knoxville requesting him to return. But he decided to stay with his new practice in such economically uncertain times. Although recording economic hardship, doctors' daybooks spanning the war nevertheless reveal that despite postwar currency inflation and a consequent rise in barter and deferred payments, the overall pattern of income and rounds (and physicians' notation of them) was essentially unchanged by the conflict.[10]

Indeed, other basic texts arising from daily practice show a deep continuity in physicians' bedside expectations even as some doctors focused on the immediate "lessons" brought home by the war. Some former military surgeons, like A. J. Semmes, rushed to publish case studies of suturing technique, gunshot wound management, and the like, often presented with no particular argument for their relevance to peacetime community practice but brimming with the antebellum faith in "experience" nonetheless. Other physicians, however, were less certain of the lessons of the hospital and field. There is a distinct sense of hunkering down on the part of many men who expressed the need for caution and re-engagement with *southern* disease and bedside ways. Skeptical of the "restless spirit of the age in which we live," Mark Reynolds, a Statesburg, South Carolina, physician warned colleagues in 1873 against rashly adopting wartime practices, perhaps tainted by "another latitude," which would harm the core of "Southern practice." He recommended staying with "*fixed* and *settled* views . . . the result of our own experience." The war had provided no clear lessons, in this view, but had fostered a false optimism that wartime measures were easily transferred to the bedsides of neighbors. In short, although the war had been a kind of bazaar of medical information, postwar reflection revealed that shared knowledge was not necessarily sound knowledge. Thus, although he hoped for continued "association" among physicians in scattered rural communities after the war, Dr. Reynolds's anchor, like that of many of his peers, was the familiar figure of the solo practitioner, whose "individual observation with reflection must of necessity constitute the basis for all knowledge."[11]

The single greatest change in practitioners' routine mirrored the most dramatic change in southern society after the war, the end of slavery. For many white physicians, the number of black patients attended fell off sharply when no longer determined by white owners calling on them. African Americans who chose other kinds of doctors delivered a keen economic loss for some white physicians; for others, however, the change was a welcome release from a vexing aspect of practice. Adjustments to the new state of affairs were on a wholly local scale. There were white doctors who continued to treat former slaves who had stayed in the neighborhood, sometimes contracting with freed people for group care, or with white employers as part of a sharecropping arrangement. South Carolina physician S. H. Pressly, for instance, signed a contract in 1870 to care for the thirty-seven people in eight African American farm families in which he agreed "to furnish all necessary medicine and medical attention to the Freedmen and their families" for the year. Notably, he explicitly excused himself from "cases of midwifery." Other white doctors, however, refused to take on new African American patients altogether and, in some cases, would no longer treat former ones. Thomas P. Bailey seems to have excluded black families altogether from his low-country South Carolina practice in the 1870s, for he makes no racial identifications among his patients after the war.[12]

For those white physicians who did continue to treat African Americans after emancipation, however, race remained the underlying constant for grouping black patients into a general social category, a device all the more obvious as the organizing structure of slavery crumbled away. In this regard, doctors' means of recording black patients in daybook accounts vividly suggest the different ways of coming to terms with social change even as practitioners continued to divide black from white. Some M.D.s, for instance, continued to list freed people under their former owner's accounts as if nothing had happened, whether out of habit or in defiance of postwar change is not clear. Other physicians removed the names of freed people from their old plantation accounts and placed them under new "colored" accounts of their own, sometimes in separate daybooks altogether. What to call individual freed people became an issue as well, and the proliferation of naming practices suited the shaken-up times. Some physicians retained their old habit of listing African Americans by first name only, while others inserted new surnames—or new names altogether—into old patient listings. Former slave Ralph Bowman, who had George Colmer for a doctor, changed his name to Raphael Boone after the war, and Colmer did the same in his daybook. New names, suggesting new identities, made these African American patients at least somewhat visible in a new way. Too, whether reluctantly or not, physicians began to note marital unions and family relationships among their black patients as never before. And yet some lines were not redrawn; in their naming usages, as in the social relations that names signified, doctors rarely accorded single black women the title "Miss" as they did unmarried white women, and they reserved the term "lady" for the white race only.[13]

In all, it seems that a considerable number of rural M.D.s continued to minister to "their" black patients with the old mixture of condescension, suspicion, and the exchange of practical information. The immediate postwar letters and accounts of South Carolina doctor Joel Berly, for example, suggest that his own farm workers contracted for his care when they became hired labor after the war. Berly's correspondence also reveals the extent of his bartering with other local black farmhands: a confirmation from the employer of "Sarah and Robert" that they owed him a shoat; a note concerning Eusebius, urging him to have his tooth pulled and to "tell Eusebius I cooked his [bartered] rabbit for supper." But if the quotidian texture of such relations seems largely unchanged, the postwar years also permitted other M.D.s to simply write off all bedside contact with African Americans. It permitted racial hatred to boil up with new virulence from years of mutual frustration and suspicion, allowing physicians simply to exclude African Americans from the personal doctor-patient engagements at the moral heart of orthodoxy. "The more I see of the negro race now growing up," wrote Arkansas doctor Frank James with chilling candor in 1877, "the more I am persuaded of one thing—we must either educate them, or we will have them to kill. Their brutality is something frightful, and as to morality it is unknown."[14]

Physicians writing in medical journals were rarely as blunt. And yet if white racism in the 1870s was not as biologically ironclad as it would be at the turn of the century, it continued to thrive on white doctors' relative lack of curiosity about black sickness. Published articles featuring African Americans' health were markedly fewer after the war, and the essays on "Negro disease" that did appear contained much the same discussion of supposed black variations in susceptibility and immunity as before the war. Bat Smith, for example, a bright young Louisiana physician studying "miasm" in 1874, noted as if for the first time that blacks "seem to enjoy a relative immunity" against malarial fevers because they were "as a race for many centuries accustomed to the intense heat and deleterious influences" of a tropical climate. Medical topographers recapitulated without new analysis the high mortality rate among blacks and restated the conventional wisdom that fevers were shared by the races. In all of these instances, as before the war, "race" conflated biology and the environmental influences shaping it.[15]

In this regard, it is a striking comment on white orthodoxy that African Americans dropped out of general medical topographies and were much less likely to appear as individual patients in case histories. Over time this added to the likelihood that white physicians would draw conclusions about black health based on abstract ideas of "race," not on actual encounters with black patients, and continue to ignore the concept's promiscuous blend of biological, cultural, and environmental assumptions. In W. A. Cochran's 1871 topography of Orrville, Alabama, for instance, his notice of the African American community in Orrville is typically brief and dismissive in its drive to generalize in racial terms: "Since the late war, there has been built up on the southern limit of the village a negro settlement, composed entirely of huts or cabins huddled together without any regard to order or system, but perfectly in keeping with the primitive style and gregarious habits of this race." There is no suggestion that Dr. Cochran considered venturing into the settlement to conduct an empirical study. Another physician noted with somewhat more misgiving that although he had intended "to collect statistics of the mortality of the negro population," he found it impossible, "from the fact that many are taken sick and die without any medical aid afforded them." He meant, of course, white, *orthodox* aid. And that was the point: white doctors less often saw black patients or black doctors, making it all the more difficult to see the profile of black health in general. Satisfied with this distanced view, postwar white physicians were thus far more likely to fall back on "race" as a covering explanation for African American illness.[16]

These staggering problems of race aside, much about physicians' vision of postwar bedside practice is no better summed up than in a thoughtful essay on the war's lessons written at the very close of the conflict by Francis P. Porcher, then surgeon in charge of the City Hospital in Charleston, South Carolina. Writing at the behest of the surgeon general, Porcher, the author of an earlier wartime work on southern botanical "resources" for health care, articulated conventional wisdom: the need to cut back on the "stimulation" of alcohol and opium, to rely more on "expectant" treatment, and to recognize the importance of nutrition and ventilation (though, interestingly, he warned that "cleanliness" could be overdone). More compelling, however, was Porcher's view that the war had underscored the deep significance of the social context of sickness. He was profoundly impressed with the emotional "prostration" of wartime patients and linked the collapse of their mental attitude to their weakened physical stamina.

He wrote with reference to soldiers, but his words reflected on the experience of all patients. With some intensity, Porcher noted how much the patient's own thinking and emotions mattered, and told of how shocked he had been by "the fear, almost approaching to servility," with which sick soldiers approached army physicians. He particularly was struck by how physicians acting under the bureaucratic rules of hospitals utterly ignored questions of patients' suffering and hope, and thus abrogated their moral bond with them. War medicine was no model for the future.[17]

In a sense foreshadowing the bane of health bureaucracies to come, Porcher warned his colleagues against a doctor who "is willing to content himself simply with conforming to the Regulations." This might well "please all in authority over him," but such a doctor would "be far from performing his duty." And what was the physician's duty? It was to re-create the best of antebellum doctor-patient relationships, a bond of neighbors and friends whose reasons for caring flowed naturally from shared lives. The chief lesson of wartime, Porcher believed, should be that "our patients are our brethren." His ideal for the postwar physician thus had all of the marks of the antebellum country doctor transformed by the conflict into a better version of himself. A skilled man, yes, and an educated one; but, as important, a man wise in the ways of comforting his patients. Porcher could not make it any clearer: the war had taught him that the "real practical effect . . . of encouraging the sick" was as great as any drug.[18]

With the clamor of war still fresh, Porcher's attempt to read the future grew cloudy at certain points. But in writing about deep "lessons" of individual character and personal bonds he anticipated the efforts of many other doctors who would recall the war so as to strengthen these traditional qualities of doctoring. For these men, memories of war were a complex staging of stories and identities that pointed out the new, but, even more important, protected the continuity of country orthodox practice. Physicians remembered the war they needed to remember, and their modes of memory braided together antebellum ideals of a man's character, training, and individual practice into an ideal for the future.

To be sure, some doctors were bitter and despaired. Julian J. Chisolm in 1867, for instance, saw impending disaster in every facet of South Carolina's medical life: in the "useless" medical society, in the threat of epidemics, in disorganized hospitals, and, especially, in the "debauchery, filth, destitution, disease, and death" among freed people, "formerly happy and well cared for." Others sank further into Confederate jingoism, as did B. F. Ward, who roused his audience in 1880 by placing southern physicians within a kind of essentialist regional character flowing freely between doctors and generals: "the Lees, the Johnstons, the

Jacksons, Hood, Hampton, Gordon, and Forest [sic], would have been as celebrated in surgery as they are renowned in the heroism of military history."[19]

But bitterness and Lost Cause grandiosity were relatively rare among physicians when they wrote to distill the meaning of the war and to sum up its
consequences for their medicine. There was sentiment, but by no means did
most doctors write from a high pitch of emotion. Most writing, in fact, was
notable for its appeal, in multiple ways, to the physician's experience in normal,
everyday practice. The appeal of the empirical and the "real" world of the senses
retained its strength and savor. Some physicians reacted to the war's noise
by downplaying its uniqueness, even treating it with silence. Dr. Stanford E.
Chaillé, for example, orator at the 1879 meeting of the Louisiana State Medical
Society, spoke on state medicine and medical organization without once mentioning the war or Reconstruction. Similarly, other doctors, joining the tide of
personal memorialists assessing the state of the art or revisiting their careers
by the end of the 1870s, noted the war with deliberate brevity. North Carolinian
A. B. Cox, for instance, acknowledged the "unfortunate war" as if it were
something merely ill-advised, lamenting but not lingering over it. Distancing
"our great war" in another way, by placing it in a larger context, John T. Darby,
routinely took note in 1873 of medical advances in the "treatment of wounds"
and "establishment of hospitals" but pointed out to his South Carolina colleagues that much the same had happened in Crimea and the Sudan. In fact, by
the 1880s, the medical significance of the war had receded into something
simple and rather bland. "The experience in military surgery was large," R. A.
Kinloch wrote in 1884, "but [its] benefits to the profession of our State have
not, in my view, been abundant or lasting." The consensus now, he wrote, was
that in the war there were "no good surgeons or physicians who were not
trained or skilled before it," adding, "our southern military hospitals . . . were
not good schools."[20]

Combining assessments of the war with their personal memories came easily
to physicians long used to talking about doctoring in a wholly personal register.
The individual's voice featured in antebellum medical literature carried over into
postwar writing, helping physicians mend the torn fabric of their work by giving
it a continuity of familiar forms and stories. Thus, underlying a sense of both
progress and loss, a vision of medical purpose scaled to local, individual practice, continued to structure how physicians put into words what they saw and
wished to see. Medical topographies continued to flourish after the war, for
instance, once more imparting intellectual authority to the community practitioner and his country orthodoxy. Medical journals continued to feature practitioners' case narratives in full variety as the texts that best organized what was

significant to know, conceptually and practically. Although by the 1880s more authors sensed that the future of medical writing would play down the personal voice, and thus they somewhat circumscribed their claims, they presented their cases nonetheless, with much the same expectation that stories were a contribution to knowledge. One observer, writing of "Cotton South" physicians, praised them precisely for this embrace of expressive continuity with the antebellum years. Seeing their case narratives as "experience" at large, there for the taking, local doctors might avoid abstractions and engage in "original thinking and reasoning from present facts and phenomena of everyday practice." Moreover, if told simply, individual case narratives were unmatched for capturing "unbiased observation . . . [and] bold and independent action upon the responsibility of individual judgment."[21]

So powerful was this narrative mode, so profound in its implications for the art of medicine as irreplaceably personal, that by the turn of the century, many physicians subtly shifted from recalling the war as a phenomenon influencing their practice from without to seeing it as a source of anecdotes or moral tales from *within* their practice. In a triumph of doctors' subjectivity, the war was rewritten into autobiography: meeting a brave or devout soldier, encountering a well-known general, turning a disaster into an advantage, witnessing a famous battle. Physicians were not alone in writing the war this way, of course, as aging veterans everywhere transformed chaos into a few fond or hair-raising personal tales. For physicians, however, making the war a kind of personal possession was of a piece with their sense that personal experience was the essence of their work. The achievement of country orthodoxy was to affirm that all the experience a man needed to be a good doctor was available to him in his community. Thus the important story to be told was the same story as before the war, a tale of individual effort and the texture of work; a story of personal insight and moral meaning.

In this vein, Simon Baruch, writing from New York in 1910, looked back on his days in the Army of Northern Virginia and, like others, found that the lasting effects of the war were contained in small, sharp memories, not in profession-wide therapeutic or technical acquirements. Memories of personal character particularly stood out. "Military practice in the field tended to develop self-reliance if it did not always increase skill," he wrote, after noting that in the army he had amputated limbs "before I had ever drawn human blood even by lancing a boil." It was in this lasting sense of self-reliance, not the in irony of its battlefield origins or the clinical skills it fostered, that the war had made him a better physician. As well, memories of the fraternity of medical men had strengthened through the years, as Baruch recalled the cooperation—"courteous, *yes, broth-*

erly"—between himself and Union medical officers at the battle of South Mountain in 1862. Memorable above all was their mutual bedside effort sweeping aside partisan passions, a kind of pure test of character that caused his "heart to beat high with pride in being a member of a calling that could so completely obliterate the beastly animosities of warring men."[22]

∽ Notes ∽

ABBREVIATIONS USED IN THE NOTES

ADAH	Alabama Department of Archives and History, Montgomery, Alabama
AS	George P. Rawick, ed., *The American Slave: A Composite Autobiography* (Westport, Conn.: Greenwood Publishing Group, 1978)
CP	College of Physicians, Philadelphia, Pennsylvania
Duke	William Perkins Library, Duke University, Durham, North Carolina
Emory	Robert W. Woodruff Library, Emory University, Atlanta, Georgia
Filson	The Filson Club, Louisville, Kentucky
FSL	Florida State Library, Tallahassee, Florida
GSWBFP	Gaston, Strait, Wylie, and Baskin Family Papers
HTML	Howard-Tilton Memorial Library, Special Collections, Tulane University, New Orleans, Louisiana
LSU	Louisiana and Lower Mississippi Valley Collections, King Library, Louisiana State University, Baton Rouge, Louisiana
Matas	Rudolph Matas Medical Library, Tulane University, New Orleans, Louisiana
MCG	Medical College of Georgia, Athens, Georgia
MCSSC	Medical College of (the State of) South Carolina, Theses, Waring Historical Library, Medical University of South Carolina, Charleston, South Carolina
NLM	National Library of Medicine, Bethesda, Maryland
SCHS	South Carolina Historical Society, Charleston, South Carolina
SCL	South Caroliniana Library, University of South Carolina, Columbia, South Carolina
SHC	Southern Historical Collection, University of North Carolina, Chapel Hill, North Carolina
TSL	Tennessee State Library, Knoxville, Tennessee
TSM	Transylvania School of Medicine, Transylvania University, Lexington, Kentucky
UK	University of Kentucky, Special Collections, Lexington, Kentucky
UL	University of Louisville, Louisville, Kentucky
UMiss	University of Mississippi, Special Collections, Oxford, Mississippi
UNCC	University of North Carolina, Special Collections, Charlotte, North Carolina

Vanderbilt   Vanderbilt Medical Center Library, Special Collections, Vanderbilt University, Nashville, Tennessee
VHS   Virginia Historical Society, Richmond, Virginia
Waring   Waring Historical Library, Medical University of South Carolina, Charleston, South Carolina
Winthrop   Dacus Library, Archives and Special Collections, Winthrop University, Rock Hill, South Carolina

INTRODUCTION

1. Although they are common historical experiences, becoming sick and giving care have received less attention than most other aspects of social life in this century. Most survey textbooks still include little about sickness. Even that great exemplar of nineteenth-century studies, Alexis de Tocqueville, had virtually nothing to say about it. Thus, the definition of key terms is important. Throughout, I use "disease" and "sickness" more or less interchangeably to refer to the objective or empirical aspects of being unwell (for example, something measured by a doctor's instruments and tests). I use "illness" to stress individuals' subjective sense of their own unwellness, in which their morality and emotions are important. I use the term "malady," drawing on Victorian sensibility, to suggest the pervasive, mysterious nature of disease. For reflections on these matters see Laurence B. McCullough, "Particularism in Medicine," 361–70, and Charon, "To Build a Case," 115–32.

2. On the breadth of this change, see Starr, *Transformation of American Medicine*. I use the term "physician" to refer specifically to doctors who held M.D.s, and "doctor," "healer," and "practitioner" more generally. Historians have used a variety of terms to further distinguish M.D.s from other kinds of healers in the nineteenth century: "regular," "learned," "scholastic," and "orthodox." I choose "orthodox" both because people at the time used it and because calling physicians' competitors "unorthodox" does not seem as disparaging as calling them "unlearned" or "irregular."

Before the 1960s, medical historiography featured many M.D. historians and was governed largely by the hindsight that orthodoxy would achieve twentieth-century success. Almost invariably, this hindsight bathed orthodox medicine in a singularly positive light. For histories of medicine in the South or on the rural "frontier" written in this Whiggish vein, see, for example, Blanton, *Medicine in Virginia in the Nineteenth Century*; Flexner, *Doctors on Horseback*; and Pickard and Buley, *Midwest Pioneer*. An early essay that challenged this perspective without entirely stepping outside of it is Shryock, "Medical Practice in the Old South." On medical historiography, see Numbers, "History of American Medicine"; David Rosner, "Tempest in a Test Tube"; Leavitt, "Medicine in Context"; Rosenberg, "Medical Profession"; and Rosenberg, Introduction to *Explaining Epidemics*, 1–6.

3. Broadly influential works on health and medicine in the nineteenth-century South include the pathbreaking Savitt, *Medicine and Slavery*; Cowdrey, *This Land, This South*; Horsman, *Josiah Nott of Mobile*; Sally McMillen, *Motherhood in the Old South*; Kiple and King, *Another Dimension*; and Fett, *Working Cures*. Important collections of essays include Savitt and Young, eds., *Disease and Distinctiveness*, and Numbers and Savitt, eds., *Science and Medicine*. On disease and southern regionalism in particular, see, for example, Warner, "Idea of Southern Medical

Distinctiveness, and James O. Breeden, "Disease as a Factor in Southern Distinctiveness," in Savitt and Young, eds., *Disease and Distinctiveness*, 1–28.

4. On southern fevers in the nineteenth century, see Margaret Humphreys, *Malaria* and *Yellow Fever in the South*; Savitt, *Medicine and Slavery*, 17–34; Kiple and King, *Another Dimension*, chs. 1–3; John Duffy, "The Impact of Malaria on the South," in Savitt and Young, eds., *Disease and Distinctiveness*, 29–54; and K. David Patterson, "Disease Environments of the Antebellum South," in Numbers and Savitt, eds., *Science and Medicine*, 152–65. Disease perceived as a strikingly protean entity created conceptual difficulties in physicians' diagnostic goals and language. Excellent, broad discussions of this problem are in Rosenberg, *Care of Strangers*, ch. 3; Warner, *Therapeutic Perspective*, ch. 3; and James H. Cassedy, "Medical Men and the Ecology of the Old South," in Numbers and Savitt, eds., *Science and Medicine*, 166–78. On popular views of natural ecology and health, see Valencius, *Health of the Country*.

5. On race, diet, and susceptibility to sickness, see Kiple and King, *Another Dimension*, 11–20, 53–58, 188–203, and Savitt, *Medicine and Slavery*, 17–34, 86–103, 117–20, 200–201. On the eighteenth and early nineteenth century, see Morgan, *Slave Counterpoint*, 85, 321–25, 441–46.

6. For an overview of ideas about health, work, and lifestyle, see Cassedy, *Medicine in America*, ch. 2. See also, Kiple and King, *Another Dimension*, chs. 6 and 13, and Savitt, *Medicine and Slavery*, chs. 3, 4, 8. A usefully broad view of mental illness in a southern setting is McCandless, *Moonlight, Magnolias, and Madness*. On the literature of sex and sexuality, see Horowitz, *Rereading Sex*.

7. Suggestive for vernacular medicine in the South are Moss, *Southern Folk Medicine*, and Snow, *Walkin' over Medicine*. See also Elliot J. Gorn, "Black Magic: Folk Beliefs of the Slave Community," in Numbers and Savitt, eds., *Science and Medicine*, 295–326; Cadwallader and Wilson, "Folklore Medicine," 217–27; and Fett, *Working Cures*, esp. chs. 2 and 3. On women's domestic caregiving, see Stowe, "Writing Sickness," 257–86, and, more generally, Abel, *Hearts of Wisdom*.

8. Nineteenth-century America was awash in popular health advice and in a new, middle-class audience for it. For a sense of this world as it influenced ideas about illness and medicine, see Gevitz, ed., *Other Healers*; Risse, Numbers, and Leavitt, eds., *Medicine without Doctors*; Murphy, *Enter the Physician*; Haller, *Medical Protestants* and *Kindly Medicine*; Whorton, *Inner Hygiene*; Rosenberg, ed., *Right Living*; Albanese, "Body Politic," 131–51; and Elizabeth Barnaby Keeney, "Unless Powerful Sick: Domestic Medicine in the Old South," in Numbers and Savitt, eds., *Science and Medicine*, 276–94.

9. A good overview of the broad, public context for sectarian differences is Rothstein, *American Physicians*; Joseph F. Kett, *Formation of the American Medical Profession*; Pernick, *Calculus of Suffering*, ch. 2; and Starr, *Social Transformation of American Medicine*. Additionally, southern medicine was influenced by a burgeoning sectionalist ideology after 1830; see Duffy, "Note on Ante-bellum Southern Nationalism"; Breeden, "States-Rights Medicine"; Warner, "Southern Medical Reform"; and Kilbride, "Southern Medical Students."

10. On therapeutics and on science as orthodox medicine's basis and goal, see Rosenberg, "Therapeutic Revolution"; Warner, "From Specificity to Universalism"; Beeson and Maulitz, "Inner History of Internal Medicine"; and Shryock, "Empiricism and Rationalism." On aspects of allopathy and physicians' ideas of science, see Numbers and Warner, "Maturation of American Medical Science"; Thomas G. Dyer, "Science in the Antebellum College: The University of Georgia, 1801–1860," in Numbers and Savitt, eds., *Science and Medicine*, 36–54;

Brieger, "History of Medicine"; Stephens, *Science, Race, and Religion*; Geison, *Michael Foster*; Conser, *God and the Natural World*; and Warner, *Therapeutic Perspective*. On use and action of various nineteenth-century drugs, I have found indispensable Estes, *Dictionary of Proto-pharmacology*. On the history of pharmacology, see Parascandola, *Development of American Pharmacology*.

11. For a close-up sense of physicians' mode of treatment and how they labored to set limits and possibilities, see Cleaveland, *Sacred Space*; Stowe, ed., *Southern Practice*; and Duffin, *Langstaff*. For a fascinating look at a practitioner's web of thought and work, see Duden, *Woman Beneath the Skin*.

12. See U.S. Bureau of the Census, *Historical Statistics of the United States*, 76. Between 1860 and 1870, the number of physicians in the South declined by 7 percent even though the war-torn population grew by more than 5 percent, suggesting that competition for patients lessened overall. Historians' view of the overall supply of physicians tends to vary. Kenneth Kiple and Virginia King (*Another Dimension*, 172) tentatively suggest a "relative scarcity" of regular physicians in many areas of the antebellum rural South; James Cassedy (*Medicine and American Growth*, 67, 232 n. 16) highlights an "apparent surplus" and an "alleged new abundance" of doctors by the 1840s. Certainly some southern cities were saturated with doctors. In other communities, however, people who wanted a doctor often could not dependably find one. See also Rothstein, *American Physicians*, 344–45, and Kett, *Formation of the American Medical Profession*, 185–86.

On the hardships of competition, see Duffy, "American Perceptions"; Warner, "Science, Healing"; and Rosenberg, "Making It in Urban Medicine." For interesting comparison to Britain, see Inkster, "Marginal Men."

13. African Americans established ten medical schools in the South between 1868 and 1899, but blacks were not admitted in any significant numbers to white orthodox schools and state medical societies in the South until the 1970s. See Savitt, "Straight University Medical Department." Also suggestive of black professionalism is Savitt's "Four African-American Proprietary Medical Colleges"; Walker, *Negro in the Medical Profession*; Morais, *History of the Afro-American in Medicine*; and Gamble, *Making a Place for Ourselves*.

White women in the South did not begin entering and graduating from previously male medical schools in considerable numbers until the 1920s, a generation later than outside of the region. For women and the medical profession generally, see Morantz-Sanchez, *Sympathy and Science*; Brodie, *Contraception and Abortion*; and Leavitt, *Brought to Bed*.

14. Examination of Robert M. Pearse, April 24, 1820; examination of Daniel Tompkins, January 7, 1820, Mississippi Board of Medical Censors Minute Book, 1819–35, LSU. For the importance of Louisiana's mixed French, Spanish, and English heritage in its relative open-ness to regulation, see Duffy, ed., *Rudolph Matas History*, esp. 1:327–38 and 2:105–9. The Louisiana board survived the national deregulation trend of the 1830s, but other attempts at control fell to widespread popular pressure. South Carolina established two licensing boards in 1817 that, like Louisiana's, had no enforcement power and in fact appear to have rarely met; the state did away with all "pains and penalties" of the law after 1838. Georgia repealed its mild licensing act outright in 1826, as did Mississippi in 1834. Alabama passed a law in 1823 with so many exemptions that even at the time no one took it seriously; it was abolished in 1834. In 1849, the newly born American Medical Association found only three jurisdictions in the nation with comprehensive licensure laws, New Jersey, Washington, D.C., and Loui-

siana. The AMA finding is cited in Kaufman, *American Medical Education*, 68. For the situation in South Carolina, see Waring, "Charleston Medicine," 320–42, and his *History of Medicine*, 95–100. For the Georgia act, see Spalding, *History of the Medical College of Georgia*, 38. For Alabama, see Holley, *History of Medicine in Alabama*, 257. On the struggle over law and licensure generally, see Starr, *Social Transformation*, ch. 1; Rothstein, *American Physicians*, chs. 4, 16; and Kett, *Formation of the American Medical Profession*, ch. 6.

15. E. Brooks Holifield ("Wealth of Nineteenth-Century American Physicians") found that the median wealth for certain elite urban southern doctors far outstripped that of their northern counterparts, and he attributed the difference to southern physicians' investment in slaves and planting. Holifield computed the median wealth of selected southern urban physicians as $7,300, compared to $1,500 for northern doctors. But urban physicians in this income bracket were a tiny minority among doctors. More broadly on income, see Rosen, *Fees and Fee Bills*.

CHAPTER ONE

1. Throughout midcentury, formal schooling was not a necessary requirement for becoming an M.D. For broad histories of medical education and its reform in this period, see Ludmerer, *Learning to Heal*, ch. 1; Starr, *Social Transformation of American Medicine*; and Rothstein, *American Physicians*.

2. Sims, *Story of My Life*, 115–16; Lafayette Strait to [Richard or Alexander] Wylie, January 13, 1856, GSWBFP, SCL; Nathan C. Whetstone to William C. Whetstone, November 17, [1852], Whetstone family papers, SCL; D. W. Whitehurst to Hamilton Weedon, November 13, 1851, Weedon family papers, ADAH. The logic of career "paths" in medicine did not gain a modern clarity until the end of the century, even in the professional crucibles of large northern cities. For a discussion, see Rosenberg, "Making It in Urban Medicine," 125–54.

3. Lafayette Strait to his parents, June 2, 1856, GSWBFP, SCL; Ivy diary, October 8, 1878 (entry out of sequence in the back of the volume), Waring; Sims, *Story of My Life*, 116; Lafayette Strait to Alexander Wylie, September 7, 1856, GSWBFP, SCL. See also Joseph LeConte autobiography, 141, LeConte-Furman papers, SHC, and Hentz diary, November 19, 1845, in Stowe, ed., *Southern Practice*, 57.

4. Lunsford Yandell diary, 1824–43, 402, Yandell family papers, Filson; Stowe, ed., *Southern Practice*, 439–40; Cunningham, "Autobiography," 23, ADAH.

5. Hentz diary, November 28, 1845, in Stowe, ed., *Southern Practice*, 66; Charles D. Drake, ed., *Pioneer Life*, 233; David H. Dungan to William Wylie, January 21, 1857, GSWBFP, SCL; Charles Harrod to Sara Evans, March 1, 1845, Evans family papers, LSU.

6. Lafayette Strait to his parents, June 2, 1856, GSWBFP, SCL; Charles D. Drake, ed., *Pioneer Life*, 233; LeConte, "Philosophy of Medicine," 262–63.

7. Hentz diary, November 19, 1845, in Stowe, ed., *Southern Practice*, 57. Lunsford Yandell recalls his early reading in his diary, 1824–43, 398, Yandell family papers, Filson, as does William Holcombe in his *How I Became a Homoeopath*, 4. Excellent sources for young men's reading are Jones student notebook, 1851, Jones collection, HTML, and Porcher commonplace book, 1843–45, SCHS. On medicine as opening up the study of the sciences in general, see Joseph Jones to "Dear Cousin," June 16, 1853, Jones collection, HTML;

Joseph A. S. Milligan to Joseph Milligan, September 8, 1844, Milligan family papers, SHC; and Horton, "Education of a Physician," Vanderbilt. On this same issue, see Kohlstedt, *Formation of the American Scientific Community*, 14–16; Ben-David, "Scientific Productivity"; and Beaver, *American Scientific Community*.

8. LeConte, "On the Science of Medicine," 458.

9. Charles Hentz autobiography, in Stowe, ed., *Southern Practice*, 409; Still, *Early Recollections*, 16; Lunsford Yandell diary, 1824–43, 393, Yandell family papers, Filson. See also Frances Sage Bradley autobiography, 21, Bradley papers, Emory.

10. On medical education generally and reformers' efforts to bring it into line with new discoveries in the physical sciences, therapeutics, and institutional power, see, in addition to the citations in note 1, above, Kaufman, *American Medical Education*; Warner, *Against the Spirit of System*; Rothstein, *American Medical Schools*; Kett, *Formation of the American Medical Profession*; and Numbers, ed., *Education of American Physicians*. On the South, see Spalding, *History of the Medical College of Georgia*; Duffy, ed., *Rudolph Matas History*; Waring, *History of Medicine*.

11. On the founding of medical schools nationally, see Rothstein, *American Physicians*, and Cassedy, *Medicine and American Growth*. The extensive correspondence of Dr. Samuel Brown in the 1810s and 1820s is an excellent window on the thinking of physicians who set up new schools; see the Brown papers, Filson. Philadelphia set the standard for orthodox medical education largely because of the University of Pennsylvania medical school, esteemed since the eighteenth century, but also because of Jefferson Medical College; both schools enrolled large numbers of southerners well into the 1850s; see Daniel Kilbride, "Southern Medical Students." On individual southern schools, in addition to works cited in n. 10, above, see Cox and Morison, *University of Louisville*; Ellis, *Medicine in Kentucky*; Bridgforth, "Medicine in Antebellum Mississippi"; Peter, *History of the Medical Department*; John D. Wright, *Transylvania*; Duffy, *Tulane University Medical Center*; Shryock, "Medical Practice in the Old South;" Sewell, *Medicine in Maryland*; Gay, *Medical Profession in Georgia*; and Holley, *History of Medicine in Alabama*.

Two other early southern schools should be mentioned. The University of Maryland Medical College was founded in 1807 as a proprietary school with a nominal academic link. Although it never became as large as the major schools, it was a model for them, with direct ties to the founding of the University of Louisiana school. The Medical Department of the University of Virginia was included in the founding of the university but did not graduate its first class until 1828. Virginia, too, remained a small school throughout the years covered here, not simply because of its proximity to the huge Philadelphia schools, but also because it remained tied to ideals of a liberal education rather than diversifying into practical science and clinical treatment. See Blanton, *Medicine in Virginia in the Nineteenth Century*.

In terms of tuition and fees, most schools in the South and the North charged students not inconsiderable fees, ranging from $110 to $140 per term, plus $20–30 for cadavers and, sometimes, an extra $10 for both "library" and "graduation." See also the brief discussion of the costs of training a physician in Cooper, *Lectures on the Elements*, 72 (thanks to Michael O'Brien for this reference).

12. Ludmerer, *Learning to Heal*, 3; Dickson, "Introductory Lecture" (1826), 17; Daniel Drake, "Inaugural Discourse," 16; Cozart, "Southern Students," 10, Theses, MCSSC. For historians who characterize mid-nineteenth-century medical education largely in terms of schools' shortcomings by modern standards, see Starr, *Social Transformation of American Medi-*

cine, 40–44, and Rothstein, *American Physicians*, ch. 5. They only partially soften disparaging criticism of contemporary reformers. One such critic was embarrassed that schools "scramble for students as boys for marbles or ginger cakes"; see "Medical Ethics," 395; compare Jerome Cochran, "Address," 60. John Harley Warner (*Against the Spirit of System*, ch. 1) tips the balance toward appreciating schools on their own terms, seeing them as important sources of professionalization.

13. Perhaps the most notable rivalry between two southern schools was that between Kentucky's Louisville Medical Institute (later the University of Louisville Medical Department) and the Transylvania School of Medicine, located ninety miles away in Lexington. In 1836–37, more than half of the Transylvania faculty was lured to Louisville by that city's business and civic leadership, in large part because the latter city's key position on the Ohio River gave it a larger transient, poor population and thus a more ready supply of cadavers used for anatomical dissection; see Cox "Louisville Medical Institute;" John D. Wright, *Transylvania*, 147–50; and Ellis, *Medicine in Kentucky*, 13–18. For contemporary accounts, see Lunsford P. Yandell, "Narrative"; and "Medical Intelligence," *Southern Medical and Surgical Journal* 2 (August 1837): 63–64.

The path to the modern medical school, which peaks with Abraham Flexner's 1910 Carnegie Foundation report exposing the shortcomings of most American medical schools, is discussed in Ludmerer, *Learning to Heal*, 88–90 and ch. 9, and Starr, *Social Transformation*, 90–101. My view of this change is that it was less clearly tied to big-picture ideals; reformers' actions often took shape from their immediate need to define how their own schools fit into their communities.

14. Schools' annual circulars neatly document the flow of both material and ideological change in schools over the century, their avid, argumentative quality revealing more than their authors probably intended. According to one doctor, "To lie like a college catalogue" was an adage that should govern all readers of these circulars. However, he and other doctors avidly read catalogs as we might: as brief, rhetorical samplings of ideals, as well as self-promotion. For the adage, see Dowler, "Historical Retrospective," 491; see also, "Word about Catalogues."

15. Schools' annual circulars appear in manuscript collections cited here throughout. Especially large collections of circulars are at the Medical College of South Carolina, the University of Louisville Medical School, and the Medical College of Georgia; smaller collections are at Tulane University and Vanderbilt University.

16. For the Medical College of Georgia's 1830 experiment, which received national notice by other schools (much of it critical), see Spalding, *History of the Medical College of Georgia*, 28, and Norwood, *Medical Education*, 277. For the flurry of reform that followed the AMA's advocacy of longer terms, see Medical College of Georgia, "Annual Announcement," 1848, [2]; Medical College of the State of South Carolina, "Catalogue," 1848, [8]; University of Louisville, "Annual Catalogue," 1849, 12–13; Lunsford P. Yandell, "Introductory Lecture" (1848); and "Medical Convention of the State of South Carolina."

17. Along these same lines, the major schools limited their thirst for students by accepting transfer students only from other orthodox institutions and by agreeing not to permit mid-term transfers between schools. These various requirements may be found in most of the large schools' annual circulars throughout the antebellum years.

18. Wilson Yandell to Lunsford P. Yandell, November 22 and 24, 1824, and Charles

Caldwell to Lunsford P. Yandell, May 8, 1831, Yandell family papers, Filson. For a good discussion of private teaching in the Charleston, S.C., medical scene, see Waring, "Charleston Medicine," 331. As some reformers knew, the extracurricular offerings recapitulated an orthodox tradition of urban medical education in eighteenth-century Britain; see Susan Lawrence, *Charitable Knowledge*; on the role of the Paris clinics, see Warner, *Against the Spirit of System*.

19. Medical College of Georgia, "Annual Announcement," 1858, 12; University of Nashville, "Second Annual Announcement," 1852, 10; University of Louisville, "Annual Catalogue," 1862, 4. For similar developments at the Medical College of the State of South Carolina, see "Catalogue," 1853, 9–10, and "Annual Circular," 1858, 14.

Interestingly, schools took notice of each other's extra courses in what seems a tentative effort to create a general movement toward curricular expansion. For example, a New Orleans journal linked to the University of Louisiana commented favorably on courses associated with the Medical College of the State of South Carolina; see "Charleston Preparatory Medical School." This reform-on-the-margins has not been given much positive notice by historians. Even so keen a student of nineteenth-century medical education as Kenneth Ludmerer (*Learning to Heal*, 17) sees the growth of "extramural" courses as merely "a testimony to the inadequacy of conventional medical education."

20. University of Nashville, "Catalogue," 1860, 4. As a mark of distinction, Nashville noted "university" by the names of new students who had attended college; see, for example, "Annual Announcement," 1855, 11–12. Similarly, starting in the 1850s, the Medical College of South Carolina noted "literary opportunity" beside the names of graduates with university experience; see, for example, Medical College of the State of South Carolina, "Catalogue," 1851, 12–13, and "Annual Circular," 1860, 9–12. For discussion of whether premedical education was elitist, see John Berrien Lindsley, "Table Talk," in his diary, 1860, TSL, 6, 28–29; "American Medical Association"; and John Davis, "Thoughts on the Medical Convention."

21. [University of Louisville], "Louisville Medical Institute [Circular]," 1838, 7. A discussion of the thesis' place in students' work is in Chapter 2. Historians have differed widely on the significance of the thesis; some ignore it, while others look at it as a window on institutional life, as I do here. For the former view, see Ludmerer, *Learning to Heal*, and Rothstein, *American Physicians*. A brief, balanced mention is in Spalding, *History of the Medical College of Georgia*, 34–35, and Warner, *Against the Spirit of System*. Susan Wells uses theses to shed light on the learning of women M.D.s; see her *Out of the Dead House*, esp. ch. 4. A thoughtful overview of one collection of theses is Warner's foreword to *Bibliography of Inaugural Theses*.

22. Apprenticeship was thoroughly freelance and, in the view of reformers, embarrassingly unprofessional. Terms of service differed widely. Some students paid their mentors room and board; others were given both free. In some cases, mentors actually paid apprentices a small cash stipend; in other arrangements, apprentices paid tuition, by the month or by the year. Some agreements stipulated payment in cash, but, as one former apprentice recalled, some students paid in "nominal" amounts of eggs, vegetables, and butter. Some apprentices lived in the doctor's house, others came and went each day; some worked alone, others worked in tandem. For a sampling of apprenticeship terms and conditions, see William Whetstone to Margaret Boatwright, January 10, March 12, and October 14, 1853; and William Whetstone to Nathan C. Whetstone, March 24, 1853, Whetstone family papers, SCL; Russell Cunningham, "Autobiography," 64, ADAH; Dunlap account book, 307, 309, SCL; David H.

Dungan to Miss H. Wylie, April 3, 1861, GSWBFP, SCL; and Hentz diary, May 13, 1846, in Stowe, ed., *Southern Practice*, 93.

23. Caldwell, *Autobiography*, 77; Ward, "Medicine in the Cotton States," 12. For other nineteenth-century critiques of education that implicated apprenticeship, see Wright, "On the Qualifications Requisite for a Medical Student," 13, TSM, and Sutton, "Medical Reform." Historians of American medicine have not looked at apprenticeship closely, often echoing nineteenth-century critiques of it as merely slipshod. The approach taken here suggests that what apprentices learned was more varied and useful than we have thought. See Rosenberg, *Care of Strangers*, 60–61; Ludmerer, *Learning to Heal*, 16; Starr, *Social Transformation*, 41; Rothstein, *American Physicians*, 85–87; and Rothstein, *American Medical Schools*, 27. Compare Lane, "Role of Apprenticeship."

24. Samuel H. Dickson to James A. Milligan, August 27, 1844, Milligan family papers, SHC.

25. George Logan to [Robert Lebby], April 4, 1826, Lebby family papers, SCL; John E. Montgomery to J. S. Copes, May 11 and May 29, 1841, Copes papers, HTML.

26. Lunsford Yandell diary, 1824–43, 402, Yandell family papers, Filson; Richardson diary, March 24, June 14, 1854; June 6, 1853, SHC. As student Thomas Wade read anatomy, physiology, and surgery, he also was reading the Bible, Sir Walter Scott, and Lord Byron; see Wade diary entries for April through December, 1851, Matas. Other fairly comprehensive lists of student reading are found in Hentz diary, throughout 1845–46, in Stowe, ed., *Southern Practice*; Porcher commonplace book, 1843–45, SCHS; and Charles Bonner to John Young Bassett, October 21, 1842, Bassett papers, SHC. Orthodox texts frequently mentioned include Bell, Bell, and Godman, *Anatomy and Physiology of the Human Body*; Dewees, *Compendious System of Midwifery*; Eberle, *Treatise on the Practice of Medicine* (1830 and 1831); Eberle, *Treatise of the Materia Medica*; Gross, *Elements of Pathological Anatomy*; and Gross, *System of Surgery*.

27. William Whetstone to his mother, April 15, [1853], Whetstone family papers, SCL; J. A. S. Milligan to James Milligan, September 8, 1844, Milligan family papers, SHC; Charles Hentz autobiography, in Stowe, ed., *Southern Practice*, 438.

28. See, for example, Richardson diary, July 22, 1853, SHC; Wade diary, June 2, 1852, Matas; and Hentz diary, June 24, 1846, in Stowe, ed., *Southern Practice*, 110. The Henry Clay Lewis sketches are darkly humorous tales of a willful young physician. Lewis received his M.D. in 1846 from the University of Louisville, and he practiced in northern Louisiana until 1850, when he drowned crossing a river while out on a call. On apprentices, see Lewis's sketches "Getting Acquainted with the Medicines" and "Cupping on the Sternum," in John Q. Anderson, ed., *Louisiana Swamp Doctor*, 83–91.

29. William Whetstone to his mother, April 15, [1853], Whetstone family papers, SCL; Jobe, "Autobiography," 116, TSL; William Whetstone to Nathan C. Whetstone, May 13, [1855], Whetstone family papers, SCL; Richardson diary, November 2, 1853, SHC. It seems that most apprentices did not observe many childbirths involving white women, quite likely because women and families did not want young, local men in the birthing room. The supervision of apprentices was a tangled issue. Apprentices were not supposed to practice unsupervised, but clearly some did so once they had gained the trust of their mentors and patients. For an instance of an apprentice threatened with punishment for practicing on his own, see James H. Hall to J. S. Copes, June 27, 1832, Copes papers, HTML. For instances of apprentices doing their own work, see Susan Yandell to Lunsford Yandell Jr., April 19, 1859,

Yandell family papers, Filson; W. M. Meador to John Robinson, May 28, 1867, Robinson papers, SCL; and Knox medical diary, 1843, Winthrop. Interesting issues in a mentor's legal responsibility for his apprentice are raised in a Canadian context in Jacalyn Duffin, " 'In View of the Body of Job Broom.' " On the birthing room, see Leavitt, *Brought to Bed*, ch. 4, and McMillen, *Motherhood in the Old South*, ch. 4.

30. See Wade diary, May and June 1852, Matas, and Hentz diary, September 30, 1846, in Stowe, ed., *Southern Practice*, 141.

31. William Whetstone to Nathan C. Whetstone, March 23, 1855, and William Whetstone to his mother Margaret Boatwright, May 12, 1854, Whetstone family papers, SCL; Edward Armstrong to J. S. Copes, July 14, 1834, Copes papers, HTML.

32. Daniel Drake, "Strictures on Some of the Defects," 5–12; Fayette Baker Spragins to Thomas M. Spragins, April 6, 1841, Clark family papers, VHS; F. M. Jones to "Dear Wife," November 6, 1885, Jones papers, Emory. See also J. H. Parker to Josiah Hawkins, March 31, 1883, Hawkins papers, LSU. Boarding expenses were remarkably stable throughout the century, save for immediate postwar inflation in the South; for students listing typical expenses, see Charles Bonner to John Young Bassett, October 21, 1842, Bassett papers, SHC, and Lafayette Strait to Jacob Fox Strait, December 13, 1856, GSWBFP, SCL; see also Duffy, *Tulane University Medical Center*, 18. On individual students' experience, see Barlow and Powell, "Dedicated Medical Student"; Victor H. Bassett, "Georgia Medical Student"; and Atlee, "Education of a Physician."

33. William Bonner to [Samuel Bonner?], February 24, 1850, Bonner family papers, LSU; Wade diary, December 7, 1851 (see also January 13, 1852, and February 28, 1852), Matas. See also [W. M. Meador?] to John A. Robinson, November 16, 1873, Robinson papers, SCL. For the intellectual touring of churches, see Hentz diary, July 31, 1847, in Stowe, ed., *Southern Practice*, 173, and Joseph Jones to Mary Sharpe Jones, November 24, 1853, Jones collection, HTML.

34. Thomas M. McIntosh to Emma McIntosh, October 23, 1874, McIntosh papers, Duke; [W. M. Meador?] to John A. Robinson, May 28, 1867, Robinson papers, SCL; Wade diary, January 20, 1852, Matas; Marmaduke D. Kimbrough to Nathan Hunt, August 29, 1860, Hunt papers, Duke; J. Williman to J. A. S. Milligan, September 3, 1843, Milligan family papers, SHC; Charles Colcock Jones to Joseph Jones, January 31, 1855, Jones collection, HTML; James W. Copes to J. S. Copes, March 7, 1832, Copes papers, HTML. For other letters about these moral issues, see, for example, Adaline Evans to Joseph Heard, February 28, 1842, Heard papers, ADAH, and Thomas Furman to Ann Armstrong, January 8, 1832, Furman papers, Emory. The diaries of Charles Hentz for 1847–48 (in Stowe, ed., *Southern Practice*) and Thomas Wade, 1851–52 (Matas), give especially rich accounts of student life.

35. J. H. Parker to Josiah Hawkins, March 31, 1883, Hawkins papers, LSU; Charles Hentz autobiography, in Stowe, ed., *Southern Practice*, 458; Hentz diary, [June 14], 1847, in ibid., 165; A. V. Carrigan to "Dear Bro.," December 23, 1854, Carrigan papers, SCL; Charles Johnson to Lou McCrindell, April 5, 1860, Johnson family papers, LSU. See also Lafayette Strait to "Dear Anna," December 9, 1856, GSWBFP, SCL.

The daily routine in most schools consisted mainly of lectures, with perhaps a few demonstrations, which took up five to six hours a day at the larger schools, usually from nine o'clock in the morning to noon, and then from three to five or six o'clock in the evening. With the expansion of the "shadow" curriculum in the 1840s, students also spent time accompanying faculty on rounds to nearby homes of patients or to lecture-demonstrations at clinics or hospitals.

36. A. V. Carrigan to "Dear Bro.," December 23, 1854, Carrigan papers, SCL; Charles Johnson to Lou McCrindell, January 12, 1860, Johnson family papers, LSU; Ivy diary, October 14, [1878; entry out of chronological order, appearing near the end of the volume on an unnumbered page marked "Cash Account. May."], Waring; Charles Johnson to Lou McCrindell, April 5, 1860, Johnson family papers, LSU; Lunsford Yandell to Wilson Yandell, January 15, 1824, Yandell family papers, Filson. The students betting on patient survival appear in "Medical Department of Louisville University," 545.

37. Allen student notebook, 1874 (quotation from loose sheet in Allen's handwriting), MCG; "Tribute of Respect," 127–28; Lunsford Yandell diary, 1824–43, 407, Yandell family papers, Filson; Jeptha McKinney to Adeliza McKinney, January 25–27, 1857, McKinney papers, LSU. For other accounts of student funerals, see Jeptha McKinney, ms. page beginning "1857—Mr. Tinsley, of Alabama . . . ," McKinney papers, LSU, and Albert Bachelor to Cornelia Steward, March 2, 1874 (draft), Bachelor papers, LSU.

38. Wade diary, December 24, 1851, Matas; Jeptha McKinney to Adeliza McKinney, January 25, 1852, McKinney papers, LSU; I. H. Blair to William Mobley, December 26, 1853, GSWBFP, SCL. Charles Hentz became seriously ill just after his arrival at the Louisville school; see Hentz autobiography, in Stowe, ed., *Southern Practice*, 460.

39. Louisville Medical Institute, "Circular," 1839, p. [3]. Medical journals were a forum for discussion of faculty careers and competition among schools, and faculty correspondence also gives a sense of how inward looking medical education was. For good examples of the latter, see the Yandell family papers and the Brown papers, both at the Filson Club, the Jones collection, HTML, and the Short papers, SHC. Noting great or well-loved faculty became the chief way for schools to claim a place in history; older histories of medicine in general similarly use esteemed practitioners as a way of tracing a "genealogy" of respected physicians who had passed through the school. For examples, see the Medical College of Georgia, "Annual Announcement," [1881]; University of Louisiana, "Catalogue from 1834 to 1872"; and Chaillé, "Historical Sketch."

40. J. E. Walthall to Dr. Joseph Heard, December 26, 1842 (typed copy), Heard papers, ADAH; Charles Bonner to John Young Bassett, October 21, 1842, Bassett papers, SHC; Charles Hentz autobiography, in Stowe, ed., *Southern Practice*, 459–60; Peter, *History of the Medical Department* (quoting David W. Yandell), 42; Caldwell, *Autobiography*, 409; Clark lecture notes, 1841, 1, Clark papers, Duke; Lewis, "Being Examined for My Degree," in John Q. Anderson, ed., *Louisiana Swamp Doctor*, 171; ? to John A. Robinson, November 16, 1873, Robinson papers, SCL. Drake's quacking gallery of students is in Charles Hentz autobiography, in Stowe, ed., *Southern Practice*, 459. Drake was Harriet Beecher Stowe's doctor in Cincinnati in the 1830s, and she once characterized him as "stiff as a poker" and as writing "very polite, ceremonious" directions for taking medication (see Fields, ed., *Life and Letters of Harriet Beecher Stowe*, 79). Henry Clay Lewis lampoons Drake as excessively vain; see "Frank and the Professor," in John Q. Anderson, ed., *Louisiana Swamp Doctor*, 121–25.

41. Dunglison, *Medical Student*, 175; Porcher, "Personal Reminiscences," 3–4, Waring; Joseph Jones to [Mary Sharpe Jones], November 24, 1853, Jones collection, HTML; Lunsford Yandell to Sarah Wendel, December 3, 1831, Yandell family papers, Filson; Hentz diary, in Stowe, ed., *Southern Practice*, 266. On faculty entertaining students, see also Charles Johnson

to Lou McCrindell, November 12, 1859, Johnson family papers, LSU. An example of published expressions of gratitude to the faculty are the resolutions of appreciation printed in the annual circulars of the Medical College of South Carolina for most years in the 1850s and late 1860s. The University of Louisiana class of 1874 bought Dr. Frank Hawthorn a "locket inlaid with diamonds" in gratitude for his teaching; see the receipt dated March 14, 1874, for $67.50 from I. C. Levi jewelers, 108 Canal St., New Orleans, in Bachelor papers, LSU.

42. Charles Hentz autobiography, in Stowe, ed., *Southern Practice*, 478; Lunsford Yandell to Wilson Yandell, January 15, 1824, Yandell family papers, Filson; Lunsford Yandell diary, 1824–43, 406, Yandell family papers, Filson; Knox medical diary, January 15, 1843, Winthrop; Wade diary, January 13, 1852, Matas; Hentz diary, January 6, 1848, in Stowe, ed. *Southern Practice*, 189.

43. ? to John A. Robinson, November 16, 1873, Robinson papers, SCL; Joseph Jones to Charles Colcock Jones, February 20, 1854, Jones papers, HTML; Milf[ord] Woodruff to Charles Hentz, November 27, 1847, Hentz family papers, SHC. Ecclesiastes 11:9 reads, in part, "Rejoice, O young man, in thy youth; and let thy heart cheer thee in the days of they youth . . . but know thou, that . . . God will bring thee into judgment." On sermons aimed at medical students, see also William C. Wright to Benjamin A. Wright, February 6, 1848, Wright papers, Duke. On temperance activities, see Physiological Temperance Society of the Medical Institute of Louisville, "Proceedings of the Physiological Temperance Society," and "Physiological Temperance Society." The faculty of the Medical College of Georgia warned one student about his habitual drunkenness and "resolved to expell him from the College should the offence be repeated" (Faculty Minute Books, December 9, 1834, MCG). On the widespread sensitivity to drink, see Tyrrell, "Drink and Temperance."

CHAPTER TWO

1. Although now told with greater sophistication, the history of medical education has remained largely a tale of how its modern organization and rationale emerged from a less sound nineteenth-century model. This perspective, while sharpening our sense of change, tends to portray nineteenth-century education as merely failing to achieve modern standards rather than as a world built on its own rewards and insights. For histories that take daily routine seriously, see John Harley Warner's look at the "French impulse" in American medical learning in *Against the Spirit of System* and Charles E. Rosenberg's view of hospital training in *Care of Strangers*.

2. Ernest Sydney Lewis, "Reminiscences," 749; Clark lecture notes, 1841, 199, Clark papers, Duke; Hentz diary, December 20, 1849, in Stowe, ed., *Southern Practice*, 270. The memory of Dudley is in Peter, *History of the Medical Department*, 19. For other commentary of this kind, see E. L. McGehee to Albert Bachelor, March 21, [18]73, Bachelor papers, LSU; Keller student notebook, 1847–48, Keller papers, ADAH; and Thomas Copes (written jointly with Barkley Townshend) to J. S. Copes, November 11, 1835, Copes papers, HTML; for a critical faculty view, see Short, *Duties of Medical Students*.

3. Joseph Jones, "Suggestions on Medical Education," 14; Moultrie, "Introductory Address," 29; Porcher, ms. lecture notes, "Materia Medica and Therapy delivered 1854–5–6–7–8 again 1873–74," Porcher papers, Waring. On nature in various guises during this century,

see Conser, *God and the Natural World*; Albanese, *Nature Religion in America*; and Keeney, *Botanizers*.

Oliver Wendell Holmes used the term "nature-trusting heresy" in his *Currents and Counter-Currents in Medical Science* to describe the efforts of those physicians, himself included, who gave new—that is, practical—attention to what had long been called the *vis medicatrix naturae*, the healing power of nature. Other influential texts in the advocacy of nature-trusting were the 1835 address by Jacob Bigelow, "On Self-Limited Diseases," and Elisha Bartlett's influential text advocating bedside observation, *Essay on the Philosophy of Medical Science*. The significance of this debate is thoroughly explored in Warner, " 'Nature-Trusting Heresy' "; see also Rosenberg, "Therapeutic Revolution," and his concise discussion in *Care of Strangers*, 86–93.

4. Arnold, "Random Thoughts," 490; see also Breckenridge, "Address," 11.

5. Keller student notebook, 1847–48, 263–64, Keller papers, ADAH. The Randolph-Macon student was Philip Southall Blanton; see his "Modus Operandi," VHS. For other examples of this kind, see Huronymous student notebook, 1833–35, Matas; Clark lecture notes, 1841, esp. 155–98, Clark papers, Duke, and the medical notebook, University of Nashville, of an unknown member of the Sneed family, 1860–61, Sneed family papers, TSL. The observation of Charles Short was by Louisville student Charles Hentz in the mid-1840s; see Stowe, ed., *Southern Practice*, 459.

6. Porcher, undated ms. (in file headed "Notes on Clinical Lectures & Examinations"), Porcher papers, Waring.

7. Allen student notebook, 1874, MCG; ? to John A. Robinson, November 16, 1873, Robinson papers, SCL.

8. Huronymous student notebook, 1833–35, 47, Matas.

9. Kennon student notebook, lecture notes, 1866, Matas.

10. Knox medical diary, January 27, 1843, Winthrop; Kennon student notebook, lecture notes, January 29, 1866, Matas. For other examples of this universal anecdotal style, see Baruch medical notebook, 1860–61, 14, Baruch papers, Emory; Keller student notebook (especially Daniel Drake's lectures), and Huronymous student notebook, 1833–35, 70–78, Matas; and McKinney student notebook, January 20–22, 1857, McKinney papers, LSU.

11. Lectures on obstetrics became a distinct subject area by the mid-1830s, and by the 1860s they were usually defined as covering "obstetrics and the diseases of women and children," which meant that the teacher said a great deal about pregnancy, labor, and delivery, with a few remarks about the care of women and newborns immediately after delivery. As for conception, William Potts Dewees's definition of it in his much-used textbook is typically unspecific: "We employ this term [conception] to signify, the successful application of the male semen to whatever is furnished by the female" (*Compendious System*, 75). Compare Denman, *Practice of Midwifery*, 94, and Churchill, *Theory and Practice*, 98–100. For a representative M.D. thesis focusing solely on women's reproductive anatomy, see DuPont, "Peculiarities of the Female," MCSSC; for one on femininity, see Hill, "Treatise on Women," MCSSC. On both of these matters, see Angus McLauren, "Pleasures of Procreation."

Climate and diet are other topics that tended to be dispersed throughout the curriculum, depending on a given teacher's interests. Climate, of course, was an ancient interest of physicians, but by the mid-nineteenth century its study was in awkward transition from earlier correlations of ill health to ill winds to a new, empirical meteorological emphasis that became part of modern epidemiology. Diet also received frequent but episodic mention in lectures and, even more than climate, drifted without its own home in the curriculum. Samuel Dickson told his class in Charleston in 1854 that "cooking . . . is truly an important science and it is an absurd affectation to disparage it." But, as he suggests, this view cut against the orthodox grain; see Hunter, "Preservation of Health," 8, MCSSC.

12. Hunter, "Preservation of Health," 22, MCSSC; Huronymous student notebook, [Benjamin Dudley lecture], 1833–35, 47, Matas. See also Jones, "Peculiarities of the Female," MCSSC.

13. Allen student notebook, 1874, MCG. Teachers were wary of schools being seen as hotbeds of salaciousness. When a Transylvania student in his thesis on venereal disease referred to a sexually available young woman as "a *fresh snap*" he was reprimanded by the faculty for his "indecent and inappropriate" language; see Parker, "Gonorrhoea," 2, TSM.

14. There was a distinct literature on slaves in medical periodicals by the 1850s, paralleling discussion of slavery in the larger society. So it is all the more striking that these did not shape textbooks or school curricula more forcefully. The orthodox view in periodical literature is taken up in more detail in Chapter 7. But, in the context of school, it is notable that only 10 of more than 4,000 extant antebellum medical theses (from South Carolina, Transylvania, and Nashville) dealt with blacks or slaves as such. Even home health care books for a southern audience mentioned blacks only in passing. For examples of home health care books' in-passing mention of slaves, see John Hume Simons, *Planter's Guide*, 207; Goodlett, *Family Physician*, 630; and Jennings, *Compendium of Medical Science*, 493. See also Savitt, *Medicine and Slavery*, ch. 1.

15. McLoud, "Hints on the Medical Treatment of Negroes," 17–18, MCSSC; see also Pope, "Professional Management of Negro Slaves," and Moore, "Plantation Hygiene," both in MCSSC. Compare Kiple and King, *Another Dimension*, esp. pt. 3; Savitt, *Medicine and Slavery*; and Fett, *Working Cures*.

16. Gilmer, "Pathology and Treatment," 9, MCSSC. For other examples of M.D. theses on this subject, see Briggs, "On Cachexia Africana," and Coleman, "On Cachexia Africana," both in TSM; and Gresham, "On the Subject of Cachexia Africana," MCSSC.

17. Pope, "Professional Management," 7, 9, MCSSC. Similar in style are McLoud, "Hints on the Medical Treatment of Negroes," and Moore, "Plantation Hygiene," both MCSSC. Compare Westmoreland, "Anatomical and Physiological Difference," Vanderbilt, which is rare among theses for having no social context for the discussion of African Americans. Instead, the author simply asserts racist clichés: Africans have thicker skulls than whites, little family feeling, no chastity, etc.

18. McCaa, "Manner of Living and Diseases of the Slaves," 1–2, Waring. These themes run throughout the theses by McLoud, Pope, Moore cited above; see also Broyles, "Life of a Physician," Vanderbilt. The agricultural press took a similar tack; see James O. Breeden, *Advice among Masters*.

19. Lunsford Yandell to David Wendel, January 18, 1826, Yandell family papers, Filson. For other students excited by the prospect of bedside rounds, see Thomas Furman to Ann Armstrong, [August?] 1832, Furman papers, Emory, and Nathaniel Siewers to "Dear Parents!" January 7, 1866 (typed copy), Siewers letters, UNCC. Looking back on his student experience in "these magazines of misery and contagion,—these Babels of disease and sin," John Young Bassett ("Climate and Diseases," 319) nonetheless praised the ward's blunt message: "this is Pathology."

Here the term "ward" generally refers to hospital or institutional settings for contact with patients, while "clinic" is the broader term, including patients seen in their homes or in mentors' offices. Opportunities for students to see at least a few sick people arose in apprenticeships, but in a way limited by the social relations of practice, as noted in Chapter 1. The definitive overview of the rise of the American general-care hospital from its beginnings in a farrago of almshouses, charity institutions, and private teaching clinics is Rosenberg, *Care of Strangers*. Also suggestive about medical students' role in clinics are Lawrence, *Charitable Knowledge*; Warner, *Against the Spirit of System*; Ludmerer, *Learning to Heal*, esp. chs. 1, 2, and 8; and Rothstein, *American Medical Schools*, chs. 2 and 3.

20. University of Louisville, "Announcement," 1864, 6. The size and number of hospitals in a given city, of course, importantly shaped clinical opportunities. In a city with more than one medical school, New Orleans, for instance, competition for student places on the wards was intense throughout most of the century. Even in one-school cities, such as Charleston, the small size of hospitals, along with rivalries between hospital administrators and medical faculty, led to restrictions on students. In Charleston, the small City Hospital and the Marine Hospital were the major sites until the college faculty set up a "college hospital" in the 1850s, followed by the larger Roper Hospital, which took in resident physicians in 1857. The Medical College of Georgia, in Augusta, constantly struggled to place students in the small City Hospital, which was supplemented in the 1850s by an even smaller black hospital and a city dispensary. Similarly, Louisville distributed its students to the small (fifty-bed) Marine Hospital and to a scattering of dispensaries until just before the war, when the City Hospital took in more students.

New Orleans' Charity Hospital was comparatively so large through the antebellum years that it received national notice as an institution. See, for example, [Fenner], "Report on the New-Orleans Charity Hospital," and "Statistics of the Charity Hospital." For a nonmedical view, see the interesting mixture of admiration and disgust in "New Orleans Charity Hospital." A useful recent study is John Salvaggio, *New Orleans Charity Hospital*, esp. chs. 4 and 6; see also Duffy, ed., *Rudolph Matas History*, vol. 1, chs. 7–8, and Waring, *History of Medicine*, chs. 3 and 5.

The annual circulars of all large schools also give an excellent sense, year-by-year, of how schools wished to portray their hospital connections to prospective students, patients, and to supporters of the school. Organizational issues and evidence of faculty battles with hospital trustees run throughout the Faculty Minute Books (1833–52), MCG; University of Nashville Trustees' Minute Books (4 reels microfilm, including various years in the 1850s through the 1870s and into the twentieth century), TSL; and Waring, ed., *Excerpts from the Minute Book*.

21. Traill Green to J. S. Copes, January 29, 1834, Copes papers, HTML; Huronymous student notebook, 1833–35, 65, Matas; he notes the surgical strapping on p. 28. Whetstone's notes are in his letter to his brother Nathan C. Whetstone, May 13, 1854, Whetstone family papers, SCL. See also Lewis, "Cupping an Irishman," in John Q. Anderson, ed., *Louisiana Swamp Doctor*, 158.

22. I. S. Blair to Lafayette Strait, April 15, 1857, GSWBFP, SCL; T. L. Laws to Thomas Lee Settle, November 3, 1867, Settle papers, Duke; William Bonner to [Samuel Bonner?], February 24, 1850, Bonner family papers, LSU; Francis Jones to Cleopatra Jones, n.d. (probably 1885 or 1886), Jones papers, Emory. Supervision of students seems to have varied greatly, mentor by mentor. In addition to surgery, students also wrote about experimenting with

drugs—sometimes on themselves, sometimes on patients; see, for example, Thomas Furman to Ann Armstrong, August 11, 1831, Furman papers, Emory, and Charles Wilkins Short to Jane Wilkins, June 27, 1814, Short papers, SHC. On experimentation, see Martin Pernick, *Calculus of Suffering*, ch. 3, and Lederer, *Subjected to Science*, ch. 1. On bedside witnessing as a traditional pedagogical technique in medical education, see Lisa Rosner, "Eighteenth-Century Medical Education."

23. Medical College of Georgia, "Annual Announcement," 1859, 5. Schools acknowledged the antebellum scarcity of African American patients only after the war, as when the Medical College of the State of South Carolina noted in 1866 the new postwar influx of "an immense colored pauper population, who, in former times, were never found in Southern Hospitals"; see Medical College of the State of South Carolina, "Annual Circular," 1866, 8.

24. Medical College of the State of South Carolina, "Annual Announcement," 1840, 5; Medical College of Georgia, "Annual Announcement," [1855], 10; see also Faculty Minute Books, January 16, 1838, MCG. On the particular vulnerability of slaves to the blurred distinction between therapy and experimentation, especially in surgery, see Savitt, "Use of Blacks for Medical Experimentation."

25. Medical College of Georgia, "Annual Announcement," [1852], 4; Marmaduke D. Kimbrough to Nathan Hunt, December 17, 1859, Hunt papers, Duke; Hentz diary, April 6, 1848, in Stowe, ed., *Southern Practice*, 199.

26. Nathaniel Siewers to "Dear Father and Mother," August 17, 1866 (typed copy), Siewers letters, UNCC; Hentz diary, August 9, 1847, in Stowe, ed., *Southern Practice*, 178–79. Siewers spent some time at the University Pennsylvania and was outraged that "Northern philanthropists can lavish their sympathy on our negroes in the South and let their own poor die uncared for at their very door" (Siewers to "Dear Father and Mother," July 25, 1866, Siewers letters, UNCC). For Lewis, see "Cupping an Irishman," in John Q. Anderson, ed., *Louisiana Swamp Doctor*, 158–64.

27. Nathaniel Siewers to "Dear Mother and Father," July 25, 1866 (typed copy), Siewers letters, UNCC; Traill Green to J. S. Copes, October 19, 1833, Copes papers, HTML; Thomas M. McIntosh to Emma McIntosh, November 11, 1876, McIntosh papers, Duke; Hentz diary, December 15, 1849, in Stowe, ed., *Southern Practice*, 267; Solomon Mordecai to Ellen Mordecai, January 15, 1820, Mordecai family papers, SHC; Lewis, "Cupping an Irishman," in John Q. Anderson, ed., *Louisiana Swamp Doctor*, 158. See also Thomas Wade's diary accounts of rounding with surgeon Warren Stone at Charity Hospital, December 1851 through February 1852, Matas.

28. Ernest Sydney Lewis, "Reminiscences," 758–59; Billingslea, "Appeal on Behalf of Southern Medical Colleges," 216. Clark lecture notes, 1841, Clark papers, Duke, gives an excellent sense of a serious student going on rounds.

29. E. L. McGehee to Albert Bachelor, May 15, [18]73, Bachelor papers, LSU; Cozart, "Place Where Southern Students," 4, MCSSC; Albert Bachelor to Cornelia Stewart, December 6, 1873 (draft), Bachelor papers, LSU. On teachers' enthusiasm for focusing on things "rarely or never met with" outside the wards, see Dunglison, *Medical Student*, 204.

30. [Fenner], "Report on the New-Orleans Charity Hospital," 283.

31. Descriptions of anatomy as the most basic medical science are common among medical educators in this era. See also Dickson, "Introductory Lecture" (1846), 8, and Dunglison, *Medical Student*, 168–70. On anatomy in the school curriculum, see Blake, "Anatomy:" At-

water, "Protracted Labor"; Warner, *Against the Spirit of System*, esp. 20–28; Rothstein, *American Medical Schools*, 34–35; and Sappol, *Traffic of Dead Bodies*, chs. 3 and 4.

32. University of Louisiana, "Annual Circular," 1838, 5; University of Louisville, "Annual Catalogue," 1842, [3]; "Practical Anatomy," 187–88; Medical College of the State of South Carolina, "Catalogue," 1845, 4. Where schools' circulars in the 1830s tended to focus on a the excellence of a school's wax models or drawings of the body, later circulars touted the well-lighted rooms, large "pit" arenas, and ample space for multiple dissecting tables.

33. Chaillé, "Historical Sketch," 5; Medical College of Georgia, "Annual Announcement," [1852], [3]; see also Medical College of the State of South Carolina, "Catalogue," 1852, 19. The language describing the aims and outcomes of anatomy classes is similar from school to school and does not vary much from year to year until the 1890s. Here the examples are from Medical College of Georgia's announcement for 1855 ("intimate structure," "morbid specimens," "primary tissues") and from Medical College of the State of South Carolina's announcement for 1840 ("private dissections," "minute knowledge").

34. Charles Hentz autobiography, in Stowe, ed., *Southern Practice*, 458; Medical College of the State of South Carolina, "Annual Announcement," 1840, [7]; Charles Hentz autobiography, in Stowe, ed., *Southern Practice*, 458. Compare Elizabeth Blackwell's memory of learning that a man of her acquaintance "could not look at my long slender fingers without thinking of the anatomical work in which they had been engaged" (Blackwell, *Pioneer Work*, 74). For notice of medical schools highlighting anatomy and dissection, see, for example, the review of the new medical department at Hampden-Sidney College in Richmond in the *Southern Literary Messenger* 5 (1839), 827 (cited in Blanton, *Medicine in Virginia*, 1933, 39), and Chaillé, "Historical Sketch," 4–5. Popular views of the teaching of anatomy ranged from enlightened approval to horror; see Alcott, *House I Live in*, an approving anatomical book for youth, and compare the harsh criticism in "Editor's Table." See also Richardson, *Death, Dissection, and the Destitute*; Jordanova, *Sexual Visions*, esp. ch. 5; Stafford, *Body Criticism*; and Sappol, *Traffic in Dead Bodies*, ch. 3.

35. Timmerman, "Difficulties and Privileges," 13, MCSSC; Joseph Jones to Charles Colcock Jones, February 10, 1854, Jones collection, HTML; Todd, "Young Physic," 7, TSM; Hicklin, "Necessary Connexion," 17, MCSSC; Broyles, "Life of a Physician," 15, Vanderbilt.

36. Hentz diary, August 13 and 14, 1847, in Stowe, ed., *Southern Practice*, 181; Miller, "Diagnosis," 10, 3, Vanderbilt. Teachers understood that anatomy was, in Robley Dunglison's words, "decidedly the most attractive" subject in school; but students needed to be warned against the idea that medicine was "nothing but the knife"; see Dunglison, *Medical Student*, 147, 149. For a similar view, see Dickson, "Introductory Lecture" (1826), 23. For students who grasped this point, see Furman, "Impediments," MCSSC, and Broyles, "Life of a Physician," Vanderbilt. For typical critiques of French physicians as excellent anatomists but indifferent or worse bedside doctors, see Lunsford P. Yandell, "Address on the Improvement of the Medical Profession," and Crumpton, "State and Utility of the Medical Science," MCSSC; see also David Wendel Yandell, *Notes on Medical Matters*, and Warner, *Against the Spirit of System*, esp. ch. 8.

37. Ivy diary, November 15, 1878, Waring; Russell Cunningham, "Autobiography," 67, ADAH; Wade diary, December 18, 1851, Matas; Joseph LeConte autobiography, 67, LeConte-Furman papers, SHC; Benjamin Lucas to "Dear Dr" [William Wylie], November 16, 1853, GSWBFP, SCL; Solomon Mordecai to Ellen Mordecai, January 1, 1820, Mordecai

papers, Duke. Although schools charged students a fee of ten dollars for cadavers through most of this period, Thomas Wade notes buying limbs for fifteen to twenty-five cents apiece. On changing fees and requirements in anatomy, see Robert Lovett to "My Dear Parents," November 16, 1843, Lovett papers, Emory.

38. Solomon Mordecai to Ellen Mordecai, January 1, 1820, Mordecai papers, Duke; Wade diary, January 22, 1852, Matas; Lunsford Yandell, student notes, ca. 1856, Yandell family collection, UL; Hentz diary, May 2, 1847, in Stowe, ed., *Southern Practice*, 159; Lewis, "Stealing a Baby," in John Q. Anderson, ed., *Louisiana Swamp Doctor*, 153; J. Williman to James A. Milligan, March 13, 1844, Milligan family papers, SHC; Ernest Sydney Lewis, "Reminiscences," 745. Henry Clay Lewis doubtless was not alone in his fantasy of recharging beautiful dead women; Edgar Allen Poe did not write in a cultural vacuum. A beautiful cadaver brought back to life by electrical shock is exactly what happens in one weirdly serious piece of fiction, and the experimenting medical student marries the girl. See Robinson, *Marietta*; see also the discussion in Sappol, *Traffic of Dead Bodies*, 216–20. On the dissection room jokes, sexual and otherwise, and the emotional climate of dissection, see Cohen, "Anatomy and the Dirty Philosopher."

39. Ivy diary, 1878, n.d., Waring; William Whetstone to Margaret Boatwright, February 24, 1854, Whetstone family papers, SCL; Bibb, "Essay on the Effects," 2–3, MCSSC.

40. Charles Colcock Jones to Joseph Jones, n.d., [1853], Jones papers, LSU; Joseph Jones to Charles Colcock Jones, December 13, 1853 (typed copy), Jones collection, HTML.

41. Mary Sharpe Jones to Joseph Jones, December 17, 1853, Jones collection, HTML; Mary Sharpe Jones to Joseph Jones, n.d., [1853 or 1854], Jones papers, LSU; Mary Sharpe Jones to Joseph Jones, December 17, 1853, Jones collection, HTML. Three years later, Joseph still was reassuring her (in a letter of February 21, 1856) that he believed that "the Creator governs all things."

42. Nathaniel Siewers to "Dear Father and Mother," March 2, 1866 (typed copy), Siewers letters, UNCC; Charles Hentz autobiography, in Stowe, ed., *Southern Practice*, 467–68. On grave-robbing as a social and medical phenomenon, see Shultz, *Body Snatching*; Blake, "Development of American Anatomy Acts"; Breeden, "Body Snatchers"; Spalding, *History of the Medical College of Georgia*, 36; Warner, *Against the Spirit of System*, 25–26; and Marshall, *Murdering to Dissect*.

43. Louis A. Dugas [1860], quoted in Spalding, *History of the Medical College of Georgia*, 69; James Riddell [1852], quoted in Duffy, *Tulane University Medical Center*, 32; J. H. Parker to Josiah Hawkins, March 11, 1883, Hawkins papers, LSU.

44. Knox medical diary, February 5, 1843, Winthrop.

45. Charles Hentz autobiography, in Stowe, ed., *Southern Practice*, 513–14.

46. Changes in the status of the M.D. thesis in medical education are noted in Chapter 1. Many of the copybook-sized, handwritten texts have survived, all from the antebellum years; the largest collections (from the Medical College of South Carolina, Transylvania, and Nashville) total just over 4,000. Each is typically twelve to fifteen pages in length, some obviously penned by the student himself and others inscribed by people with better handwriting, probably most often a female friend or family member. Nearly one-fifth of the extant theses concern "fever" of some sort. Certain diseases appear and disappear over the decades, especially epidemics such as cholera; others topics, such as "dysentery" and "typhoid," remained relatively constant choices. "Pneumonia" as a topic arose to stay in the 1840s,

suggesting a new agreement on its specificity as a disease. As in lecture notes, women are singled out as the only social group deserving solo study, and African Americans are rarely mentioned except in the general terms of the "public health" of slaves. Useful introductions to collections include Burkett, Sawyer, and Worthington, comps., "Bibliography of Inaugural Theses," and *Catalogue of the Transylvania University Medical Library*, Appendix A; see also Risse and Warner, "Reconstructing Clinical Activities."

47. Lafayette Strait to "Anna," June 25, 1857, GSWBFP, SCL; William C. Wright to Benjamin Wright, February 6, 1848, Wright papers, Duke; Jeptha McKinney, M.D. thesis (draft), "Pneumonia" (University of Louisiana, 1857), 1, McKinney papers, LSU; see also Todd, "Young Physic," 1, TSM. For other examples of the many students who obviously used the thesis to sort through professional or intellectual issues important to them, see McSwain, "Some of the Discrepancies," MCSSC, and Maddin, "Problem of Man's Proclivity to Live," Vanderbilt. Even students who joked about their thesis (such as the Nashville student who dedicated his thesis to the faculty, "provided they grant me a Diploma") betray an anxiety about doing well. See Coleman, "Physical Education," Vanderbilt.

48. Shackleford, "Gossipium," 2, Vanderbilt; Smith, "Hygiene of Mississippi," 1, TSM; Ewing, "On Theses," 5–6, TSM.

49. Lebby, "Lycopus Virginicus," 2, MCSSC; Greene, "Profession of Medicine," 10, MCSSC. See also, Maddin, "Problem of Man's Proclivity to Live," Vanderbilt.

50. Nesbit, "Rise and Progress of Medicine," 4, TSM. For other examples of this historical vision, see Tarlton, "Progress and Separation," 2, 10–11, TSM; Wilson, "Fashion in Medicine," 1–3, 6–11, MCSSC; and Guerard, "Science of Medicine," 10–11, MCSSC.

51. Hardin, "Physic and Physicians," 1, MCSSC; Timmerman, "Difficulties and Privileges," 2, MCSSC; Wright, "Qualifications Requisite," 6, TSM. For the fabric and pabulum tropes, see Moseley, "Duties of a Physician," 4–5, MCSSC. For typical descriptions of fellow doctors, see Bruce, "Medical Science," 7, 13, TSM; Todd, "Young Physic," 14, TSM; Moody, "Responsibility and Duty," 2–6, Vanderbilt; and Taft, "Medical Experience," 8, TSM. For patients, see Miller, "Diagnosis," 15–16, Vanderbilt; Sartor, "Medical Ethics," 9, TSM; Philips, "Qualifications," 12, TSM; and Timmerman, "Difficulties and Privileges," 8–9, MCSSC.

52. Stewart, "Doctor," 10, TSM; Hardin, "Physic and Physicians," 26–27, MCSSC. For the motif of physicians as domestic men desiring the bosom of family but called to grapple with disease, see also Sartor, "Medical Ethics," 3, TSM, and Keitt, "Duties of the Physician," 5, MCSSC.

53. Elliott, "Medical Etiquette," 10–11, TSM; Woolridge, "Medical Student," 12–13, Vanderbilt; Philips, "Qualifications," 15, TSM. See also Stewart, "Doctor," 8–9, TSM, and Crutcher, "Medical Student," 5–6, Vanderbilt.

CHAPTER THREE

1. Samuel Maverick Van Wyck to his wife, January 22, 1860, Maverick and Van Wyck papers, SCL.

2. William Bernard Harrell autobiography, [1903], part II, 219, Harrell family papers, UNCC; *Louisville Morning Courier*, March 9, 1848, 3; Wilson Yandell to Lunsford Yandell, February 6, 1824, Yandell family papers, Filson; Charles Colcock Jones to Joseph Jones,

March 31, 1856, Jones collection, HTML; James W. Copes to J. S. Copes, March 7, 1832, Copes papers, HTML; John B. Davidge to Wilson Yandell, April 4, 1825, in Yandell scrapbook (photocopy), n.p., Yandell family collection, UL; Porcher, "Personal Reminiscences," 4–5, Waring; Oliver Stout to James Taliaferro, May 4, 1823, Taliaferro papers, LSU. Schools' annual circulars highlight graduation, advertising it as a day of public celebration. Augusta, Georgia, resident Ella Clanton Thomas, like many who lived in medical school cities, looked forward to attending commencement and was disappointed when bad weather prevented it; see her diary, March 2, 1852, Duke. For other typical student commentary blending pride and nostalgia on graduation day, see Traill Green to J. S. Copes, April 25, 1833, Copes papers, HTML; Knox medical diary, February 24, 1843, Winthrop; and Wade diary, February 28, 1852, Matas.

3. Dickson, "Introductory Lecture" (1846), 13; Robert Lovett to "My Dear Parents," January 22, 1844, Lovett papers, Emory; Faculty Minute Books, April 10, 1835, and March 2, 1842, MCG; Joseph LeConte autobiography, 110, LeConte-Furman papers, SHC. For other instances of conflict, see Charles Caldwell to Lunsford Yandell, November 11, 1830, Yandell family papers, Filson, and Charles Johnson to Lou McCrindell, February 18, 1860, Johnson family papers, LSU. See also the notice by the University of Louisville ("Addendum," Annual Announcement, Medical Department, University of Louisville, 1872) confirming the degree of one Jacob Geiger, which was published to counter "a statement . . . in circulation" to the effect that Geiger had failed to graduate.

4. Bibb, "Essay on the Effects," 1, 8–9, MCSSC.

5. Taft, "Medical Experience," 10, TSM; Dismukes, "Physician," 7–8, Vanderbilt; Keitt, "Duties of the Physician," 9, MCSSC.

6. Wilson Yandell to Lunsford Yandell, in a letter, 1823, quoted in Lunsford Yandell diary, 1824–43, 329, Yandell family papers, Filson.

7. Lewis, "Being Examined for My Degree," in John Q. Anderson, ed., *Louisiana Swamp Doctor*, 172. The professor here is modeled after Samuel Gross, who taught Lewis surgery at Louisville in 1844–46.

8. Robert Battey to Mary Halsey, March 15, 1857, Battey papers, Emory; Samuel H. Dickson memoranda book, ca. 1841, 17, Waring; Jones student notebook, 1855–56 (vol. 15), 172–73, Jones papers, LSU; M. M. Lewis to J. S. Copes, November 11, 1833, Copes papers, HTML. On the supposed advantages of practicing medicine in war, see the thoughts of Alexander Campbell in his letter to J. S. Copes, June 29, 1847, Copes papers, HTML. On the appeal of Europe, see the Paris letters of John Young Bassett to his wife, Isaphoena, in 1835–36, Bassett papers, ADAH. On the West, see Thomas Furman to Ann Armstrong, [October 1831], Furman papers, Emory, and Traill Green to J. S. Copes, October 19, 1833, Copes papers, HTML.

9. Alfred T. Hamilton to his father, December 18, 1858, Hamilton papers, TSL; Frederick Egan to Mrs. J. S. Egan, May 8, 1853, Egan family papers, LSU; Hentz diary, September 18, 1846, in Stowe, ed., *Southern Practice*, 138.

10. William Whetstone to Margaret Boatwright, April 20, [1854], Whetstone family papers, SCL; S. C. Corkern to Jeptha McKinney, June 23, 1858, McKinney papers, LSU; Jobe, "Autobiography," 96, TSL.

11. Alfred T. Hamilton to his father, December 18, 1858, Hamilton papers, TSL. Samuel Dickson tells of his arrangement in his memoranda book, ca. 1841–50, 17–18, Waring; see

also Jobe, "Autobiography," 95, TSL. Such word-of-mouth prospecting led to many disappointments. A young Tennessee doctor anticipated taking over the practice of a senior man rumored to be retiring; but "it now appears that he expected to receive the Presidency of a Bank. Failing to get this position, he continues his practice." See A. VanHoose to John A. Robinson, May 1, 1869, Robinson papers, SCL.

12. Richard Davidson to Antonio Walsh, January 11, 1820, Walsh papers, LSU; [Jn?] W. Mabry to Joseph W. Tucker, February 25, 1860, and James Creswell to [whom it may concern], March 2, 1860, Maverick and Van Wyck papers, SCL. See also Thomas Y. Prioleau to [whom it may concern], May 3, 1826, Lebby family papers, SCL.

13. Thomas Copes to J. S. Copes, June 11, 1833, Copes papers, HTML. Detailed advice of all sorts abounds in correspondence; for other good examples, see Thomas Wright to William C. Wright, October 6, 1846, Wright papers, Duke; Benjamin McKenzie to Thomas Mitchell, September 30, 1844, ADAH; and William Whetstone to Margaret Boatwright, March 26, 1856, Whetstone family papers, SCL.

14. James W. Copes to J. S. Copes, July 25, 1833, and Thomas Copes to J. S. Copes, October 7, 1833, Copes papers, HTML.

15. William Whetstone to Margaret Boatwright, December 7, 1855, Whetstone family papers, SCL; J. R. Manning to William Reedy, January 17, 1883, Reedy and Beacham family papers, SCL; John A. Robinson to H. S. Shirk, July 19, 1873, and W. E. Tynes to John A. Robinson, July 28, 1873, Robinson papers, SCL.

16. James Milligan to James A. S. Milligan, September 10, 1846, Milligan family papers, SHC; J. Y. Henderson to Joel Berly, November 20, 1856, Berly family papers, SCL; Fairey, "Medical Student," 11, MCSSC. For similar experiences, see Ryland, "Note," in his account book, n.p., Ryland papers, LSU; Harry [Kilbourne] to "Dear Mama," September 14, [18]88, Kilbourne family papers, LSU; and Lewis, "Seeking a Location," in John Q. Anderson, ed., *Louisiana Swamp Doctor*, 176.

17. J. Marion Sims to Theresa Jones, March 3, March 13, March 3, 1835, Sims papers, SHC; Hentz diary, December 17, 1848, in Stowe, ed., *Southern Practice*, p. 218; Leland diary, autobiographical note, 1851, 30, SCL.

18. Jobe, "Autobiography," 96, TSL. The opinion that people held to their own judgment in medicine is well expressed in Timmerman, "Difficulties and Privileges," 6, MCSSC.

19. Moseley, "Duties of a Physician," 10, MCSSC; Keitt, "Duties of the Physician," 16–17, MCSSC; see also Handley, "Medical Man," 24, Vanderbilt. For similar rhetoric in the context of an older doctor's career, see Ernest Sydney Lewis, "Reminiscences," 772, in which the doctor is memorialized as serving in "the palace of the prince and the hut of the peasant alike." The long-lived appeal of this arch language is striking and suggests a lasting uneasiness over how to express emotional engagement with suffering.

20. Handley, "Medical Man," 12, Vanderbilt; J. Marion Sims to Theresa Jones, November 13, 1835, Sims papers, SHC; J. E. Clark to Josiah Hawkins, February 14, 1883, Hawkins papers, LSU; Howard Reedy to William Reedy, July 18, 1883, Reedy and Beacham family papers, SCL; Jobe, "Autobiography," 101, TSL. Also on rivalry, see DeGraffenreid, "On Brotherly Love," and Hardin, "Physic and Physicians," MCSSC.

21. Jobe, "Autobiography," 100, TSL.

22. Some young doctors found themselves subordinated to senior men in a way that in effect prolonged their apprenticeships. In describing his practice to a doctor interested in

buying it, for instance, B. C. Smith said that one of the assets of the location was a nearby practitioner who was "a clever young man . . . [who] has very little territory and cannot remain, except in a sort of cooperative way. He is an advantage to me." See B. C. Smith to J. A. Reedy, August 25, 1881, Reedy and Beacham family papers, SCL.

23. Jobe, "Autobiography," 100–101, TSL.

24. Ibid., 101.

25. Moody, "Responsibility and Duty," 2–3, 5–6, Vanderbilt. Though he was earning his M.D., Moody was an experienced physician who was here recalling his first days in practice.

26. Leland diary, autobiographical sketch, 1851, 33, SCL; Lewis, "Valerian and the Panther" and "Seeking a Location," John Q. Anderson, ed., *Swamp Doctor*, 125, 176. See also J. P. Thomas to Samuel Brown, June 20, 1824, Brown papers, Filson; W[illia]m Bonner to his mother, June 10, 1851, Bonner family papers, LSU; and Hentz diary, in Stowe, ed., *Southern Practice*, 213–15.

27. Richardson diary, December 21, 1853, SHC; Hentz diary, November 26, 1849, in Stowe, ed., *Southern Practice*, 254; Leland diary, autobiographical sketch, 1851, 35, SCL; Leland notes the dates of these events as April 22 and 27, 1849. See also S. Moffat Wylie to John A. Robinson, March 9, 1868, Robinson papers, SCL.

28. James M. Hundley to John M. Hundley. October 8, 1849, Hundley family papers, VHS; Daniel Drake, "Inaugural Discourse," 26. On the deaths of early patients, see also Risk, "Medical Education," 9–11, TSM, and Richardson diary, November 2, 1853, SHC. A certain mystique attached to first failures and first successes; one medical student was convinced that "should we be successful in the early part of our career, it matters but little what may befall us in our subsequent practice" (S. G. Twitty, "Importance of a Thorough Medical Knowledge," 10–11, MCSSC).

29. Porcher, ms. lecture notes, "Materia Medica and Therapy delivered 1854–5–6–7–8 again 1873–74," Porcher papers, Waring; J. Marion Sims to Theresa Jones, December 31, 1835, Sims papers, SHC; Hort, "Medical Education &c," 315.

30. Algernon Sydney Allan, "Popular Objections," 7, TSM; Nesbit, "Rise and Progress of Medicine," 1, TSM.

31. Hardin, "Physic and Physicians," 26–27, MCSSC; Horton, "Education of a Physician," 7, Vanderbilt; Broyles, "Life of a Physician," 13, Vanderbilt.

32. S. Carswell Ely to J. S. Copes, January 27, 1834, Copes papers, HTML; Philips, "Qualifications," 17, TSM. See also Alexander Campbell to J. S. Copes, January 7, 1834, Copes papers, HTML; Porcher, ms. lecture notes, "Materia Medica and Therapy delivered 1854–5–6–7–8 again 1873–74," Porcher papers, Waring; and Hentz diary, December 8, 1848, in Stowe, ed., *Southern Practice*, 213.

33. Crutcher, "Medical Student," 2, Vanderbilt; "G" to James Gage, March [1837?], Gage papers, SHC.

34. Todd, "Young Physic," 8, TSM; Woolridge, "Medical Student," 12–13, Vanderbilt. See also David W. Yandell, "Progress of Medicine," 5.

35. Huronymous student notebook, Transylvania Medical College, 1833–35, n.p., Matas; Porcher, ms. lecture notes, "Materia Medica and Therapeutics delivered 1854–5–6–7–8 again 1873–74," Porcher papers, Waring.

36. Bruce, "Medical Science," 7, TSM; Albert Bachelor to Cornelia Stewart, August 31,

1873 (draft), Bachelor papers, LSU; William L. Torrance to James G. Torrance, December 20, 1846, Torrance-Banks family papers, UNCC; Broyles, "Life of a Physician," 26, Vanderbilt.

37. James M. Hundley to John M. Hundley, November 10, 1849, Hundley family papers, VHS; Hentz diary, February 7, 1849, and December 17, 1848, in Stowe, ed., *Southern Practice*, 242, 218.

CHAPTER FOUR

1. Colmer daybook, November 27–28, 1873, 55, Colmer papers, HTML.

2. George Colmer was born in London, England, in 1807, received his M.D. from the Medical College of Louisiana in 1838, and practiced in Springfield until his death in 1878. Colmer had at least one publication, "Paralysis in Teething Children," *American Journal of the Medical Sciences* 5 (January 1843): 248. Albert E. Casey and Eleanor H. Hidden ("George Colmer and the Epidemiology of Poliomyelitis," *Southern Medical Journal* 37 [September 1944]: 471–77) suggest that this publication is the earliest, if unwitting, clinical description of epidemic poliomyelitis in American medical literature. See also Duffy, ed., *Rudolph Matas History*, 2:78, 80.

3. I am drawing on Joan Scott's discussion in "Experience," 22–40.

4. Colmer daybook, Gillespie account, 82, and Spiller account, 66, Colmer papers, HTML.

5. Examples of this style are legion throughout the nineteenth century. In addition to the wording here, other doctors wrote "various medicines," "Medicine, box of," and, most commonly, "visit and medicine." A few physicians, however, kept meticulous notes on their prescriptions; for an example, see the daybooks of E. Belin Flagg, 1847–53, SCHS.

6. Thomas Davis diary, 1820s–38, entry for June 17, [1835], and passim, Duke. For Armstrong, see Armstrong notebook, 1839–47, LSU. For an earlier example of this kind of mixture of diary and notes, see the Blanding diary, 4 vols., 1807–23, Blanding papers, SCL. The tie between diary-keeping and a doctor's life is explored in Leavitt, "'Worrying Profession.'"

7. Thomas McCarty obstetrical record, 1869–91, McCarty papers, UL. For other physicians who comment on unmarried, pregnant women, see Charles Hentz, obstetrical record, 1849–91, entry for September 22, 1867, in Hentz family papers, SHC, and O'Dwyer diary, March 16–21, 1825, SHC. One blind spot of rural physicians' daybooks is that most do not make it possible to tell where patients actually were located in the neighborhood, unlike the daybooks of some city practitioners; for an example of the latter in which working-class patients' residences are noted ("Centre St." "above jail," for example), see Eve account book, 113, 118, 178, 197, 337, 342, MCG.

8. Jenkins daybooks, entries for Pinckney account, vol. 1, February 27 to March 7, 1844, Waring. See also anonymous account book, entries for February 19 to August 11, 1845, MCG.

9. For instance, William Jenkins, who attended slaves on a plantation, noted their names but noted their owners only as "self" and "wife"; see his daybook, Chapman account, October 12 and 13, 1850, Waring. For other examples of this style, see the daybooks of Andrew Hasell, 1841–50, and Flagg, both at SCHS.

10. Butler account book, Ellis account, September 17, 1860, and Guion account, September 21, 1860, Butler papers, LSU.

11. Anonymous account book, E. Dalby alias Sharpe account, October 31 and November 27, 1845, MCG; Colmer daybook, Davidson account, April 5 and July 31, 1862, 72–73, Colmer papers, HTML; anonymous account book, account for "Sally . . . Freewoman," MCG; Knox casebooks, vol. 2, November 2, 1852, UK; W. W. Anderson medical account book, 1818–27, account for "William Ellison—colored man," Borough House papers, SHC. I am indebted to James Roark for pointing out this collection to me. See also Carter account book, vol. 1, 1859, account for Catherine (free Negress), UK.

12. See Cox account book, Abner Ellis account, vol. 2, September 25 to October 12, 1848, SHC, and Flagg daybook, Wilkinson account, November 14 to 25, 1848, SCHS. See also the week's close attendance on a "negro child" by Dr. William Jenkins, in his daybook, "Estate, Col. Thos. Pinckney" account, May 13–19, 1843, Waring. Physicians, not surprisingly, argued that money spent on slaves' health was money well spent. One medical journal calculated that the "loss of a single adult negro . . . would counterbalance the bill of [a physician], for at least two years' attendance on a plantation, say of one hundred and fifty slaves." See "People's Medical Gazette," *Charleston Medical Journal and Review* 9 (March 1854): 125.

13. The "distressingly healthy" quotation is from S. L. Strait to William Mobley, February 22, 1856, GSWBFP, SCL. For other doctors who typically equated a community's good health with their bad luck, see, for example, Thomas W. Castle to Jeptha McKinney, August 24, 1859, McKinney papers, LSU, and Robert H. Carson to John A. Forsyth, August 30, 1839, Forsyth papers, Duke.

For fees generally, see Rosen, *Fees and Fee Bills*. On urban physicians' wealth, see Holifield, "Wealth of Nineteenth-Century American Physicians"; Grob, *Edward Jarvis*, 45–46; and Horsman, *Josiah Nott of Mobile*, 61. On "booked" income, see the letter from Dr. James Milligan to his physician son J. A. S. Milligan where the father notes that "if out of $170 you have booked, you received $40 or 50, *very well*. . . . keep in mind that this is your first month. I consider you truly a lucky dog" (June 11, 1846, Milligan family papers, SHC). Compare Dr. William Holt's delight at having collected one-half of the $6,000 he booked (Holt to Louis A. Dugas, October 29, 1872, Holt papers, SCL).

Particularly detailed daybooks include those of J. W. Brigham, Joseph and Joseph A. S. Milligan, Benjamin and Benjamin West Robinson, and James Strudwick Smith, all SHC; Jeptha McKinney, LSU; Joseph A. Eve, MCG; S. D. Davis, Duke; Robert Burns Pusey and John Coleman Carter, both UK; Joseph L. Lee, Waring; and Josiah E. Hawkins, LSU. For analyses of individual daybooks and account books, see Flesher and Schumacher, "Natchez Doctor's Ledgers," and Irvine Loudon, "Doctor's Cash Book." For comparison outside of the South, see Coombs, "Rural Medical Practice"; Barlow and Powell, "Malthus A. Ward"; and Duffin, *Langstaff*, 46–49.

14. Dunlap account book, SCL. For the rain notations, see Southall account book, May 1, 1823, April 27, 1824, and March 18, 1827, VHS; Hawkins daybook, Carpenter account, July 20, 1871, Hawkins papers, LSU. Typical charges at the low end of fee bills are seen throughout the daybooks cited in n. 13, above. John Duffy makes the same observation in *Rudolph Matas History*, 2:352–54. For a sampling of fee bills and discussion of them, see "Medical Attendance on Families by the Year" and Medical Society of Columbia, "Constitution." See also two Kentucky fee bills (Louisville, 1859, and Henderson County, 1862) in *Medicine and Its Development in Kentucky*, 81 n. 20; 84 n. 20; and the Smyrna [Tennessee] Medical Society fee bill, adopted November 17, 1876, in the Smyrna Medical Society By-laws and Minutes, TSL.

It should be noted that some physicians supplemented their incomes in various ways as they made their rounds, carrying mail or making other kinds of deliveries. A few physicians sold drugs to neighbors, but I have not found many doctors doing a full-scale pharmaceutical business. Especially by midcentury, the orthodox view was that supplying patients with drugs not only undercut practice but also was ethically irresponsible. For doctors discussing this, see, for example, W. A. Shands to William Anderson, July 22, 1880, Anderson papers, SCL; Louis A. Dugas to William J. Holt, May 7, 1868, Holt papers, SCL; and Doniphan daybook, 1819–22, Filson.

Some physicians established themselves in "plantation practices," in which they contracted with large slave owners to give regular care for an annual fee. However, as noted in Chapter 3, such practices were neither as numerous nor as secure as rumor had it; for discussion of this, see Savitt, *Medicine and Slavery*, 198–99; Duffy, ed., *Rudolph Matas History*, 2:100; and Fisher, "Physicians and Slavery," 38–39. For examples of different kinds of contract arrangements, see the ms. contract dated July 23, 1841, in Lebby family papers, SCL, and Meek diary, January 15, 1814, Meek papers, ADAH.

15. See James Spann medical accounts, 1830–35, Spann papers, SCL, and Colmer diary, e.g., 61, 69, Colmer papers, HTML.

16. James D. Trezevant to Gerhard Muller, n.d. [ca. 1852], Muller papers, SCL; Eve account book, 141 (for a similar example, see the Shehan account, 189), MCG; Holcombe diary, January 19, 1855, SHC; Baird, ed., *Years of Discontent*, September 29 and October 18, 1877, 12–13, 21–22; Eve account book, 214, MCG; Ryland account book, accounts for McDaniel, 1850, [n.p], Gibbons, 1850, [n.p.], and Taylor, 1850, 1, Ryland papers, LSU. See also McKinney diary, May 16, 1865, McKinney papers, LSU.

17. Mary A. Peterson to John Young Bassett, "May the fifteenth," [no year], Bassett papers, ADAH; Baird, ed., *Years of Discontent*, September 29, 1877, 13; G. F. Steifer to John A. Robinson, December 29, 1870, January 26, 1871, and John A. Robinson to G. F. Steifer, February 7, 1871, Robinson papers, SCL. Steifer included a list of fourteen white and six black patients, though he noted that "Freed People (Negroes)" were especially vexing.

18. Colmer diary, ca. 1874, sheet attached to p. 79, Colmer papers, HTML; Alexander Campbell to J. S. Copes, June 29, 1847, Copes papers, HTML. For other examples of the web of credit, see J. Settoon to George Colmer, February 24, 1878 (letter pasted in Colmer's diary, p. 64), Colmer papers, HTML, and William J. Holt to [Louis A. Dugas], February 5, 1867, Holt papers, SCL.

19. John Hainey Davis account book, Mulligan account, August 22, 1829, SCL; the grey horse is in the Stephen Duncan ledger, April 25, 1805, UMiss; Ryland account book, Henning account, [1850, n.p.], Ryland papers, LSU; Colmer diary, ca. 1872–73, 76, Colmer papers, HTML; Ms. account sheet, October 24, 1827, Weeks family collection, LSU; Pusey account books, vol. 1, pp. 42, 47, 49, 55, 62, 126, 190; vol. 2, pp. 10, 21, 40, 155, UK. For other examples of much in-kind activity, see Eve account book, MCG, and Campbell account book and diary, VHS.

20. Eve account book, Ansley account, January 4, 1866, MCG. For physicians discussing charity, see J. A. Reedy to William Reedy, August 6, 1883, Reedy and Beacham family papers, SCL; Alexander Baron Williman to Mitchell King, February 28, 1857, Mitchell King papers, SHC (I am indebted to Michael O'Brien for this reference); and William Neill to Andrew MacCrery, December 19, 1842, MacCrery family papers, LSU.

21. William C. Wright to Thomas W. Wright, September 19, 1846, Wright papers, Duke; Leland diary, December 2, 1853, SCL.

22. Charles Hentz to Thaddeus Hentz, February 23, 1868, Hentz family papers, SHC; Holcombe diary, May 4, 1855, SHC. For similar comment, a strong theme in doctors' writing, see Robert E. Peyton to Richard Peyton, August 25, 1828, Peyton family papers, VHS; Mark M. Shivers to Joseph Heard, n.d. [ca. 1841], Heard papers, ADAH; Edward Armstrong to J. S. Copes, July 14, 1834, Copes papers, HTML; Samuel H. Dickson to Joseph Milligan, February 10, 1835, Milligan family papers, SHC; and Nathaniel [Siewers] to "Dear Parents!" January 7, 1866 (typed copy), Siewers letters, UNCC.

23. Conevery Bolton Valencius (*Health of the Country*, 5) also uses the term "health talk" to describe the people's ordinary conversations about their health. For a range of different ways to approach the historical meaning of such conversations, see Cassedy, *Medicine in America*, 44–53; Wells, *Out of the Dead House*, ch. 2; and Rothman, *Living in the Shadow of Death*, chs. 6 and 7.

24. David Campbell to Maria H. Campbell, April 19, 1801, Campbell family papers, Duke; Jane Barr to "Dear Brother & Sister," September 30, 1854, Berly family papers, SCL; Elizabeth Bell to Elizabeth Yates, July 8, 1834, Yates family papers, SCHS. For a typical child's letter using health as an "adult" topic, see Sarah Rutherfoord to John Rutherfoord, June 10, 1810, Rutherfoord papers, Duke.

25. William Tillinghast to Sophie Tillinghast, October 21, 1880, Tillinghast family papers, Duke; Davis W. Clark to Samuel Lewis, April 1, 1836, Burge-Gray family papers, Emory.

26. Virginia Shelton to David and Maria Campbell, January 18, 1852, Campbell family papers, Duke; Mary Henderson diary, October 5, 1856, and August 12, 1855, Henderson papers, SHC; Maria Campbell to David Campbell, February 25, 1809, and David Campbell to Virginia Shelton, November 6, 1851, Campbell family papers, Duke. On children, see also Ellen [Campbell] to "My Dearest Mother," September 19, 1868; on youth "crowding us off the stage of action," see Mary Kelley to "My dearest friend," March 3, 1887, both in Campbell family papers, Duke.

27. Daniel Grant to John Owen, September 15, 1791, and October 4, 1788, and Margaret [Campbell] to Mary Kelley, January 25, 1870, Campbell family papers, Duke.

28. Archibald Henderson to Mary Henderson, August 16, 1854, Henderson papers, SHC; Virginia Shelton to Maria Campbell, February 6, 1850, Campbell family papers, Duke. The letters of Anna King to her husband, Thomas Butler King, in the 1840s and 1850s are in the Thomas Butler King papers, SHC. For similar writing, see Ann S. Rutherfoord to John Rutherfoord, March 30 [1858?], Rutherfoord papers, Duke, and C. Quitman to Louisa Quitman, February 20, 1852, Quitman family papers, LSU.

29. Lucila McCorkle diary, July [5], 1847, McCorkle papers, SHC; Robert Lovett to Robert Lovett Jr., November 28, 1841, Lovett papers, Emory; Adaline Evans to Joseph Heard, September 13, 1842 (typed copy), Heard papers, ADAH. See also Sarah Newell to Robert Newell, April 2, 1863, Newell papers, LSU. See the discussion of whites' sense of "soundness" as an overall measure of African American health in Fett, *Working Cures*, ch. 1.

30. Lucy Skipwith to John H. Cocke, May 30 and August 29, 1856, and [July 25, 1862], in Miller, ed., *"Dear Master,"* 206, 208, 245.

31. Quoted in Snow, *Walkin' over Medicine*, 34; Lizzie Williams, in *AS*, ser. 1, vol. 10.5, p.

2336; Rachel Santee Reed, in *AS*, ser. 1, vol. 9.4, p. 1815; Smith Simmons, *AS*, ser. 1, vol. 10.5, p. 1939. For a former slave who recalled the spirit world as well known, see LaSan Mir, in *AS*, ser. 2, vol. 7.6, p. 2708. As for former slaves who maintained to WPA interviewers that sickness was rare, WPA interviewers typically inquired about health by asking, "Who took care of you when you were sick?" Many respondents seem to have assumed that the interviewer wanted to hear about white doctors and equated "sickness" with the times a white doctor was called in. Since these times were relatively rare, "sickness" became rare. For discussion of the spirit world, see Snow, *Walkin' over Medicine*, 47–54. I have drawn on twentieth-century cultural anthropologists and ethnographers for a sense of the traditions of African American medicine. In addition to Snow, see Watson, ed., *Black Folk Medicine*; Jones-Jackson, *When Roots Die*; Fontenot, *Secret Doctors*; and Holloway, ed., *Africanisms in American Culture*. See also Moss, *Southern Folk Medicine*, and Sharla Fett's concise discussion of the antebellum plantation context in *Working Cures*, chs. 2–4.

32. Frank Jackson, in *AS*, ser. 1, vol. 12.1, p. 183. See also in *AS*, William Byrd, ser. 2, vol. 3.2, p. 578; Maggie Pinkard, ser. 1, vol. 12.1, p. 257; Callie Washington, ser. 1, vol. 10.5, pp. 2192–93; and Squire Irvin, ser. 1, vol. 8.3, p. 1087.

33. O'Dwyer diary, April 3, 1825, Wheeler papers, SHC; Hentz diary, November 3, 1857, in Steven M. Stowe, ed., *Southern Practice*, 321; Leland diary, October 23, 1854, SCL.

34. Holcombe diary, January 28 and February 17, 1855, SHC; Hentz diary, November 3, 1857, in Stowe, ed., *Southern Practice*, 321; Hawkins daybook, 1857–64, frontispiece, Hawkins papers, LSU.

35. Wilson Yandell to Lunsford Yandell, January 17, 1825, Yandell family papers, Filson; McKinney student notebook, 1857, 1864–68, n.d. (he notes he bought the horse on October 25, 1864), McKinney papers, LSU; J. A. Reedy to William Reedy, September 10, 1883, Reedy and Beacham family papers, SCL. For Hentz's expensive horse, see his diary, December 13 and 22, 1848, in Stowe, ed., *Southern Practice*, 216, 222–23; on his memories of horses, see his autobiography in ibid., 553–54, 571–72. Medical periodicals took up horse lore, often as a form of humor. One journal deflated self-important doctors by implying that they judged a horse by its appearance, seeking a horse that would "excite attention without attracting ridicule" regardless of the actual quality of the mount. This same journal, however, also published serious obituaries for horses: "A Venerable Horse—The Western Lancet mentions the death of a horse owned by Dr. F. Dorsey of Hagerstown, Md., at the advanced age of 45 years. . . . He has done the profession some service" ("Medical Ethics in Virginia," 7:254 and 9:263). For other typical comment on horses, see W. A. Peoples to Joel Berly, January 18, 1855, Berly family papers, SCL; Ogilvie daybook, [February 15?], 1875, MCSSC; and Leland diary, April 27, 1856, "December 1858," SCL. Also see Duffin, *Langstaff*, 40–42.

36. William Reedy to Lydie McLure, June 8, 1883, Reedy and Beacham family papers, SCL; Henry W. Ravenel, quoted in Haygood, *Henry William Ravenel*, 51; Knox medical diary, July 6, 1844, Winthrop; Weedon diary, May, 1823 (typed copy), ADAH; for the tobacco-craving boy, see Hentz medical diary, November 11, 1868, Hentz family papers, SHC.

37. Isaac M. Comings to Samuel Lewis, June 1, 1843, Burge-Gray family papers, Emory; R. E. Manson to J. D. Davidson, August 14, 1857, Davidson papers, Duke. Although Dr. James Still practiced in the North, his experience is suggestive of white doctors' opposition to black practitioners elsewhere; see his *Early Recollections*. For mention of slave healers by former

slaves, see, for example, in *AS*, Ophelia Whitley, vol. 15.2 (N.C. pt. 2), pp. 373–74; James Lucas, ser. 1, vol. 8.3, pp. 1346–47; Charity Jones, ser. 1, vol. 8.3, p. 1201; Lucretia Brown, ser. 1, vol. 6.1, p. 267; Rube Brown, ser. 1, vol. 6.1, p. 287; Frances Banks, ser. 1, vol. 12.1, p. 11; and Sarah Louisa Augustus, vol. 14.1 (N.C., pt. 1), p. 54. For slaves writing to their master on such issues, see Miller, ed., *"Dear Master,"* 165, 175, 228. Thomsonians were followers of the medical ideas of Samuel Thomson (1769–1843), who achieved a popular following for his largely botanical regimen of tonics and purges.

38. B. T. Neill to J. S. Copes, December 10, 1835, Copes papers, HTML; Oliver Stout to James Taliaferro, September 27, 1825, Taliaferro papers, LSU; Wilson Yandell to Lunsford Yandell, December 28, 1824, Yandell family papers, Filson. Samuel Leland describes an eccentric colleague whom he respected nonetheless because the man was interested in collecting specimens; see Leland diary, November 12, 1856, SCL. As for physicians who were dis-esteemed drunkards, see, for example, Hentz diary, September 22, 1860, in Stowe, ed. *Southern Practice*, 341; Frank James diary, October 4, 1877, in Baird, ed., *Years of Discontent*, 16; and Jobe, "Autobiography," 114, TSL. For professional bonds cemented by the language of personal esteem—a request for the "honor" or "favor" of a consult, for instance—see Alfred Fowler to J. S. Copes, [1836], Copes papers, HTML, and J. A. J. Hildebrand to Gerhard Muller, July 2, 1856, Muller papers, SCL. Compare other requests for consultations: for example, J. P. B. to Robert Butler, n.d. (probably 1860s), Butler papers, LSU, and F. J. Smith account book, August 19, 1840, Mary Ruffin Smith papers, SHC.

39. Leland diary, February 16, 1856, and March 20, 1852, SCL; Clark medical notebook, 1844–74, entries for April 4, July 4, August 21, September 16, 1844, and January 19, 1845, Clark papers, Duke; Wilson Yandell to Lunsford Yandell, January 2 and 4, 1825, Yandell family papers, Filson; Holcombe diary, May 11, 1855, SHC. For other examples of the pace and variety of work, see Knox medical diary, June 20, 1843, Winthrop; Thomas Wright to William C. Wright, October 6, 1846, Wright papers, Duke; David H. Dungan to Lafayette Strait, September 20, 1859, and William Mobley to Hannah Wylie, November 12, 1859, GSWBFP, SCL; and Blanding diary, July 17–20, 1807, Blanding papers, SCL.

40. J. A. Reedy to William Reedy, August 13, 1883, Reedy and Beacham family papers, SCL.

41. Knox casebook, vol. 2, May 21, August 14, September 25, 1852, January 11 and 26, 1853, UK; Wilson Yandell to Lunsford Yandell, December 28, 1824, Yandell family papers, Filson; J. M. Steamson to William Reedy, September 12, 1884, Reedy and Beacham family papers, SCL; Frank James diary, October 5, 1877, in Baird, ed., *Years of Discontent*, 17. For other accounts of accidents, see Leland diary, October 6, 1855, SCL, and Elizabeth M. Izard to Alice Izard, August 12, 1816 (holograph copy), Izard family letters, Cheves-Middleton papers, SCHS.

42. Frank James diary, December 22, 1877, January 21 and 23, 1878, in Baird, ed., *Years of Discontent*, 48, 58–59; Arnold diary, December 4, 1832, Arnold papers, Duke; see also his entries for August 17 and December 7, 1832.

43. Wilson Yandell to Lunsford Yandell, November 22 and 24, 1824, Yandell family papers, Filson; J. A. S. Milligan to James Milligan, May 15, 1849, Milligan family papers, SHC; Leland diary, August 3, 1853, SHC. Leland seems more than a little incurious as to the cause of death, and he attempts to avoid the seriousness of the deadly occasion by making a joke that only serves to raise more questions: the deceased slave "was heard to say after the

whipping, that he would never do another stroke of work for [his owner] Chappel. And he kept his word!" For a doctor involved in assessing competence, see Dr. Levin Joynes, ms. case notes [1851], Joynes family papers, VHS. Work that today would be considered "expert testimony" sometimes was done pro bono, either by agreement or by default, and some physicians thought that such "expert testimony" work should have more systematic standards and fees; see the action proposed by the *Savannah Journal of Medicine* in 1858, described in Fisher, "Physicians and Slavery," 39–41. See also the discussion of physicians in contested sales of slaves in Walter Johnson, *Soul by Soul*, 208–10, and the excellent overview of physicians' legal testimony in Ariela Gross, *Double Character*, ch. 5.

44. Charles Ball, quoted in Norrece Jones, *Born a Child of Freedom*, 88. The instance of the Virginia doctors' testimony against a murdering slave owner is in Faulkner, "Case of Homicide," 485–90. However, in a more typical South Carolina case, three doctors joined the other nine men on a jury in acquitting a slave owner of a similar murder charge; one juror privately said the murder was "death by inhumane treatment"; see Rosengarten, *Tombee*, 456–58 (quote from 457).

45. Robert Battey to Mary Halsey, November 29, 1857, Battey papers, Emory; James Milligan to J. A. S. Milligan, June 25, 1846, Milligan family papers, SHC; Thomas Fearne to Samuel Brown, October 18, 1820, Brown papers, Filson; S. Moffat Wylie to John Robinson, May 18, 1870, Robinson papers, SCL. See also James Milligan to J. A. S. Milligan, June 11, 1846, Milligan family papers, SHC, and Wilson Yandell to Lunsford Yandell, January 2 and 4, 1825, Yandell family papers, Filson; and compare to Dr. Jonathan Woolverton's experience in Charles Roland, "Diary of a Canadian Country Physician."

46. McSwain, "Some of the Discrepancies," 19, MCSSC; E. W. Thomason to Robert Lebby, September 19, 1866, Lebby family papers, SCL; Daniel Ryan Sartor, "Medical Ethics," 9, TSM; Stanford E. Chaillé, "Medical Colleges," 833. For similar comment on these themes, see James Milligan to J. A. S. Milligan, January 4, 1846, and E. R. Calhoun to J. A. S. Milligan, June 4, 1847, Milligan family papers, SHC; Holcombe diary, January 24, 1855, SHC; Traill Green to J. S. Copes, January 29, 1834, Copes papers, HTML; Frank James diary, September 22, 1877, in Baird, ed., *Years of Discontent*, 8; and Caldwell, "Valedictory Address."

47. Martha Battey to Mary Halsey, September 19, 1857, Battey papers, Emory; William Anderson to "Miss Georgie," June 12, 1881, Anderson papers, SCL; Lydie McClure to William Reedy, February 17, 1883, Reedy and Beacham family papers, SCL; Arnold diary, September 13, 1838, Arnold papers, Duke; Josiah Nott to James Gage, July 28, 1836, Gage papers, SHC. Lydie McClure was not shy about her needs as she contemplated marriage with Reedy. "We cannot live in the country," she wrote him. "I don't like it. I hope you won't want me to" (March 17, 1883; see also March 26, 1883, Reedy and Beacham family papers, SCL). One doctor's wife, Julia A. Jones, accented her diary pages with notations "Dr. is absent" and "Dr. home awhile" (Julia A. Jones diary, 1843–71, Jones family papers, SHC). For observations on the drawbacks of marrying a doctor, see Nancy P. Lawrence to "My Dear Mother," August 21, 1819, Lawrence family papers, TSL; J. A. S. Milligan to Octavia Camfield, December 20, 1847, Milligan family papers, SHC; and Leland diary, August 22, 1855, SCL.

48. James Milligan to Margaret Milligan, April 13, 1835, Milligan family papers, SHC. See also "Elliott" to James Milligan, August 8, 1835, ibid., and Joshua Whitridge to William Whitridge, November 14, 1819, Whitridge papers, SCHS.

1. The summoning of the "horseback" doctor is a set piece in sentimental literature on the "frontier." See, for example, Pickard and Buley, *Midwest Pioneer*, esp. chs. 2 and 3. For a sense of M.D.s' essential diagnostic vision as they undertook care in the mid-nineteenth century, see Warner, *The Therapeutic Perspective*, ch. 1; Rosenberg, "Therapeutic Revolution"; and Duffin, *Langstaff*, ch. 3.

2. Sallie Price to Robert Lovett, May 6, 1858, Lovett papers, Emory; M. L. McMurran to L. P. Conner, September 7, 1853, Conner family papers, LSU; Davies diary, July 23, 1854, Davies papers, Duke. This popular talk drew from, and found its echo in, popular health advisers. This literature is vast; for books circulated in the South, see, for example, Goodlett, *Family Physician*; Jennings, *Compendium of Medical Science*; and Joseph Johnson, "Advice to Persons"; compare Murphy, *Enter the Physician*.

3. Harriott Pinckney to Eweretta Middleton, n.d., Cheves-Middleton papers, Middleton letters, SCHS; *American Gentleman's Medical Pocket-Book*, 22. The seed ticks and bark jackets are mentioned in Alexander, *Reminiscences*, 226, 465. On the general dosing with quinine for fever, see J. Marion Sims to Paul F. Eve, April 25, [18]74, Eve papers, TSL, and Thomas Rutherfoord to John Rutherfoord, June 19, 1810, Rutherfoord papers, Duke. For self-medication generally, see Whorton, *Inner Hygiene*, and Stowe, "Conflict and Self-Sufficiency." For typical talk about scrutinizing bodies, see "Your affectionate Sister" to J. A. Berly, June ?, 1871, Berly family papers, SCL; Mahala Roach diary, February 23, 1853, Roach and Eggleston family papers, SHC; Mary Ann Shields to Andrew MacCrery, July 11, 1842, MacCrery family papers, LSU; Murphy diary, December 27, 1817, ADAH; and Eliza Izard to Alice Izard, December 8, 1816 (holograph copy), Izard family letters, Cheves-Middleton papers, SCHS.

4. Fannie Moore, in *AS*, 15.2, p. 134; Agnes MacRae to Donald MacRae, September 19, 1879, MacRae papers, Duke; "Sister" to Eweretta Middleton, November 30, 1832, Middleton letters, Cheves-Middleton papers, SCHS; Brandon diary/memoir, June 21, 1860, 235, ADAH. On dosing with harsh medicines, see James Reed Branch letter, April 1, 1866, VHS; Fanny Hodges, *AS*, supp. 1, 8.3, p. 1026; James Franklin Torrance to James G. Torrance, February 28, 1847, Torrance-Banks family papers, UNCC; and Mary Campbell to "Dear Mother," May 16, 1803 (on the reverse of her December 7, 1803, letter addressed "Dear Aunt"), Campbell family papers, Duke.

Some changes occurred during the nineteenth century in all of this self-medicating. Certain drugs passed in and out of favor, especially among white southerners. Calomel seems to have dwindled in domestic use after the 1840s; quinine and bromides are mentioned more often. But such trends are difficult to map. Commercial patent medicines certainly became more plentiful after the Civil War and appear to have been employed in some white households in place of older, homemade remedies. And yet it still was not uncommon to find southerners preparing their own decoctions, teas, and tinctures into the 1880s, as well as using the old standbys castor oil, ipecac, and whiskey or wine. Self-remedies among African Americans, especially, through preference and necessity, persisted during and after slavery.

5. Lunsford Yandell to Susan Yandell, April 9, 1860, Yandell family papers, Filson; Victoria Thompson, in *AS*, supp. 1, 12.1, p. 322. See also Alabama physician Courtney Clark's notation of slave therapy in his medical notebook, 1844–74, 57, Clark papers, Duke. On slave practitioners in domestic settings, see, for example, Savitt, *Medicine and Slavery*, ch. 5; Morgan,

Slave Counterpoint, ch. 10; Fett, *Working Cures*, esp. ch. 2; Chireau, "Uses of the Supernatural"; and Schweninger, "Doctor Jack."

6. Mary Henderson diary, July 8, 1855, Henderson papers, SHC; McCorkle diary, October 10, 1847, McCorkle papers, SHC; Davies diary, August 8, 1852, Davies papers, Duke. See also M. H. Campbell to Maria Campbell, November 18, 1851, Campbell family papers, Duke; McCorkle diary, September 27, 1846, McCorkle papers, SHC; and Mahala Roach diary, March 6, 1853, Roach and Eggleston family papers, SHC. For Smedes's recollection, see Susan Dabney Smedes, *Memorials of a Southern Planter*, esp. ch. 4. Some former slaves recalled mistresses giving care, sometimes with praise, other times with the implication that such work was merely self-interest; see, for example, Andrew Jackson Fill, in *AS*, supp. 1, 8.3, p. 841, and Lucretia Brown, *AS*, supp. 1, 6.1, p. 267.

7. N. W. Whetstone to William Whetstone, July 28, 1850, Whetstone family papers, SCL; Louisa Muller to Gerhard Muller, September 23, 1852, Muller papers, SCL; R. Fletcher to Elizabeth Yates, February [14?], 1825, Yates family papers, SCHS; James Franklin Torrance to James G. Torrance, February 28, 1847, Torrance-Banks family papers, UNCC; "Antonia" to Louisa Quitman, February 1, 1848, Quitman family papers, LSU; Mary Henderson to "Ann," November 15, 1852, Henderson papers, SHC; Isabella P. Porcher plantation prescription book, ca. 1834, Waring; Davies diary, December 14, 1852, Davies papers, Duke; M. L. McCurran to L. P. Conner, September 7, 1853, Conner family papers, LSU; Thomas and Mary Boulware diary, October 13, 1867, Winthrop. For other examples of this kind of talk, which is everywhere in people's letters and diaries, see Sarah Bruce to Ann Rutherfoord, August [12?], 1857, Rutherfoord papers, Duke; Emily Liles Harris diary, August 17, 24, 1860, Winthrop; and R[obina Tillinghast] to "My Dear Brother," January 5, 1880, Tillinghast family papers, Duke.

8. Murphy diary, July 15, 1816, ADAH; C. Quitman to Louisa Quitman, October 4, 1855, Quitman family papers, LSU. See also William Martin to Lunsford Yandell, January 2, 1845, Yandell family papers, Filson, and "Eweretta" to Eweretta Middleton, December 14, 1832, Middleton letters, Cheves-Middleton papers, SCHS.

9. McCorkle diary, May 29, 1847, McCorkle papers, SHC. For similar examples, see William B. Yates to Elizabeth Yates, May 30, 1828, Yates family papers, SCHS; W. B[arnewall] to Eweretta Middleton, September 11, 1838, Middleton letters, Cheves-Middleton papers, SCHS; and Brandon diary/memoir, May 11, 1860 (on loose sheet), ADAH.

10. Davies diary, August 2, 1852, Davies papers, Duke. Skepticism of doctors runs throughout people's letters and advice literature as well; see, for example, Joshua Whitridge to "Dear Brother," September 19–21, 1817, Whitridge papers, SCHS, and R[oswell] King Jr., "On the Management of the Butler Estate," quoted in Breeden, ed., *Advice among Masters*, 164.

11. Lewis Davis to J. S. Copes, August 28, 1836, Copes papers, HTML; V. LaFasta to Joseph Heard, n.d., probably 1840s (typed copy), Heard papers, ADAH; Thomas Brewer to J. S. Smith, May 4, 1833 (attached to James Strudwick Smith account book, vol. 2, p. 155), SHC; A. B. Johnston to Beverley Jones, August 17, 1854, Jones family papers, SHC. For mention of strange symptoms and uneasy turning points, see also [Charles Carpenter] to George Colmer, January 19, 1860 (attached to Colmer diary, p. 119), Colmer papers, HTML, and Mary Field to John Robinson (attached to Robinson account book, vol. 4, between pp. 112 and 113), SHC. On requests for medicines, see also Patrick O'Hare (writing on behalf of Andrew Ward) to Robert Butler, April 16, 1866, Butler papers, LSU; and R. S. Izard (on

behalf to June Wilson) to J. R. Sparkman, March 7, 1871, and N. P. Boney (on behalf of "Bacchus's wife") to Sparkman, January 18, 1872, Sparkman family papers, SHC.

12. ? Cummings to James K. Chapman, "Sunday morning," n.d. (attached to the inside of the back cover of Chapman's account book, vol. 6, 1874–82), SCL. For summoning letters that show the range of information people chose to include, most of it terse, see Nancy Love to John Mettauer, n.d., Mettauer papers, VHS; George Work to J. S. Copes, September 20, 1843, Copes papers, HTML; M. Speer to J. S. Smith, n.d. (attached to James Strudwick Smith account book, vol. 2, p. 90), SHC; and Sallie G. Adams to Thomas Settle, [October 16, 1868], Settle papers, Duke.

13. McCorkle diary, April 25, 1847, McCorkle papers, SHC; Pendleton, "Comparative Fecundity," 353–54.

14. Thomas Holloway to Joel Berly, May 12, 1859, Berly family papers, SCL. For the "prescription" of violent means in order to "cure" slave willfulness, see also McLoud "Hints on the Medical Treatment of Negroes," MCSSC. See also Fett, *Working Cures*, 189–90.

15. Alexander Yuille to John Mettauer, August 9, 1839; James Neal to Mettauer, August 1, 1839; James Fretwell to Mettauer, November 29, 1832, all Mettauer papers, VHS. See also Nancy Thompson to Mettauer, January 19, 1843; Thomas Clark to Mettauer, September 18, 1843; and Alfred Eggleston to Mettauer, September 27, 1835, all ibid.

16. Nancy Jeffress to John Mettauer, June 15, 1839, Mettauer papers, VHS.

17. Mary Henderson diary, December 21, 1854, Henderson papers, SHC.

18. Mitchell, "Diagnosis," [2], TSM; see also Ford, "Remarks," 340. Although closely examining the body may seem an obvious measure, it is important to recall that many non-M.D.s did not do so, relying on visual observation or on a single substance taken from the body, usually blood or urine. The medical notes of Nathan A. Hixon, a Thomsonian practitioner in Kentucky in the 1830s, are suggestive in this regard; see Hixon casebook, 1834–38, UL. Interesting on how nineteenth-century diagnosis was not the clinical imperative it was a century later is Warner, *Therapeutic Persuasion*, 92, and Rosenberg, *Care of Strangers*, 72; see also Beeson and Maulitz, "Inner History of Internal Medicine," and Kunitz, "Classifications in Medicine."

19. Eve, "Essay on Expectation," 328. By the 1840s, particular methods of physical examination, some of ancient origin, began to be more systematically employed. These were the techniques of palpation (feeling areas of the body for abnormal organ growths or anomalous growths), percussion (using rhythmic tapping to detect fluids or blockages), and auscultation (heightened listening to body sounds). For examples of physicians speaking of these techniques, see McLean, "'Medical Progress,'" MCSSC; Stanford Chaillé, "Anniversary Oration"; and Price, "Physical Diagnosis," TSM. There is a compelling discussion of the visualized body in Duden, *Woman Beneath the Skin*, esp. 35–36.

20. For examples of these categories in use, see Joseph Jones clinical chart, in vol. 8, 1868–69 (small notebook bound between pp. 146–47), Jones collection, HTML, and O'Keeffe, "Experimental Researches."

21. Hentz medical diary, November 27, 1858, Hentz family papers, SHC; for the inspection of stool, see Lunsford P. Yandell, "Cases of Dysentery," 246–47, and Duffin, *Langstaff*, 67.

22. Vandergriff, "Southern Practice of Medicine," 335, Matas. See also Wragg, "Report on Closing the Roper Hospital," and Joseph Jones, Savannah Marine Hospital record, 1857, Jones collection, HTML.

23. For the healthy body as a kind of absence of signals, see Leder, *Absent Body*, esp. 1–2, 39–45, 81. On the privileged place of the pulse in diagnosis, Jacalyn Duffin found much the same thing in her study of a Canadian doctor; see Duffin, *Langstaff*, 62–64.

24. See the pulse terms (which are nearly identical) in two typical sources: Massie, *Treatise*, 72–75, and Vandergriff, "Southern Practice of Medicine," 331–34.

25. Walke, "Continued Fever," 21; [Boyd], "Finale of Twenty Years Study," 4, MCSSC. See also Baruch medical notebook, 1860–61, 24, Baruch papers, Emory.

26. James E. Smith, "Cases Illustrating the Practice of Medicine," 167; Dungan, "Report on the Topography," 194; Westmoreland, "Anatomical and Physiological Difference," 1, Vanderbilt; C. H. Jordan, "Thoughts on Cachexia Africana," 23. For white Americans' fascination with skin "color" from the eighteenth century on, see Melish, *Disowning Slavery*, 141–51. In this regard it is significant that "skin, color of" and "skin, discoloration of" are separate subcategories under "skin" in the major catalog of medical periodical literature in the nineteenth century; see *Index-Catalogue*, 13:68–70. With regard to the pulse and blood, traditional African American medicine privileged ideas of "high" or "low" blood, which dovetailed to some extent with M.D.s' notion of blood's "congestion"; for African American ideas, see, for example, Snow, *Walkin' over Medicine*, 120–28, 134–41. This physiological sense of blood also resonates in its larger, metaphorical meaning, in both black and white experience, through its relation to courage, kinship, sexuality, and Christ's passion. On these matters, see Camino, "Cultural Epidemiology of Spiritual Heart Trouble," 118–36, and Mathews, "Doctors and Root Doctors," 68–98.

27. Louis A. Dugas to William Holt, September 10, 1878, Holt papers, SCL; Ford, "Remarks," 355. Also expressing reservations about the stethoscope as useful are Williams, "Physical Diagnosis," 4–5, Vanderbilt, and Hazen, "Physical Diagnosis," [9], TSM. For a general discussion of physicians' (and patients') skepticism of the stethoscope, thermometer, and other instruments, see Reiser, *Medicine and the Reign of Technology*, chs. 2 and 5; see also the discussion of one physician's cautious adoption of new instruments (as opposed to his eager adoption of new medicines) in Duffin, *Langstaff*, ch. 3.

28. T. B. T. to William Anderson, October 22, 1875, Anderson papers, SCL; Allen student notebook (Lewis D. Ford lecture on the Institutes and Practice of Medicine), 1874, MCG; see also Mitchell, "Diagnosis," [10–11], TSM.

29. Sharpe, "Report on the Diseases," 282–83; Galt medical student notebook, [ca. 1860], 36–37, Galt family papers, Filson; medical notebook, University of Nashville, of an unknown member of the Sneed family, 1860–61, 1, Sneed family papers, TSL; Musser student notebook, 1843–45, November 10, 1845, Matas. The posture of the body often is remarked upon; see, for instance, Gatewood, "Importance of a Correct Diagnosis," 9, TSM, Porcher, "Clinical Examination" (ms. notes, n.d.), Porcher papers, Waring.

30. John Terrill Lewis, "Remarkable Case of Hemorrhage," 261; J. R. Freese, "Healing Art vs. the Knife," 13; Camden, " 'Missed Labor,' " 152; C. H. Jordan, "Thoughts on Cachexia Africana," 25; Charles Chester, "Four Cases of Cerebro-Spinal Meningitis," 315; Walke, "Continued Fever," 20.

31. Hentz medical diary, September 16, 1860, Hentz family papers, SHC; Schmidt, "Observations on Diphtheria," 270; N. Coles to Ann S. Rutheroord, April 27, 1857, Rutheroord papers, Duke; Farrar, "General Report," 358. For similar comment on closely watched disease and naming, see P[atteson], "Patterson's Cases," 323; William Anderson, "On the Uses

of Cold Water," 193; Rumph, "Thoughts on Malaria," 445; and Baruch medical notebook, 1860–61, 112, Baruch papers, Emory. The usefulness of attempting to name a disease runs throughout professional efforts to reform orthodox medicine during this era, with mixed results. It is striking to see the widely read author John Eberle second-guess the organization of his own medical textbook in this regard. He introduced his 1830 text by saying that he probably should have organized it around organ systems rather than the "disease states" he had chosen to use. Names, he feared, conferred a false certainty: "The artificial divisions of nosology are apt to lead [the physician] to regard the group of symptoms . . . as so many distinct essences, possessing fixed and specific peculiarities of character." Although Eberle altered the organization of his text the very next year, he continued to name diseases as he discussed them. See Eberle, *Treatise on the Practice of Medicine* (1830), vi–vii; compare his *Treatise on the Practice of Medicine* (1831).

32. Scruggs, "Clinical Notes from Private Practice," 34; Bates, "Prevailing Diseases," 310; see also Barnes account book, vol. 2, p. 12, SCL. On the usage "something like," see, for example, Richardson diary, March 1, 1854, SHC.

33. This vision of the "experience" to be gained at the bedside appears with special clarity in two kinds of texts. One is the M.D. thesis, with its blend of mentors' assurances and students' doubts; see, for example, Price, "Physical Diagnosis," 6, and Taylor, "Privileges and Responsibility," [4], TSM. The other is the kind of hybrid textbook and memoir, such as that by Texas physician J. C. Massie, in which one's own practice is the basis for huge generalizations. The sheer personal richness of Massie's observations defy his ability to organize his volume around a single scheme. Instead, he uses several: organs, kinds of disease, types of medicine, and more; see his *Treatise on the Eclectic Southern Practice of Medicine*.

34. Monette, "Essay on the Summer and Autumnal Remittent Fevers," 88.

35. Historical attention to changes in orthodox therapeutics has focused on how physicians and patients used many of the same drugs, and how M.D.s, especially those in institutional settings and in cities, began to innovate with new therapeutic ideas to the point of critiquing both vernacular and orthodox ways. My sense is that many country and small-town physicians shared similar concerns. But a look at rural practice emphasizes the slow and uneven nature of the shift among physicians away from diagnostic terms shared with patients; indeed, rural southern physicians remained solidly planted in vernacular understandings throughout this period. Rosenberg raised the meaning of the shared therapeutic world in "Therapeutic Revolution"; he has an excellent brief discussion of broad continuity and change in therapeutics in his *Care of Strangers*, 86–94. Also important here is Warner, *Therapeutic Perspective*, esp. ch. 4, and his *Against the Spirit of System*, esp. ch. 7.

36. Sterrett, "Medical Topography," 24, TSM; Cooke, "Essay on Autumnal Diseases," 398; Eve, "Essay on Expectation," 325. Opponents typically attacked expectancy as if it were an outcome, rather than a method; see, for example, Ford, "Remarks," 340, and William Fletcher Holmes, "Two Cases of Pneumonia," 179.

37. Porcher, ms. lecture notes, "Materia Medica and Therapeutics delivered 1854–5–6–7–8 again 1873–74," Porcher papers, Waring. See also Warren Stone, quoted in Duffy, ed., *Rudolph Matas History*, 2:21; Duzan, "Rudiments and Practice," 11, TSM; and Gatewood, "Importance of a Correct Diagnosis," 13, TSM.

38. Phillips, "Plate of Artificial Teeth," 544; N. B. Johnson, "Passage of a Half-Dollar," 343.

39. Certain potent substances appear frequently in doctors' prescriptive notes. Calomel, a

chloride of mercury in the form of a chalky powder, was the cathartic of first and last resort. Ipecac and jalap, widely used as emetics, are still in use. Opium and its derivatives were used effectively as sedatives and analgesics, as well as for their now less well known action as antidiarrheals. For general discussions of allopathic medicines, see Duffy, *From Humors to Medical Science*, 69–74, and Cassedy, *Medicine in America*, 25–33. An especially dim view of allopathy's harshness and errors runs throughout Rothstein, *American Physicians*, but see esp. ch. 2. John Harley Warner offers a sophisticated and even sympathetic reading of allopathy's permutations in both *Against the Spirit of System* and *Therapeutic Perspective*. See also Haller, *Medical Protestants*, for doctors who chose to name themselves for their willingness to borrow and combine therapies.

40. As historians have been quick to point out, the failures of this style of therapy were dramatic. At times, however, modern critics have implied that because nineteenth-century physicians did not have modern knowledge they must have had no knowledge. In one such view, "physicians seldom gave any thought to pharmacology in their use of drugs . . . prescriptions were compounded haphazardly." Such criticism, however, seems based on the low end of orthodoxy—on careless, rote prescribers—rather than on the more typical (if, by our standards, mistaken) physicians who gave careful consideration to their medicines; see Rothstein, *American Physicians*, 54. Moreover, even by modern standards, some workhorse allopathic drugs were not utterly lacking. Calomel, for instance, now is seen has having some antimicrobial effects, notably with respect to some strains of venereal disease. It is possible that physicians were seeing similar action in other allopathic drugs they prescribed. See the interesting modern clinical trial of tartar emetic in Duffin and René, "'Anti-moine; Antibiotique.'"

41. John Harley Warner has an excellent discussion of the chemical and physiological reasons for using aggressive medicines in *Therapeutic Perspective*, 91–102; see also Rosenberg, "Therapeutic Revolution," and Brieger, "Therapeutic Conflicts."

42. Blanton, "Modus Operandi," 11–13, VHS. This discussion draws on Blanton's concise descriptions, as well as on the definitions in Estes, *Dictionary of Protopharmacology*, and in Eberle, *Treatise on the Practice of Medicine* (1831). See also Warner, *Therapeutic Perspective*, esp. chs. 4 and 5.

43. McSwain, "Some of the Discrepancies," 1–2, MCSSC; Rea student notebook, ca. 1869, n.p., Matas; [Boyd], "Finale of Twenty Years Study," 3, MCSSC; see also Pendleton, "General Report on the Topography," 323.

44. Sharpe, "Report on the Diseases," 279–80; Hentz diary, June 29, 1846, in Stowe, ed., *Southern Practice*, 112. For another poetic impulse inspired by medical work, see the brief verse on the imperviousness to medicine of a "mind diseased," in Rea student notebook, ca. 1869, n.p., Matas.

45. Flagg daybook, April 10, 1850, SCHS. For other examples, which are legion, see Joseph Jones to Charles Colcock Jones, November 12, 1856, Jones papers, HTML, and Lunsford Yandell diary, 1824–43, June 24, 1830 (p. 100), Yandell family papers, Filson.

46. Dupuy commonplace book, 1845–58, VHS. See also the notes and recipes in Thomas and Mary Boulware diary, 1850–71, Winthrop; anonymous medical notebook, LSU; Isabella P. Porcher plantation prescription book, ca. 1834, Waring; Cook memorandum book, Duke; Bagby commonplace book, VHS; and Middleton household accounts, Cheves-Middleton papers, SCHS. On particular southern syntheses of healing agents, see Weymouth T. Jordan,

"Martin Marshall's Book" and *Herbs, Hoecakes, and Husbandry*. On books of secrets, see Eamon, *Science and the Secrets of Nature*.

Physicians' daybooks frequently show the mingling of popular and orthodox drugs, but see, especially, Knox casebooks, UK; Hentz medical diary, Hentz family papers, SHC; J. A. S. Milligan "Formulae," ms. vol. 5, 1846, Milligan family papers, SHC; and Robert Lovett prescription book, ms. vol., 1844, Lovett papers, Emory. See also the combinations of basic medicines (including, apparently, one Thomsonian mixture) in the leather carrying case belonging to Robert Burns Pusey, in the Pusey papers, UL. For especially substantive accounts of like medicines recalled by former slaves, see August Smith, in *AS*, supp. 1, 2.4, pp. 250–54, and Sally Brown, *AS*, supp. 1, 3.1, pp. 98–99; and see Croom, "Herbal Medicine." Most physicians seem not at all reluctant to credit slaves with using effective local drugs; see, for instance, William Gilmore Simms to Francis P. Porcher, April 14, 1863, Porcher papers, SCL; Cauthorn, "New Anti-Periodic"; and Porcher, *Resources of the Southern Fields*.

Physicians also constantly traded prescriptions with each other, and sometimes the medicines themselves; see, of many possible examples, R. Duer to William S. Hamilton, August 2, 1841, Hamilton papers, LSU; Simon Baruch to James R. Sparkman, February 18, 1874, Sparkman papers, SCL; and Coleman Rogers to Samuel Brown, January 17, 1824, Brown papers, Filson.

47. Bachelor student notebook, 1873, 22, Bachelor papers, LSU; Rea student notebook, ca. 1869, n.p., Matas; Armstrong notebook, 1839–47, 4, LSU; McKinney student notebook, 1857, 1864–68, 47–48, McKinney papers, LSU. For a similar slave "ash-cake" remedy, see Clark medical notebook, 1844–74, 57, Clark papers, Duke. For a medical recommendation of flannel, much advocated by caregiving women, see Porcher commonplace book, 1843–45, 48, SCHS, and for pure water, Hunter, "Preservation of Health," 9, MCSSC. For a typical recommendation of a slave antidote, see Musgrove, "Poisoning by Phytolaccoe Radix," 230–31.

48. Sterrett, "Medical Topography," 14, TSM; Macon, "Diuretic Virtues," 21; L. B. Anderson, "Treatment of Cancer," 50–51.

49. Eberle, *Treatise on the Practice of Medicine* (1831), 2:213–21. The standard shorthand for the directions in giving medicines (today, as well as in the nineteenth century) also privileges the subjective judgment of individual practitioners. For example, directions to give a drug "P.r.n." (*pro re nata*—"as occasion may arise") and "q.p." or "q.s." (*quantum placeat*—"as much as may please" and *quantum sufficiat*—"as much as may suffice") invite healers to rely on their previous experience. Thus, even a careful physician worked within a set of practices that might easily blur the line between therapy and experimentation. For prescription notations, see Dunglison, *Medical Student*, 112–13.

50. Patrick Todd to Joel Berly, October 28, 1848, Berly family papers, SCL; Frank James diary, November 18, 1877, in Baird, ed., *Years of Discontent*, 35. Systematic medical experiments did not become widespread until the turn of the century, and then only in the urban and academic centers possessing the concentrations of people and money that fueled a research based on well-financed laboratories and well-stocked hospitals. Occasionally, though, individual rural doctors engaged in piecemeal, freelance efforts at testing drugs comparatively. See, for example, O. P. Mayers to Joel Berly, November 23, 1853, Berly family papers, SCL. On the advent of the modern context of medical experimentation, see Lederer, *Subjected to Science*. Within limits established by the master's interests, doctors clearly felt more at ease

experimenting on slaves than on white neighbors, or, as they sometimes did, on themselves. If the doctor were himself the master, however, as in the case of J. Marion Sims's infamous surgical experiments on Anarcha and other slave women, the only limits were the doctor's self-imposed ones. On Sims, see McGregor, *Sexual Surgery*, and Barker-Benfield, *Horrors of the Half-Known Life*.

51. J. A. Reedy to William Reedy, June 9, 1884, Reedy and Beacham papers, SCL; Holcombe, *How I Became a Homoeopath*, 6; Turner, "Record of Two Singular Cases," 681. For this kind of trial and error, see also Leland, "Inflammation," 1, MCSSC; Meek diary, [March] 4, 1814, Meek papers, ADAH; Wooten, "Topography and Diseases," 339; and Pusey, *Doctor of the 1870's and 80's*, 96. For an excellent example of a young doctor puzzling over what to do with three different textbook authors recommending three different courses of action in cases of scarlatina, see McSwain, "Some of the Discrepancies," MCSSC.

52. On pain as both a sign of disease and a sign of healing in the nineteenth century, see Pernick, *Calculus of Suffering*. The now-classic work on the phenomenology of pain is Scarry, *Body in Pain*; see also Bakan, *Disease, Pain, and Sacrifice*.

53. Frank James diary, January 9, 1878, in Baird, ed., *Years of Discontent*, 55; Dickson, "Essay on Mania a Potu," 17. See also John Y. Bassett, "Report on the Topography," 271–72.

54. Van Bibber, "Fatal Poisoning by Alcohol," 101–3. For a similar case, in which two well-trained physicians subject a middle-class woman to extreme treatments and subsequently attribute her turn for the worse to "the atmosphere," see Lebby, "Tetanus."

55. Samuel Van Wyck to "Dear Ma," February 18, 1861, Maverick and Van Wyck papers, SCL; Frank James diary, January 1, 1878, in Baird, ed., *Years of Discontent*, 55; Dr. Billings on veratrum viride, quoted in Norwood, *Medical Education*, 143; Pressly Bolar Ruff to James M. H. Ruff, May 23, 1885, Ruff and Caldwell papers, SCL; Grant, "Case in Which the Placenta Was Retained," 196. Many doctors applauded their drugs' "noble effects" and their working like "a charm"; see, for example, Day, "Obstetrical Cases," 225; Long, "Eleven Years of Practice," 22, Vanderbilt; and Dugas, "Purulent Ophthalmia of Infants," 81.

56. Wharton, "Account of Epidemic Erysipelas," 282; see also Bates, "Prevailing Diseases," 314.

57. D. P. Calhoun, "Trismus Nascentium," 124–25; Joseph Johnson, "Some Account of the Origin," 165.

CHAPTER SIX

1. Levin Smith Joynes medical notes [1851], n.p., Joynes family papers, VHS.

2. Ibid. In cupping patients, doctors placed small, heated glass hemispheres over an incision, creating a vacuum that "gently" drew blood or "poisons" from an affected area of the body.

3. James E. Smith, "Cases Illustrating the Practice of Medicine," 446; Kilpatrick, "Report on the Medical Topography," 180. A seton is a strip or string, usually of silk or linen, drawn through a wound so as to keep it open and discharging. For a variety of assertive patients, see, for example, Mary Ann Shields to Andrew MacCrery, November 1840, MacCrery family papers, LSU, and Frances Wall to Jeptha McKinney, "Sabbath morn," n.d. (probably late 1850s), McKinney papers, LSU. For more cooperative, ally-type patients, see, for example,

Scruggs, "Clinical Notes," 31; Lunsford Yandell to Sally Yandell, June 1, 1860, Yandell family papers, Filson; C. F. Pearson to T. G. Richardson, January 26, 1860, Pearson letter, LSU; Laban Taylor to J. S. Copes, October 2, 1845, Copes papers, HTML; and Mary Henderson diary, August 18, 1855, Henderson papers, SHC. For other examples of doctors who appear only as marginal figures, see Mahala Roach diary, May 17, 1860, Roach and Eggleston family papers, SHC, and Davies diary, July 13, 1852, Davies papers, Duke. Patients often noted their skepticism of a physician's prognosis. Thomas Rutherfoord was not sorry he called a doctor to visit his sick slave Septima, but he was certain the man had "flattered himself she was mending" when she was not (Thomas Rutherfoord to John Rutherfoord, August 15, 1811, Rutherfoord papers, Duke).

4. Pusey, *Doctor of the 1870's and 80's*, 96, 92; Blanding diary, October 16, 1810, Blanding papers, SCL. For practitioners acceding uneasily to patients, see also Bates, "Prevailing Diseases," 314, and Wilson Yandell to Lunsford Yandell, October 14, 1824, Yandell family papers, Filson, where the former regrets not challenging a woman's conviction that "some evil would befall" her family because she had heard hens crowing.

5. Bailey, "Essay on Medical Faith," 20; Hentz diary, September 30, 1846, in Steven M. Stowe, ed., *Southern Practice*, 141; Buchanan, "Remarks on Negro Consumption," 407. For other examples of slaves, doctors, and masters negotiating the type and timing of treatments, see M. D. McLoud, "Hints on the Medical Treatment of Negroes," 5, MCSSC; Boykin, "Observations on the Medical Topography," 502; and, for an unusually attentive physician to a slave, William R. King, "Diseases of Franklin County," 10–11.

6. Philips, "Qualifications," 3–4, TSM; Hort, "Enquiry," 61. For other examples of doctors countering noncompliant patients, see Barnes account book, vol. 2, p. 12, SCL; Nathaniel Siewers to "Dear Father and Mother," August 17, 1866, Siewers letters, UNCC; and Samuel Cartwright, "The One Dose Cure for Camp Dysentery," ms., n.d. (ca. 1846), Cartwright papers, LSU.

7. Reese, "Proceedings of the Medical Association," 328; Wilson Yandell to Lunsford Yandell, October 12, 1824, Yandell family papers, Filson. On childbirth as a young practitioner's most feared call, see "Dick" to John A. Robinson, October 20, 1874, Robinson papers, SCL. That fears of disaster sometimes came true, see Armstrong notebook, 1839, 24–29, LSU, and Blanding diary, November 14–21 and December 6, 1810, Blanding papers, SCL. Women seeking to abort pregnancies appear occasionally in physicians' notes but seem not to have been a focus of much conflict. Physicians responded as their personal moralities dictated. Some, like Frank James, were appalled when asked by women for abortifacients— "both . . . are strict church members," James wrote in astonishment at two such requests. But other M.D.s were less affronted; though noting that "the prejudices of the profession" did not support abortion, M. A. Shackleford personally used gossipium herbaceum "in many cases with much success." See Frank James diary, September 21, 1877, in Baird, ed., *Years of Discontent*, 7, and Shackleford, "Gossipium," 4, Vanderbilt.

8. Lecture notes (probably Warren Stone's lectures), University of Louisiana, Kennon student notebook, 1866, n.p., Matas; Colmer diary, n.d., James H. Bailey account, 87, Colmer papers, HTML; Baruch medical notebook, 1860–61, 177, Baruch papers, Emory; Rouanet, "Popular Errors Exposed," 199. On children's tenuous health and their difficult nature as patients, see also H[enry] H. Jones to Joseph Jones, June 25, 1857, Jones collection, HTML;

R. A. Edmonston to John Lyle, November 2, 1851, Lyle and Siler family papers, SHC; Allen student notebook, 1874, MCG; and anonymous student notebook, Transylvania Medical College, 1833–35, 76, Matas.

9. Baruch medical notebook, 1860–61, 179, Baruch papers, Emory; Holcombe diary, May 6 and February 3, 1855, SHC. See also James R. Sparkman to Benjamin Allston, March 10, 1858, quoted in Waring, *History of Medicine*, 8; Charles Hentz autobiography in Stowe, ed., *Southern Practice*, 500.

10. McLoud, "Hints on the Medical Treatment of Negroes," 12–13, MCSSC (this M.D. thesis has much to say about ways to expose feigning, which the author attributes to slaves' laziness but at the same time to their "anger and malevolence," [p. 9]); Dunglison, *Dictionary of Medical Science*, 316–17. Medical advice given to slave owners often recommended dosing suspected feigners with harsh medicine; see, for example, Gage, "Plantation Hygiene." For other feigning cases, see P[atteson], "Patterson's Cases," 325–26, and [Review of] "On the Treatment of Cholera," 212. As James Mohr (*Doctors and the Law*, 20–21, 157–58) points out, many nonsouthern doctors' experience in detecting feigning arose largely from their being asked by military officials who suspected it in soldiers. For interesting discussion of slave feigning, see Ariela J. Gross, *Double Character*, ch. 5, and Fett, *Working Cures*, ch. 7; see also Stepan, "Race, Gender, Science."

11. For the slave who appeared to vomit up pins, see Hopkins, "Remarkable Case of Feigned Disease." For a similar instance of a slave using knotted thread that seemed to come from her body, in this case in order to obtain opium from the doctor, see Brown, "Curious Case of Malingering." At the same time, physicians and masters recognized that slaves might, for various reasons, seek to conceal that they actually were ill; see, for example, C. H. Jordan, "Thoughts on Cachexia Africana," 23, and Boykin, "Observations on the Medical Topography," 503.

12. Mary Henderson diary, November 3, 1855, Henderson papers, SHC.

13. Hentz medical diary, August 20, 1860, Hentz family papers, SHC; Ella Gertrude Clanton Thomas diary, August 18, 1856, in Burr, ed., *Secret Eye*, 150. Contests of will between masters and slaves did not always divide along lines of race or servitude. Suspecting a slave named Jarret of feigning, a physician received confirmation from a "slave nurse" who maintained Jarret was faking; see Clark, "Remarks on the Existence of Typhoid Fever," 467.

14. Wilson Yandell to Lunsford Yandell, October 12, 1824, Yandell family papers, Filson.

15. Occasionally, Knox uses more vivid language—a man's injured foot "had near thrown him into jaundice"—but for the most part his descriptions depict sickness evenly, as something manageable. Like many other physicians, Knox was comfortable using approximate names for the ailments he saw, appropriately denoting disease's propensity to change at any moment. Thus one patient suffered "something like Erecipelas or bilboes" and another had "something like pneumonia." See Knox casebooks, vol. 2, May 8, September 28, and November 21, 1852, UK.

16. A rare exception to the usual doctor-patient couple in Knox's writing is his note on Mr. Gourley's sickness in which the doctor "gave him a vomit—& bled him & Mrs. Sterling steamed his head" (Knox casebooks, vol. 1, February 2, 1848, UK). The isolation of patients is sharpest with regard to slaves, whose very individuality is vague in a way typical of most doctors' bedside notes.

17. Knox casebooks, vol. 2., November 23, [1851], September 20, 1852, UK.

18. Ibid., vol. 1, January 13, 1851, April 22 through May 5, 1847.

19. Knox relied heavily on certain premixed compounds, many of which were readily available to families. This would have made his medicines familiar and thus reassuring to patients, along with giving him some flexibility should he need to draw on a family's medicine chest. Knox was partial to Dover's powders, for example, a mixture of ipecac and opium, an orthodox medicine also found in many home medicine chests. The same was true for Seidlitz powder, a blend of cream of tartar and sodium bicarbonate used as a mild "cooling" cathartic. In the various cases featured here, it is not clear what Tulley's powder and Wright's pills consisted of, but whatever they were, they were further from the allopathic mainstream; Keeley's Cordial has the ring of a patent medicine.

20. Hentz medical diary, November 16–20, 1860, Hentz family papers, SHC. Hentz's course of therapy is a classic allopathic orchestration of drugs and symptoms. Calomel, of course, was the workhorse purge, mercurous chloride; it reliably activated a wide range of the body's visible secretions in a swift and thorough way. Though calomel itself might induce vomiting, Hentz adds the surefire emetic ipecac as well. The scillae syrup was a compound of medicines made chiefly from the bulb of squill, or sea onion; Hentz probably used it, in combination with the boneset tea, as a diuretic, further "opening" Mrs. Goodson's body to expose and unsettle disease. Veratrum viride was a relative newcomer among drugs that many physicians had been enthusiastically adopting since the 1850s and that Hentz administers here in an alcohol-based form. Veratrum, a form of false hellebore, widely known to domestic healers as poke root, was admired as a drug with swift "operation." Nevertheless, Hentz appears somewhat wary of veratrum; here he believes it responsible for a sort of vomiting that displeased him.

21. Hentz medical diary, November 21–24, 1860, Hentz family papers, SHC.

22. Hentz obviously used the well-known ear-ringing side effect of quinine as a sign of its appropriate operation, much as he pushed mercurials to the point of salivation, and sometimes a bit beyond. Although he does not recount his clinical reasoning on the twenty-first, he adds yet another mercurial mixture, hydrargyrus cum creta (a mercury base combined with "chalk," or calcium carbonate), that was known as a milder purge than calomel and one, somewhat paradoxically, that acted as a antidiarrheal (he is troubled by his patient's "too free" bowels). Throughout the course of treatment, Hentz's case-note style shows how he imagined drugs as operating in waves, each adding a tone or harmonic to the symphony of medicines he aimed to create.

23. After the first two days of treatment, Hentz's therapeutic style illustrates how an allopath easily merged domestic and orthodox remedies, once again suggesting that under the pressure of a case, M.D.s did not find the distinction between the two kinds of medicine a meaningful one. The substances he prescribes on the final two days of treatment here (apart from the quinine) were employed widely as tonics and stimulants, substances used as much to lift the spirits (brandy and the wine whey) as to fine-tune secretions with "diaphoretic" action, that is, action that enabled the body to constrict and release both the remnants of disease and the effects of the more powerful drugs. The vitriol acted as an astringent, for example, the cohosh and seneca teas (derived from different varieties of snakeroot), as mild diuretics and expectorants, and the asclepias tea, as a carminative, that is, something to expel gas from the intestines.

24. Hentz medical diary, March 31 to April 3, 1861 (the entire case extends through an entry for April 11), Hentz family papers, SHC. Although the notes for Jim's case appear on the page in Hentz's usual rapid-fire, sprawling style, it seems (mostly from the way Hentz refers retrospectively to certain days, as in the entries for April 1–3) that he might have written the case retrospectively, possibly transcribing a set of immediate bedside notes into this "interesting cases" volume. Even so, he wrote in a way that retained the usual sense of immediacy and closely watched change.

25. Unusually for him, Hentz does not characterize the hue of Jim's skin as a way of establishing him as an "African" patient; more typically, Hentz described black patients as he did a man named Frank on February 2, 1859 ("a bright mullato") and a woman named Sally (a "light mullato—hair like a white person's"), whom he treated on August 22, 1860 (medical diary, Hentz family papers, SHC).

26. These considerations are made more complex by the fact that Hentz no doubt would have implicitly taken Jim's sex and age into account as well, modifying whatever he concluded on the basis of Jim's race.

27. Hentz medical diary, April 4–8, 1861, Hentz family papers, SHC.

28. Ibid., April 9–11, 1861.

29. Hentz does not linger over the details of Jim's resistance, but it appears to have been substantial. "Several men" were needed to restrain Jim and force the therapy on him in a scene that rehearsed harsh punishments inflicted on slaves and threatened to blur the line between punishment and therapy. Hentz, however, sees Jim's resistance as part of his illness and thus not a reason to disregard Jim's views once he snapped out of it. For a patient, a white man, whom Hentz thought was deliberately uncompliant, see the account of Sam Gee's fatal sickness, November 18, 1858 (Hentz medical diary, Hentz family papers, SHC), in which the patient "will not speak—nor do anything asked—spits out everything put in mouth." The fact that Gee himself was a doctor may have had something to do with his resistance.

30. This style was reinforced by the way Hentz typically concludes each case. Instead of ending with a general observation or a specific note for future reference, his case notes conclude abruptly or dramatically, like one-act plays. So in Abner Gregory's mortal disease, Hentz concludes despairingly on September 6, 1860, "Abner sinking—the above did no good—nothing did good" (ibid.). In the happy outcome of Mary Campbell's illness, on November 4, 1860, Hentz's gaze is almost that of a lover or an adoring parent: "cheeks crimson again . . . color natural—tongue much better—coating leaving it; & moist lips soft—skin moist—Better" (ibid.).

31. To a greater degree than either Hentz or Knox, however, Clark had an eye for unusual cases, ones physicians saw infrequently: "sarcoma of the eyeball," "tumor of the bladder," multiple skull fracture, the birth of twins.

32. Clark medical notebook, 1844–74, 32, Clark papers, Duke.

33. Ibid.

34. Ibid., 32–33. As Clark intensified his treatment, Mrs. White's husband appears in the notes. Clark obviously relied on Mr. White's observations, and it seems that he, too, was unsure how to judge the sense of his wife's expressions. Throughout, Clark's record of his physical examinations are mainstream orthodox; he systematically noted pulse, stool, tongue, and skin temperature and texture. As always, it is tempting to wonder whether certain signs or

symptoms might have been side effects of drugs; her delirium, for example, might have been unintentionally exacerbated by his prescription of camphor.

35. Clark medical notebook, 1844–74, 34–35, Clark papers, Duke.

36. Ibid., 35–36.

37. Ibid., 14.

38. Ibid., 14–16.

39. Ibid., 26, 83.

CHAPTER SEVEN

1. Slavery and race often figured into topographical essays, of course; these will be considered in the following section. Medical topographies were a thriving genre in medical literature well into the 1880s. Their style changed slightly over the years, becoming somewhat more quantitative and less discursive. They faded away when orthodox medicine located its science in the laboratory and its research protocols and in other ways that discouraged the voice of individual practitioners. The notes that follow refer to representative topographies, but other examples of thoughtful, personable essays include Heard, "Topography, Climate, and Diseases"; Sterrett, "Medical Topography," TSM; Boykin, "Observations on the Medical Topography"; Payne, "Hydrography, Topography"; Gaillard, "Medical Topography"; John Y. Bassett, "Climate and Diseases"; Becton, "Essay on the Topography"; Briggs, "Medical Topography," Vanderbilt; Harden, "Observations on the Soil"; and Suddarth, "Physical and Medical Topography." Daniel Drake's ambitious and somewhat unruly work on the epidemiology of the "interior valley" of the continent was perhaps the greatest topographic achievement of the midcentury; see his *Systematic Treatise*. Conevery Bolton Valencius has a good discussion of medical topographies (or medical geographies, as they also were called), although she sees them as repositories of local knowledge without stressing their implications for medical reform; see *Health of the Country*, ch. 6. On medicine and demography generally in this era, see Cassedy, *Medicine and American Growth*.

2. Wooten, "Topography and Diseases," 331; Lavender, "Topography, Climate, and Diseases," 342; Little, "Climate and Diseases," 2–3, TSM. See also Sterrett, "Medical Topography," 10.

3. Pendleton, "General Report on the Topography," 315–16; Payne, "Hydrography, Topography," 35; Boykin, "Observations on the Medical Topography," 500. See also Tennent, "Medical Topography," 7; Geddings, "Report of the Committee," 23.

4. Suddarth, "Physical and Medical Topography," 484. For Bassett, see "Report on the Topography," 272.

5. Tennent, "Medical Topography," 9–10; John Y. Bassett, "Report on the Topography," 259; see also Farrar, "General Report," 352.

6. See Posey, "Report upon the Topography." In arguing for such reform, physicians added their voices to authors and editors in southern agricultural journals. For a broad treatment of environment, agriculture, and reform in the South, see Albert E. Cowdrey, *This Land, This South*.

7. Posey, "Report upon the Topography," 108–9; Farrar, "General Report," 348.

8. Briggs, "Medical Topography," 1–2, Vanderbilt; Farrar, "General Report," 346.

9. M. Troy, "Report on the Diseases," 238; Harden, "Observations on the Soil," 555.

10. Becton, "Essay on the Topography," 164; Farrar, "General Report," 351. See also John Y. Bassett, "Report on the Topography," 265, and Suddarth, "Physical and Medical Topography," 483–84.

11. Heard, "Topography, Climate, and Diseases," 3; Gibbs, "Medical Topography and Diseases," 189–90.

12. John Y. Bassett, "Report on the Topography," 259.

13. For examples of the merely in-passing reference to slaves by southern authors, especially after 1830, when advice books were more often addressed to women in the home rather than to a man's agricultural "field" setting, see Goodlett, *Family Physician*, 630, and Jennings, *Compendium of Medical Science*, 493. For an earlier adviser who spoke to men but still included only 3 pages (out of more than 200) on "general directions for raising negroes," see John Hume Simons, *Planter's Guide*, 207–9.

14. By the 1850s, the debate over whether God created blacks and whites separately or whether he created one race that later bifurcated, was, of course, a debate of great interest to many Americans who were fascinated by links between Christianity, Romantic individualism, and the natural world. For excellent discussions of Nott, and of this debate, see Horsman, *Josiah Nott of Mobile*, and Stephens, *Science, Race, and Religion*. For typical medical journal articles by Nott, see his "Instincts of the Races," and, for the full extension of his thought, see Nott and Gliddon, *Types of Mankind* and *Indigenous Races of the Earth*. For a typically skeptical view of Nott's huge claims, see "Types of Mankind." Broadly useful in the practical and theoretical implications of the debate are Savitt, *Medicine and Slavery*, esp. chs. 1 and 9, and Kevles, *In the Name of Eugenics*. For a sampling of nineteenth-century medical literature and its bias away from theory and toward questions of practice, the catalog of the U.S. Surgeon General's library is suggestive. Most of the mid-nineteenth-century articles and books listed under the topic heading "Negroes" concern particular diseases and issues of care. Articles falling under the more inclusive heading "Race" in the catalog number less than one-quarter of the entries under "Negroes." See *Index-Catalogue*, 9:695–97; 11:975.

15. Suddarth, "Physical and Medical Topography," 82.

16. Fenner, "Acclimation," 454; Affleck, "Hygiene of Cotton Plantations," 434. See also Boykin, "Observations on the Medical Topography," 500–502; "D," Review of *Indigenous Races of the Earth*, 22. For an example of a doctor typically counting numbers of slaves, and in this case revising the U.S. Census, see Wooten, "Topography and Diseases," 332.

17. McCaa, "Observations on the Manner of Living," 5, Waring. Comparisons are part of nearly every topography that considers race, but for good examples, see "Health of Augusta"; Ketchum, "Notes on the Topography"; Pendleton, "General Report on the Topography"; and Boykin, "Observations on the Medical Topography."

18. The timing of McCaa's 1822 essay is interesting, given his Charleston affiliation. In the early summer of that year, the planned slave insurrection led by former slave Denmark Vesey came to light, to the consternation of white Charlestonians. It is not known when McCaa composed his essay, a University of Pennsylvania M.D. thesis. It is dated 1822, but the cover notes, "Passed March 11, 1823"; it is possible, therefore, that he wrote it in late 1822 with some knowledge of the Vesey conspiracy.

19. Affleck, "Hygiene of Cotton Plantations," 431, 434; Moore, "Plantation Hygiene," 13, 15, MCSSC.

20. C. H. Jordan, "Thoughts on Cachexia Africana," 29; Payne, "Hydrography, Topography," 37; Moore, "Plantation Hygiene," 12, MCSSC.

21. Moore, "Plantation Hygiene," 31, MCSSC.

22. Compare the views of Fett, *Working Cures*, esp. ch. 6, and Ariela Gross, *Double Character*, esp. ch. 5.

23. For a sampling of nineteenth-century views on "Negro disease," see the typical approach of medical topographers S. L. Grier ("Negro and His Diseases") and A. P. Merrill ("Distinctive Peculiarities"), who raise and then sidestep the question of race as an abstract "governing" factor and proceed to discuss the particulars of slave diseases without attention to race. So does John S. Wilson ("Peculiarities and Diseases"), whose main message is preventative, recommending that slave owners outfit their work force with raincoats, for instance. D. Warren Brickell ("Epidemic Typhoid Pneumonia"), like other doctors, begins with a racial context, but his case-study approach to sick slaves ends up completely ignoring race as a factor. For an additional sampling, see Morton, "Causes of Mortality"; "Vaccination from the Negro"; Sharpe, "Report on the Diseases"; Burt, "Report on the Anatomical and Physiological Differences"; Henry A. Ramsay, *Necrological Appearances*; Buchanan, "Remarks on Negro Consumption"; Forbes, "Diseases of Conecuh County"; McLoud, "Hints on the Medical Treatment of Negroes," MCSSC; Harden, "Observations on the Soil"; Lavender, "Topography, Climate, and Diseases"; Wooten, "Topography and Diseases"; Boykin, "Observations on the Medical Topography"; Payne, "Epidemics of Piedmont"; C. H. Jordan, "Thoughts on Cachexia Africana"; and McCaa, "Observations on the Manner of Living," Waring.

24. John LeConte, "Observations on Geophagy," 430. For the range of discussion on dirt-eating, see, for example, W. M. Carpenter, "Observations on Cachexia Africana"; Pope, "Professional Management of Negro Slaves," MCSSC; Gilmer, "Pathology and Treatment," MCSSC; Gresham, "On the Subject of Cachexia Africana," MCSSC; Dungan, "Report on the Topography"; Harden, "Observations on the Soil"; and C. H. Jordan, "Thoughts on Cachexia Africana." For a physician puzzling out just how exotic he thought African Americans were, see Lunsford Yandell diary, January 15, 1830, Yandell family papers, Filson, and his "Remarks on Struma Africana."

25. Cartwright, "Diseases and Physical Peculiarities" (May 1851); quotations from 707 and 709. This article is the published version of a paper Cartwright read at the March 1851 meeting of the Medical Association of Louisiana, and it became the centerpiece of the ensuing controversy over his claims about race. He published several articles with the same or similar titles, some including his responses to critics; see, for example, articles in *Southern Medical Reports* (1850, actually published in late 1851), *Charleston Medical Journal and Review*, June 1851, and two follow-up pieces in the *New Orleans Medical and Surgical Journal*, September and November 1851. Other articles on Cartwright's particular enthusiasms with regard to race include "Philosophy of the Negro Constitution," "Alcohol and the Ethiopian," and "Remarks on Dysentery among Negroes."

The controversy over the extravagance of Cartwright's claims for racial difference also was fueled by his proslavery, sectionalist polemics more generally and, one suspects, by the fact that no topic seemed beyond his expertise; see, for example, his "Canaan Identified with the Ethiopian" (an early proslavery paper), "Apoplexy of the South," "Report on the Locality of

Plants," and "Hygienics of Temperance." Cartwright's quirky interpretation of empirical evidence—or the lack of it—began to attract critics by the early 1850s, although journals continued to publish him; for critics, see [Fenner], "State Medical Society of Louisiana," and "Cartwright on the Diseases and Peculiarities." Overall, there is little question, despite his atypical views, that Cartwright contributed to an intellectual atmosphere serving white dominance in the mid-nineteenth century. But compared to the far more rigid sense of "race" by the 1890s, it is important to understand that "race" was not seen as determining health and sickness so much as presenting unique, if vague, challenges to the manipulations of the doctor. Ariela Gross takes a similar, balanced view of Cartwright in *Double Character*, 87–88. For historians publishing three decades apart who have not questioned Cartwright's representativeness, see Eugene Genovese, *Roll, Jordan, Roll*, 302, 308, and Walter Johnson, *Soul by Soul*, 136, 146.

26. Cartwright, "Report on the Diseases," 205.

27. [Fenner], "State Medical Society of Louisiana," 295, 297.

28. Wooten, "Dysentery among Negroes," 448; James T. Smith, "Review of Dr. Cartwright's Report," 233.

29. Cooper, "View of the Metaphysical and Physiological," 2, 11, 13; compare Moore, "Religion and Medicine," for a midcentury view. Many of the same notes are sounded in Joseph A. McCullough, "Effect of Religious Conceptions upon Science." Examples abound of how a religious context overlapped with medical interests throughout a practitioner's life; see, for example, William Holcombe's recollection that as a child he had a "regular desire to 'play preacher' every Sunday as I 'played doctor' all the week" (Holcombe autobiography, 63, SHC). As an adult, Holcombe likened his homeopathy to the spiritual openness of Swedenborgianism, whereas allopathy was similar to dour, old-church Calvinism; see his autobiography, 19–20, 33–35, and his *How I Became a Homoeopath*.

30. Moore, "Religion and Medicine," 95. For a similar essay that notes the many reasons for rivalry between clergy and physicians but sees the possibility of unity between them, see Powell, "True Physician." For a sense of the depth of feeling in this rivalry, see Hope, "Discourse"; Ellzey, "Life-Work of the Modern Physician"; Moody, "Responsibility and Duty," Vanderbilt; and Cowling, *Relations of Medicine to Modern Unbelief*.

31. William Martin to Lunsford Yandell, April 8, 1839, Yandell family papers, Filson. See also Boardman, *Claims of Religion*, and Quintard, "Address."

32. Moore, "Religion and Medicine," 91; Leland diary, January 23, 1853, SCL; John A. Robinson to S. Moffat Wylie, November 2, 1871, Robinson papers, SCL; Frank James diary, September 16, 1877, in Baird, ed., *Years of Discontent*, 3; Joseph LeConte autobiographical ms., LeConte-Furman papers, SHC, 143; Boardman, *Claims of Religion*, 12; Quintard, "Address," 32. See also William Forwood to S[usan] R. L[yons], July 26, 1860, Forwood papers, SHC; and Hentz diary, November 11, 1860, in Stowe, ed., *Southern Practice*, 352. For a Kentucky physician's fascinating private speculations in which he struggled, often unsuccessfully, to favor science over the "mythological system" of Christianity, see John W. King, "Letters from the Dead," ms., n.d. [probably 1840s], King papers, LSU.

33. Powell, "True Physician," 158; Caldwell, "Introductory Address," 15–16, 8; Charles Caldwell to B. H. Coates, October 27, 1826 (photocopy), UK. For a spirited conversation about Caldwell's views on religion, indicating how they were of interest to practicing physi-

cians, see Lunsford Yandell to David Wendel, January 18, 1826; Wendel to Yandell, January 30, 1826; T[imothy] Flint to Yandell, May 3, 1830; and Ch[arles] Caldwell to Yandell, October 10, 1830, Yandell family papers, Filson.

34. Lunsford Yandell diary, July 18, 1830, Yandell family papers, Filson; Holcombe diary, May 4, 1855, SHC; J. Marion Sims to Theresa Sims, December 25, 1854, Sims papers, SHC. The spiritual meaning of the work ethic hearkened back to medical school. See, for example, M.D. theses by Greene, "Profession of Medicine," MCSSC, and Dismukes, "Physician," Vanderbilt. Interesting in this regard are careers, more common early in the century, of men like Samuel Mills Meek who were both ministers and doctors; see his diary, 1814–15, Meek papers, ADAH.

35. Charles Colcock Jones to Joseph Jones, November 28, 1855, Jones collection, HTML; Hope, "Discourse," 15; John Berrien Lindsley ms. notes, November 28, 1863, Lindsley notebook, TSL; Sterrett, "Medical Topography," 13; Hardin, "Physic and Physicians," 15, MCSSC. Joseph LeConte recalled that after his religious conversion, "the sky was never before so blue, the clouds so grandly massy & white, the grass so freshly green, nor the stars so bright." See his autobiographical ms., 45, Leconte-Furman papers, SHC; see also, Ellzey, "Life-Work of the Modern Physician," and Parvin, "Physician Is a Good Man."

36. Hill, "Treatise on Woman," 3, MCSSC; Dickson, *Essays on Life*, 30; Powell, *Colloquy on the Duties*, 66.

37. Powell, *Colloquy on the Duties*, 32–33, 43; John A. Robinson to S. Moffat Wylie, April 1, 1873, Robinson papers, SCL; J[eptha] McKinney to Sybil McKinney, June 14, 1862, McKinney papers, LSU.

38. Cowling, *Relations of Medicine to Modern Unbelief*, 10; Thompson, "Address on the Curative Value of High Character," 17.

39. William Martin to Lunsford Yandell, November 21, 1838, Yandell family papers, Filson; Thomas Wood to Francis Porcher, n.d., Porcher papers, SCL; McCorkle diary, October 18, 1846, McCorkle papers, SHC; see also Mary Ann Shields to Andrew MacCrery, April 3, 1840, MacCrery family papers, LSU. Sometimes patients' exalted sense of the religious significance of their treatment comported oddly with physicians' more matter-of-fact sense of their interventions. A woman wrote Dr. Paul F. Eve praising him for the "favor" of his cure and hoping that "when your mission on earth is ended, may *angels* waft *you* to *God*, who so kindly gave you to *us*." To which Eve added a note: "I got a coffee grain from the windpipe." See Mollie F. Pale to Paul F. Eve, February 28, 1875, Eve papers, TSL.

40. McKinney diary, August 9, 1865, McKinney papers, LSU; Lunsford Yandell diary, April 19, 1824, Yandell family papers, Filson.

41. Lunsford Yandell diary [ca. 1824; the recollection is Yandell's father's], 330, Yandell family papers, Filson; Alicia H. Middleton to Eweretta Middleton, July 5, 1832, Middleton letters, Cheves-Middleton papers, SCHS; McCorkle diary, October [25], 1846, McCorkle papers, SHC; William Martin to Lunsford Yandell, July 29, 1833, Yandell family papers, Filson; "Eweretta" to Eweretta Middleton, June 17, 1842, Middleton letters, Cheves-Middleton papers, SCHS.

42. J. A. S. Milligan to Octavia Milligan, July 13, 1858, Milligan family papers, SHC; Elliott, "Medical Etiquette," 18, TSM; James Milligan to J. A. S. Milligan, July 8, 1848, Milligan family papers, SHC; Brandon diary/memoir, December 3, 1860, 245, ADAH; Richardson diary, August 10, 1853, SHC. See also Hentz diary, January 3, 1849, in Stowe, ed., *Southern Practice*;

McKinney diary, August 9, 1865, McKinney papers, LSU; and Faulkner, "Cases from My Note Book."

43. Leland diary, February 24, 1853, SCL.

44. Traill Green to J. S. Copes, April 25, 1833, Copes papers, HTML; Jobe, "Autobiography," 106, TSL. It is difficult to overstate either the widespread use of certain biblical maxims and imagery or their prevalence in all forms of medical writing. A medical journal editorial, to take one example from countless instances, celebrated the new general anesthesia with this image: "The chemist, with a rod, more potent than that which smote the rock of old, commands the unwilling elements to fraternize, and lo! we have pain-destroying chloroform!" ([Editorial on anesthesia], 130). For doctors using their favorite biblical tropes in casual conversation, see, for example, Miller, "Diagnosis," 6, Vanderbilt; Holcombe, *How I Became a Homoeopath*, 19; Rives, "Death," 11, Vanderbilt; and Risk, "Medical Education," 2–3, TSM.

CHAPTER EIGHT

1. Case narratives did not entirely disappear from medical learning, of course, but they appeared more informally by the early twentieth century, as occasions for pathological conferences carried out in medical schools and as a means of teaching clinical procedures on rounds, yielding verisimilitude and the pleasures of gossip. On the form of case narratives, see Risse and Warner, "Reconstructing Clinical Activities"; Dwyer, "Stories of Epilepsy"; Charon, "To Build a Case"; Donnelly, "Righting the Medical Record"; King and Stanford, "Patient Stories"; and Laqueur, "Bodies, Details." On stories and illness more generally, see Kleinman, *Illness Narratives*; Howard Brody, *Stories of Sickness*; and Hunter, *Doctors' Stories*.

2. Bailey, "Three Cases of Puerperal Convulsions," 144–47. By the mid-twentieth century, an "interesting" case tended to be one that presented the physician with a challenging intellectual puzzle of a diagnostic nature. Mid-nineteenth-century physicians used the term to mean something more inclusive—the entire bedside and social scene of caregiving. They clearly expected their stories to have broad, applicable value. As one rural physician observed of his case narrative, he wrote it "partly for future reference, and partly . . . [for] younger brethren"; see "W.," "Contributions of a Country Doctor." For similar commentary, see Manson, "On Malarial Pneumonia," and Ford, "Remarks." See also Warner, "Science, Healing."

3. Henry A. Ramsay, "Inflammation of the Bladder," 47.

4. Bates, "Prevailing Diseases," 313–14; Hamilton, "How Long Shall We Wait?" 33–34. See also Riddell, "Epidemic Bloody Flux." Bates's prescriptions were for a tincture of opium (laudanum), used as a sedative and an analgesic; a sinapism or mustard plaster was used to draw disease out of the body.

5. The case of fatal exhalations is in Lavender, "Anthropo-toxicologia"; the black woman turning white is in Knox casebooks, vol. 1, January 21, 1848, UK; the posthumous child is in Fessenden, "Case of Puerperal Apoplectic Convulsions"; the found bullet is in "Gun-shot Wound of Heart"; the piles remedy is in T. M. Harris, "Contribution to the Curiosities of Medical Experience."

6. Leland diary, March 1, 1852, SCL. For Hentz's praise, see, for example, his medical diary,

November 3 and 18, 1858, February 2 and 14, 1859, Hentz family papers, SHC. A physician recommending training midwives is Day, "Obstetrical Cases." Moral criticism of patients is found in Sutton, "Case of Doubtful Paternity," and Louis A. Dugas, "Clinical Lecture."

7. By the early twentieth century, when hospital practices dictated the standard for writing up a case, a "case" clearly become synonymous with "individual patient"; prior to that, a case might include several members of a household. It seems that most physicians did not ask patients for permission to publish their cases, and doctors' discretion varied greatly. For instances of physicians naming the patient outright, see Dr. M. S. Watkins's blunt discussion of his own wife, beginning, "We were married on the 15th day of May, 1828, and almost immediately thereafter, Dysmenorrhoea . . . made its appearance." For obtuseness, it is hard to surpass Dr. W. J. W. Kerr's account of treating a dropsical woman; he gives her full name, her hometown, and, after relating that he had tapped her 108 times and drawn off nearly five gallons of urine each time, he asks heartily, "Has she an equal?" as if she were his entry in a contest. See Watkins, "Case of Mrs. Watkins' Cure of Recto-vaginal," and Kerr, "Letter from Mississippi."

8. Scruggs, "Clinical Notes," 29; Macon, "Diuretic Virtues," 23; Clark, "Remarks on the Existence of Typhoid Fever," 464; P[atteson], "Patterson's Cases," 332–33; Dyer, "Twins," 47.

9. W. A. Shands to William Anderson, July 22, 1880, Anderson papers, SCL; Hort, "Enquiry," 61; Day, "Obstetrical Cases," 225. For stories of harmony between patients and the doctor, see, for example, Faulkner, "Cases from my Note Book," and Scruggs, "Clinical Notes."

10. Wooten, "Topography and Diseases," 341; Blackburn, "Case of Ruptured Uterus," 73; Lawton, "Case of Rupture of the Womb," 183.

11. Clark, "Remarks on the Existence of Typhoid Fever," 465–66. The white poor in hospital wards, seen on a regular basis by only a small minority of southern physicians, are depicted similarly in narratives. After emancipation, African American patients also appear less frequently and more anonymously.

12. Compare Fett, *Working Cures*, ch. 6, and Valencius, *Health of the Country*, ch. 8. For a discussion of sixteenth-century styles of European racial thought in the New World that both imagined and restrained racial "otherness," see Chaplin, *Subject Matter*, ch. 5.

13. See P[atteson], "Patterson's Cases." The frailty of journalism is sadly evident in the title of this article, as it is attributed to a Dr. "Patterson" (the author modestly signs himself "A.A.P."), who almost certainly was Dr. Alexander A. Patteson of Fayette County, Kentucky. I have been unable to find out much about him, except that he was an 1840 graduate of Transylvania Medical College, where he wrote his dissertation on conception, one of the murkier topics in the mid-nineteenth century.

14. P[atteson], "Patterson's Cases," 324, 335–36.

15. Ibid., 332.

16. Ibid.; all quotations from the case of Mr. K. are from pp. 329–31.

17. See Dowler, "Worms in the Urinary Bladder." Dowler (1797–1879) was born in Virginia, received his M.D. from the University of Maryland medical school in 1827, and practiced most of his career in and around New Orleans. He was the author of several books despite having what seems to have been a thriving practice.

18. Dowler, "Progress of Medicine," 220; Dowler, Review of *Types of Mankind*, 113.

19. Dowler, "Researches on Meteorology," 411; "Researches into the Natural History of

the Mosquito," 164, 187; "Experimental Researches into Animal Heat," 299; "Vital Statistics of Negroes," 174–75.

20. [Bennet Dowler], editor's note to W. L. Gammage, "Topography, Settlement, Climate," 626. See also Dowler's "Transcendental Medicine."

21. Dowler, "Worms in the Urinary Bladder," 358.

22. Ibid., 357–58.

23. Lunsford Pitts Yandell (1805–78) attended Transylvania University medical school in the early 1820s, received his M.D. from the University of Maryland in 1825, and then returned to teach and practice in Lexington. In 1837, he became one of the founding faculty of the Louisville Medical Institute and continued practicing there and in the area of Murfreesboro, Tennessee.

24. Lunsford P. Yandell, "Cases of Dysentery," 240–41, 242.

25. Ibid., 246–47.

26. Ibid., 247–50.

27. Lunsford Yandell to Sarah Wendel, June 12, 13, 1836, Yandell family papers, Filson; all citations below are from this collection. Some of the extant letters are the ones Yandell mailed to his in-laws; others appear to be drafts or copies that he saved, perhaps as part of his bedside notes on the case.

28. Lunsford Yandell to Sarah Wendel, June 13, 15, 1836; Yandell to David Wendel, June 21, 1836; Yandell to Sarah Wendel, June 15, 1836; Yandell to David Wendel, June 21, 1836; June 23, 1836.

29. Lunsford Yandell to David Wendel, June 21, 24, 1836; see also his mention of taking his wife's therapeutic advice in the letter to Wendel of June 23rd.

30. Yandell recorded Willie's words on the reverse, blank side of a printed sheet announcing the publication of the *Transylvania Journal of Medicine*; the sheet is among the letters to his in-laws in the Yandell family papers, Filson.

31. Histories of medicine in this vein, too, are many; for examples, see Blanton, *Medicine in Virginia in the Nineteenth Century*; James Thomas Flexner, *Doctors on Horseback*; and Victor Robinson, *Victory over Pain*.

32. John Young Bassett was born in Baltimore, the son of a physician. In 1831 he married Isaphoena Thompson, with whom he had eight children.

33. See Osler, "Alabama Student," *Johns Hopkins Hospital Bulletin*. Before publishing his sketch here, Osler used it as a lecture to inspire Johns Hopkins medical students, and he subsequently published it in a volume of essays, *Alabama Student*. Osler's filial attachment to Bassett was apparent some ten years later when colleague Howard Kelly asked Osler to contribute to a volume of essays on pathbreakers in medicine. Osler's choice was Bassett, the only ordinary practitioner in the collection. For later acknowledgment of Bassett, the result of Osler's attention, see Elkin, ed., *Medical Reports*. On Osler and his associates at Johns Hopkins, see Fleming, *William H. Welch and the Rise of Modern Medicine*; on Osler, see Bliss, *William Osler*.

34. William Osler to "Miss [Laura] Bassett," August 25, 1906, Bassett papers, ADAH; Osler, *Alabama Student*, 2. The two articles by Bassett that are the centerpiece of Osler's essays, "Report on the Topography" and "Climate and Diseases," both appeared in the ambitious but short-lived journal *Southern Medical Reports* in 1849 and 1850, respectively. This journal, edited by the well-known physician and educator Erasmus Darwin Fenner, aimed to

survey the health and medicine of the South as a whole but failed financially after the first two volumes.

35. Osler, *Alabama Student*, 2, 18.

36. John Y. Bassett, "Report on the Topography," 258; for the bleeding case, see 260; see also the cases on 262 and 265. Interestingly, a few surviving letters from Bassett's patients indicate that at least some of them appreciated his work. One thanks him for acting "like a gentleman and a father to us." Nonetheless, the deep sense of being unappreciated that runs through Bassett's case narratives also appears elsewhere; Bassett wrote his sister Margaret about treating a man who suddenly fell ill in Bassett's presence: "He seemed very glad of my help until I informed him I was a physician." See Mary A. Peterson to Bassett, "May the fifteenth," [no year], and Bassett to Margaret Bassett, February 28, 1836, Bassett papers, ADAH; for another grateful patient, see [?] to Bassett, March 8, 1850, Bassett papers, SHC.

37. John Y. Bassett, "Report on the Topography," 264–65, 261.

38. Erasmus Darwin Fenner to Bassett, September 18, 1849, Bassett papers, SHC; John Y. Bassett, "Report on the Topography," 270.

39. Osler, *Alabama Student*, 11.

40. Ibid., 1. For examples of Bassett's biblical allusions, see, for example, "Report on the Topography," 259, 270.

41. Osler, *Alabama Student*, 14.

42. John Y. Bassett, "Report on the Topography," 278–79. On the debate over whether childbirth pain was divine punishment, see Pernick, *Calculus of Suffering*, 48–55.

43. John Y. Bassett, "Climate and Diseases," 315.

44. John Young Bassett to Samuel Gross, November 1, 1851, Bassett papers, SHC. Gross had written Bassett hoping that the diagnosis had been wrong. In an editorial note to Bassett's 1850 topographic essay, E. D. Fenner himself recommended castor oil in publicly acknowledging Bassett's illness; see John Y. Bassett, "Climate and Diseases," 317 n.

45. John Young Bassett to George Wood, April 6, 1851, Bassett papers, SHC.

46. Ibid., June 20, 1851.

EPILOGUE

1. Warner, *Therapeutic Perspective*, 98; Rosenberg, *Care of Strangers*, 99. Kenneth Ludmerer (*Learning to Heal*, 9–10) also emphasizes how the war exposed—but did little to remedy—the shortcomings of antebellum medicine. James Cassedy agrees but stresses certain postwar developments that pointed toward the twentieth century, including the rise of hospitals, the burgeoning pharmaceutical business, and the federal government's first ventures into the organization of medical care through the Freedman's Bureau and the office of the Surgeon General. See Cassedy, *Medicine in America*, 64–66, and Leavitt, "Public Health." Paul Starr, in his influential *Transformation of American Medicine*, does not directly address the war and professional change, but in having almost nothing to say about the war he implies that the war had little or no effect. For older works that link the war to medical advances in various ways, see Duffy, *From Humors to Medical Science*, esp. ch. 10; Spalding, *History of the Medical College of Georgia*, ch. 6; and Richard H. Shryock, "Medical Perspective."

2. David Winn to Frances Winn, May 2, October 29, 1861, and June 14, 1862; see also ibid.,

November 21, 1861, Winn papers, Emory. Many physicians volunteered as an act of community loyalty. See, for example, the letters of J. A. S. Milligan to his father during the summer of 1862, Milligan family papers, SHC, and Alexander, *Reminiscences*, 80. Many other doctors, however, claimed exemptions that permitted them to stay at home tending their communities or serving the Confederacy. Dr. Levin Smith Joynes, for example, was granted an exemption because he was superintendent of a medical hospital. Some physicians obtained commissions in the army, while others, like Samuel Leland, served unofficially, coming and going in order to balance service to their home communities ("Exemption granted under Forms Nos. 1, 2 and 4," printed ms., Richmond, Virginia, March 12, 1864, Joynes family papers, VHS; Leland diary, 1861–65, SCL; Fulmer, "Civil War Diary").

3. W. W. Mobley to "My dear sister [Hannah]," July 15, 1861; Strait to "Dear Uncle and Aunt," November 30, 1862; and Strait to ? [rough draft, ca. January 1863], GSWBFP, SCL. Strait's superiors thought there was a problem with his being "so exceedingly popular" in his unit; his chief surgeon requested that Strait be reassigned "on account of [his] great leniency and familiarity with the men." See A. W. Bailey to S[amuel] P[reston] Moore, ms. dated May 30, 1863, GSWBFP, SCL. Strait's death is recounted in a telegram, dated October 21, [1863], from his uncle A. P. Wylie to S. C. Hicklin, GSWBFP, SCL.

4. Samuel Van Wyck to "Dear Wifey," October 24, 1861, Maverick and Van Wyck papers, SCL.

5. Samuel Van Wyck to "Dear Wifey," November 21 and November 1, 1861, and Van Wyck to "Bob" [D. R. Broyles], November 6, 1861, Maverick and Van Wyck papers, SCL. For a recommendation of Van Wyck as "well informed in his profession," see James L. Orr to J. A. Orr, May 13, 1861, and for his appointment to Forrest's cavalry, see Nathan B. Forrest to [Samuel Van Wyck], October 11, 1861, ibid.

6. [Mrs. Samuel Van Wyck] to Samuel Van Wyck, November 8 and 9, 1861, and Samuel Van Wyck to [wife], [October 1861], Maverick and Van Wyck papers, SCL. His last extant letter to his wife is a pencilled note, November 23, 1861: "I write in haste to say I love you love you, love you & the little ones. . . . We leave for a fight on the Ohio River in a few hours." For a sampling of other doctors who wrote in similar fashion of military medicine as a temporary occasion for learning, not a new standard, see, for example, George Peddy's letters to his wife Kate Peddy in Cuttino, ed., *Saddle Bag and Spinning Wheel*; the memoirs of Thomas Fanning Wood, in Koonce, ed., *Doctor to the Front*; and the diary of the observant apprentice physician John Samuel Apperson, in Roper, ed., *Repairing the "March of Mars."*

7. "Medical College of Georgia, Augusta," 181; Medical College of South Carolina, "Annual Circular," 1866, [6]; Medical College of Georgia, "Annual Announcement," 1874, [5]; University of Louisiana, "A Catalogue from 1834 to 1872," 1871, 9. The South Carolina and Georgia schools closed in early 1861. The University of Louisiana stayed open until 1862; Louisville closed for one year in 1863–64. Nashville remained open throughout the war, principally as a military hospital. See Duffy, *Tulane University*, 39–40; Duffy, ed., *Rudolph Matas History*, 2:530–36; and Spalding, *History of the Medical College of Georgia*, 87–89.

8. Medical College of South Carolina, "Annual Circular," 1866, [6]; Medical College of Georgia, "Annual Announcement," 1874, [5]. For a course in military surgery, see the University of Louisville, "Annual Catalogue," 1862, [3]. Students' hospital ward experience began to deepen by the mid-1870s, although the lecture format stayed virtually the same. For students seeking to take advantage of changes in hospital organization, see E. L. McGehee to Albert

Bachelor, April 10, [1873], Bachelor papers, LSU; J. H. Parker to Josiah Hawkins, May 19, 1883, Hawkins papers, LSU; and Thomas McIntosh to Emma McIntosh, November 7, 1875, McIntosh papers, Duke. See also Rosenberg, *Care of Strangers*, 181–85, and Ludmerer, *Learning to Heal*, 60–61.

9. "Editorial: Southern Medical and Surgical Journal," 165; David Wendel Yandell, "Progress of Medicine," 11, 20, 12. See also [Weatherly], "Address," 42.

10. Robert Battey to Mary Halsey, July 19, 1865, Battey papers, Emory; "Correspondence," 182. The *Nashville Journal of Medicine and Surgery* published the Ramsay correspondence as a "familiar illustration" of how "the late civil strife broke up many associations." For physicians discussing such postwar conditions, see S. Moffat Wylie to John Robinson, November 2, 1871, Robinson papers, SCL; William Berly to Joel Berly, December 17, 1866, Berly family papers, SCL; and William J. Holt to [Louis A. Dugas], February 5, 1867, Holt papers, SCL. Physicians' account books and daybooks that span the war, showing the continuity in the way they visited patients, summarized ailments, and assigned fees, are numerous; for good examples, see the account books of J. W. Brigham and an anonymous doctor in the Albemarle Sound region of North Carolina, SHC; James T. Graves and S. D. Davis, Duke; and Josiah E. Hawkins, Hawkins papers, LSU.

11. Reynolds, "Concerning Southern Medicine," 134, 133. For Dr. Semmes, see "Surgical Notes of the Late War." For another cautious view of wartime lessons, see [Weatherly], "Address," 33; and for a more hopeful if unspecific view of war "experience," see the unnamed Confederate surgeon quoted in Cunningham, *Doctors in Gray*, 269.

12. S. H. Pressly, "Articles of Agreement," ms. dated May 6, 1870, Carrigan papers, SCL. This agreement bears the signature of Pressly and the marks of several freedmen household heads. For another contract, see the "Articles of Agreement," ms., [1867], in the Berly family papers, SCL. For Bailey's practice, see Bailey account books, 2 vols., 1875 and 1878–79, and his visiting lists, 3 vols., 1869, 1875, 1877, Bailey papers, SCL.

13. Colmer diary, Ralph Bowman/Raphael Boone account, 79, Colmer papers, HTML. See also Hentz medical diary, 1858–62, and obstetrical record, 1849–91, Hentz family papers, SHC, for his adding surnames to the accounts of former slave patients. For a variety of ways in which doctors segregated black patient accounts from white, see Carter account book, vol. 3, 1868, UK; Chapman account book, 1871–81, and his "Freedman's Account Book," 1873–74, SCL; Rea student notebook, ca. 1869, Matas; and Pusey account books, esp. vol. 1, 1863–70, and vol. 2, 1870–80, UK. For a doctor who listed freed people under names of white households, see Eve account book, 41, 81, MCG.

14. William Summer to Joel Berly, February 3, 1868, and E. I. [Barre?] to Joel Berly, December 18, 1867, Berly family papers, SCL; Frank James diary, September 29, 1877, in Baird, ed., *Years of Discontent*, 13. For some of Berly's economic arrangements with his own workers, see "Articles of Agreement," ms. 1867, in Berly family papers, SCL.

15. Bat Smith, "Miasm," 524. Typical of the distant, generalizing mode among white physicians who comment on black disease are W. A. Cochran, "Topography and Diseases," and Manning Simons, "Report on the Climatology." Alabamian P. B. Minor was rare among white doctors in noting of African Americans in his locale that "their condition is truly a pitiable one, and some legislative action should be taken for their relief." See his "Diseases of the Fork of Greene [County, Ala.]," 199.

16. W. A. Cochran, "Topography and Diseases," 151; Minor, "Diseases of the Fork of

Greene [County, Alabama]," 199. See also Manning Simons, "Report on the Climatology," 13, 16–17.

17. Porcher, "Suggestions," 258, 252–54; for general recommendations, see ibid., 255–60; for specific therapies, see ibid., 280–86.

18. Ibid., 256–57, 267.

19. Chisolm, "Report on Retiring," 3–4, Waring; Ward, "Medicine in the Cotton States," 11. Lost Cause motifs appeared in health care as elsewhere; see, for example, the letterhead for "Sumter Bitters," the "great Southern Tonic," with the Confederate flag and the motto "I Still Live" on an invoice dated June 21, 1870, in the Berly family papers, SCL.

20. Chaillé, "Address on the State of Medicine"; A. B. Cox, *Footprints on the Sands of Time*, 155–56 (thanks to Martin Crawford for this reference); Darby, "Progress of Medicine and Surgery," 13; Kinloch, "Annual Address," 30. On the negative influence of wartime medicine on postwar practice, see also Baruch, "Lessons of Half a Century in Medicine," 3–4, and George Hill Winfrey genealogical notes, 1902, VHS. For other brief, dispassionate mentions of the war, see Edward McCrady, "Historical Address," 33, and "Francis Peyre Porcher, M.D.," typescript, Porcher papers, 4, SCL.

21. Ward, "Medicine in the Cotton States," 9. For doctors pondering just how much a given case illuminated, see Bemiss, "Four Cases of Albuminaria Complicating Pregnancy"; Archer, "Memoranda of Cases"; and W. B. Harvey, "Bilious Remittent Fever." See also Smyrna Medical Society, minutes for the meeting of March 6, 1877, ms. minute book, 32, TSL, and H. W. Mitchell to Thomas H. Kenan, June 7, 1870, Kenan papers, Duke.

22. Baruch, "Lessons of Half a Century in Medicine," 3–4. For other memoirs in this vein, featuring case narratives and the centrality of physicians' personal character, see Ernest Sydney Lewis, "Reminiscences"; William Bernard Harrell autobiography, Harrell family papers, UNCC; Porcher, "Personal Reminiscences," Waring; and Pusey, *Doctor of the 1870's and 80's.*

≈ Bibliography ≈

PRIMARY SOURCES

Unpublished Primary Sources

Athens, Georgia
  Medical College of Georgia
    Joseph Eve Allen Student Notebook
    Anonymous Account Book, [Augusta, Ga.] (1845–46)
    Joseph A. Eve Account Book (1866–67)
    W. B. Freeman Daybook
    Faculty Minute Books
    Charles A. Thompson Student Notebook
Atlanta, Georgia
  Robert W. Woodruff Library, Emory University
    Simon Baruch Papers
    Robert Battey Papers
    Frances Sage Bradley Papers
      Frances Sage Bradley autobiography (typescript)
    Burge-Gray Family Papers
    Lucius Holsey Featherston Papers
    Thomas F. Furman Papers
    Francis Marion Jones Papers
    Robert Watkins Lovett Jr. Papers
    David Read Evans Winn Papers
Baton Rouge, Louisiana
  Louisiana and Lower Mississippi Valley Collections, King Library, Louisiana State
      University
    Anonymous Medical Notebook (1831–49)
    A. Armstrong Notebook
    Albert A. Bachelor Papers
    Samuel C. Bonner Family Papers
    J. Dickson Bruns–T. G. Richardson Papers
    Robert Ormand Butler Papers
    Donelson Caffery Family Papers
    Samuel A. Cartwright Family Papers

Lemuel Parker Conner Family Papers
J. S. Egan Family Papers
Nathaniel Evans Family Papers
James Foster Record Books
R. Cornelius French Papers
William S. Hamilton Papers
Josiah E. Hawkins Papers
    Josiah E. Hawkins Account Books (1871–86; 1857–92)
Alexander R. Hendry Account Book
Charles James Johnson Family Papers
Joseph Jones Papers
John Ker Family Papers
James G. Kilbourne Family Papers
John W. King Papers
Andrew MacCrery Family Papers
Charles Mathews Family Papers
R. G. McGuire Diary (typescript)
Jeptha McKinney Papers
    Jeptha McKinney Account Books
Mississippi Board of Medical Censors Minute Book
Robert Newell Papers
C. F. Pearson Letter
Samuel J. Peters Jr. Diary
John A. Quitman Family Papers
Robert H. Ryland Papers
    Robert H. Ryland Account Book (vol. 1, 1849–56)
Zachariah and James G. Taliaferro Papers
Calvin Taylor Family Papers
Antonio P. Walsh Papers
David Weeks Family Collection
Bethesda, Maryland
  National Library of Medicine
    Edward Barton Papers
    William Darroch Papers
    William Elmer Student Notes
Chapel Hill, North Carolina
  Southern Historical Collection, University of North Carolina
    Anonymous Physicians' Record Books (2 vols., 1849–66; 1855–62)
    John Young Bassett Papers
    Borough House Papers
    Brashear Family Papers
    J. W. Brigham Account Books (1842–75)
    Thomas Edward Cox Account Books (2 vols., 1844–54)
    William Stump Forwood Papers
    James McKibbin Gage Papers

Ernest Haywood Collection
John Steele Henderson Papers
   Mary Henderson Diary
Hentz Family Papers
William H. Holcombe Autobiography
William H. Holcombe Diary
Bartlett Jones Papers
Jones Family Papers
Calvin Jones Papers
Mitchell King Papers
Thomas Butler King Papers
LeConte-Furman Papers
Lyle and Siler Family Papers
William Parsons McCorkle Papers
   Lucila McCorkle Diary
Milligan Family Papers
   Joseph and Joseph A. S. Milligan Account Books
Mordecai Family Papers
Thomas O'Dwyer Diary
Roach and Eggleston Family Papers
   Mahala Roach Diary
J. M. Richardson Diary
Benjamin and Benjamin West Robinson Account Books (4 vols.)
Charles Wilkins Short Papers
James Marion Sims Papers
Francis Jones Smith Account Books
James Strudwick Smith Account Books (vol. 2, 1828–33)
Mary Ruffin Smith Papers
James Ritchie Sparkman Account Books
Sparkman Family Papers
Samuel Jordan Wheeler Diaries
Charleston, South Carolina
  South Carolina Historical Society
    R. F. W. Allston Papers
      Adele P. Allston Letters
    Baker-Grimké Papers
      Alexander Garden Letters
    Cheves-Middleton Papers
      Alice Izard Family Letters
      Eweretta B. Middleton Letters
      Harriott Middleton Household Accounts
    Arthur B. Flagg Account Books
    E. Belin Flagg Daybook
    Andrew Hasell Account Book
    Andrew Hasell Daybook

Tucker Harris Genealogy
  Tucker Harris Reminiscence
Francis Peyre Porcher Commonplace Book
Joshua Barker Whitridge Papers
Yates Family Papers
Waring Historical Library, Medical University of South Carolina
  Julian J. Chisolm, "Report on Retiring from the Presidential Chair [of the Medical
      Society of South Carolina]," December 1867 (typescript)
  Samuel H. Dickson Memoranda and Notebook
  J. C. Eliason, "Notes on the Practice of Physic"
  Henry Tracy Ivy Diary
  William L. Jenkins Daybooks
  Robert Lebby, "Extracts from Various Authors, . . . and a History of Cases . . ."
  Joseph L. Lee Account Book
  Thomas Maddox Casebook
  William L. McCaa, "Observations on the Manner of Living and Diseases of the Slaves
      on the Wateree River," M.D. thesis, University of Pennsylvania, 1822
  Medical College of (the State of) South Carolina, Theses
    Dandridge A. Bibb, "Essay on the Effects of the Study and Practice of Medicine on
      the Mind and Character," 1846
    [Alfred Boyd], "Finale of Twenty Years Study and Practice of Medicine," 1856
    William W. Cozart, "The Place Where Southern Students Should Acquire Their
      Medical Knowledge," 1856
    U. T. Crumpton, "The State and Utility of the Medical Science," 1845
    Wilfred DuPont, "The Peculiarities of the Female," 1858
    G. W. B. Fairey, "The Medical Student and M.D.," 1859
    S. C. Furman, "The Impediments to the Progress of Medical Science," 1856
    Francis L. Gilmer, "The Pathology and Treatment of Cachexia Produced by Dirt
      Eating," 1847
    William J. Greene, "The Profession of Medicine," 1852
    Joel B. Gresham, "On the Subject of Cachexia Africana," 1845
    J. St. J. Guerard, "The Science of Medicine," 1845
    Thomas B. Hardin, "Physic and Physicians," 1852
    James C. Hicklin, "The Necessary Connexion between Theory and Practice in
      Medicine," 1845
    L. S. Hill, "Treatise on Women," 1857
    James M. Hunter, "The Preservation of Health," 1854
    Larkin G. Jones, "The Peculiarities of the Female, the Physiological Changes
      Produced by Conception, and the Treatment of Some of the Most Important
      Diseases Consecutive to Parturition," 1829
    J. W. Keitt, "The Duties of the Physician," 1844
    Robert Lebby, "Lycopus Virginicus or Bugle Weed," 1826
    S[amuel] W[ells] Leland, "Inflammation," 1849
    M[oses] D. McLoud, "Hints on the Medical Treatment of Negroes," 1850
    Alex McLean, " 'Medical Progress,' " 1855

Eldridge T. McSwain, "Some of the Discrepancies in the Practice of Medicine," 1859

H. W. Moore, "Plantation Hygiene," 1856

Charles R. Moseley, "Duties of a Physician," 1845

F. Perry Pope, "The Professional Management of Negro Slaves," 1837

W. H. Timmerman, "The Difficulties and Privileges of the Medical Profession," 1854

S. G. Twitty, "The Importance of a Thorough Medical Knowledge," 1846

William C. Whetstone, "Pneumonia," 1856

Alexander E. Wilson, "Fashion in Medicine," 1828

Columbus Morrison Student Notes

Jacob Rhett Motte Plantation Journal

John W. Ogilvie Daybooks

Francis Peyre Porcher Papers

Walter Peyre Porcher, "Personal Reminiscences of a Doctor's Life," n.d. (typescript)

Isabella Porcher Plantation Prescription Book

Charlotte, North Carolina

University of North Carolina, Special Collections

Clarkson Family Papers

Jane Campbell Woodruff Autobiographical Narrative

Harrell Family Papers

William Bernard Harrell Autobiography

Nathaniel Shober Siewers Letters (typescript)

Torrance-Banks Family Papers

Columbia, South Carolina

South Caroliniana Library, University of South Carolina

William Anderson Papers

Thomas Pierce Bailey Papers

C. V. Barnes Account Books (vol. 2, ca. 1860)

Berly Family Papers

William Blanding Papers

William Andrew Carrigan Papers

James K. Chapman Account Books and Medical School Notes

John Hainey Davis Account Book

George Dunlap Account Book (1829–39)

Gaston, Strait, Wylie, and Baskin Family Papers

William J. Holt Papers

Lebby Family Papers

Joseph LeConte Papers

Samuel Wells Leland Dairies

Gabriel Manigault Autobiography (typescript)

Maverick and Van Wyck Papers

Gerhard Muller Papers

John W. Ogilvie Account Books

Francis Peyre Porcher Papers

George W. Pressly Account Books
Reedy and Beacham Family Papers
John Andrew Robinson Papers
Ruff and Caldwell Papers
James Spann Papers
James Ritchie Sparkman Papers
Whetstone Family Papers
Durham, North Carolina
  William Perkins Library, Duke University
    Richard Dennis Arnold Papers
    Iveson Brookes Papers
    Campbell Family Papers
    Courtney J. Clark Papers
    Horatio R. Cook Memorandum Book
    James D. Davidson Papers
    Maria Dyer Davies Papers
      Maria Dyer Davies Diary
    S. D. Davis Account Book (1855–90)
    Thomas Davis Diary
    R. T. Dismukes Student Notebook
    John A. Forsyth Papers
    James T. Graves Account Books (1848–71)
    Nathan G. Hunt Papers
    Thomas H. Kenan Papers
    MacRae Family Papers
    Thomas M. McIntosh Papers
    Jacob Mordecai Papers
    Ogden Family Papers
    John Rutherfoord Papers
    Thomas Lee Settle Papers
    Ella Gertrude Clanton Thomas Diary
    Tillinghast Family Papers
    Thomas S. Wright Papers
Knoxville, Tennessee
  Tennessee State Library
    Paul Fitzsimons Eve Papers
    Alfred T. Hamilton Letters
    Abraham Jobe, "Autobiography or Memoirs of Dr. Abraham Jobe of Elizabethton,
      Tennessee" (typescript)
    Lawrence Family Papers
    John Berrien Lindsley Diaries and Notebook
    P. D. Sims Letters
    Smyrna Medical Society By-laws and Minutes
    Sneed Family Papers
    University of Nashville Trustees' Minute Books

Lexington, Kentucky

Medical Theses, Transylvania School of Medicine, Transylvania University

Algernon Sydney Allan, "Some of the Popular Objections to Medicine," 1846

William T. Briggs, "On Cachexia Africana," 1848

Benjamin G. Bruce, "Medical Science, Its Improvements: and the Spirit of Progress,"
1850

Francis B. Coleman, "On Cachexia Africana," 1832

Charles Wilkins Dudley, "Medicine as an Inductive Science," 1845

William Nelson Duzan, "The Rudiments and Practice of Medicine," 1847

Benjamin F. Elliott, "Medical Etiquette," 1846

Fayette Ewing, "On Theses," 1843

C[harles] W. Flanagan, "Medical Ethics," 1838

John W. Gatewood, "The Importance of a Correct Diagnosis," 1840

Charles C. Hazen, "Physical Diagnosis," 1847

Robert Edmonds Little, "The Climate and Diseases of Madison County, Kentucky,"
1842

Benjamin Robinson Mitchell, "Diagnosis," 1844

Moses E. Nesbit, "The Rise and Progress of Medicine," 1833

John Allen Parker, "Gonorrhoea," 1852

W. C. Philips, "The Qualifications, Responsibilities, and Duties of a Physician," 1847

Joel B. Price, "Physical Diagnosis," 1849

J[ames] B. Risk, "Medical Education," 1849

Daniel Ryan Sartor, "Medical Ethics," 1843

Albert H. Smith, "The Hygiene of Mississippi," 1837

James B. Sparks, "The Duties of an Obstetrician," 1857

James B. Sterrett, "The Medical Topography of Bowling Green and Its Vicinity, "
1821

James C. Stewart, "The Doctor," 1849

Willard F. Taft, "Medical Experience," 1848

Llewellyn Tarlton, "The Progress and Separation of Physick and Surgery and the
Dependence of One upon the Other," 1836

Samuel W. Taylor, "The Privileges and Responsibility of the Obstetrician," 1851

Gilbert Tennent, "The Medical Topography of Abbeville District, South Carolina,
Together with Observations on Bilious Fever as It Occurred There in the
Summer of 1828," 1829

John A. Thompson, "Medicine—Its Uses and Abuses," 1856

George R. Todd, "Young Physic," 1848

John H. Wright, "The Qualifications Requisite for a Medical Student," 1847

University of Kentucky, Special Collections

Charles Caldwell Letter

John Coleman Carter Account Books (1859–92)

Catherine and Howard Evans Papers

John Knox Casebooks (2 vols., 1847–51; 1851–55)

Lexington and Fayette County Medical Society Constitution, By-laws, and Minutes

Robert Burns Pusey Account Books (1863–89)

Louisville, Kentucky
    The Filson Club
        Samuel Brown Papers
        Anderson Doniphan Daybooks
        Galt Family Papers
            William C. Galt Medical Student Notebook
        B. S. Marshall Student Notebook
        Charles Wilkins Short Papers
        Yandell Family Papers
    University of Louisville
        George H. Cannon Casebook
        Nathan A. Hixon Casebook (typescript)
        Thomas C. McCarty Papers
            Thomas C. McCarty Diary
        David Pusey Papers
            David Pusey Diary
        Shelby County Medical Society Minutes
            "An Old-Time Country Doctor"
        Yandell Family Collection
            Lunsford P. Yandell Autobiographical Memoranda
            Lunsford P. Yandell Student Notes
Montgomery, Alabama
    Alabama Department of Archives and History
        John Young Bassett Papers
        Zilla H. Brandon Diary/Memoir
        Russell M. Cunningham, "Autobiography of Russell McWhorter Cunningham, M.D.,
            L.L.D." MS. (typescript), 1917
        Joseph Marion Heard Papers
        Thomas Fairfax Keller Papers
        Thomas Fairfax Keller Student Notebook
        Benjamin McKenzie Letter
        Samuel Mills Meek Papers
        Murdoch Murphy Diary
        Frederick Weedon Family Papers
Nashville, Tennessee
    Vanderbilt University
        Medical Theses, Vanderbilt Medical Center Library, Special Collections
            James A. Briggs, "Medical Topography and Diseases of Warren County, Ky.," 1851
            William L. Broyles, "The Life of a Physician," 1857
            Walter P. Coleman, "Physical Education," 1851
            Theophilus Crutcher, "The Medical Student," 1856
            Thomas T. Dismukes, "The Physician," 1854
            Albert G. Handley, "The Medical Man," 1853
            John Henley, "The Modes of Dying," 1855
            William D. Horton, "The Education of a Physician," 1856

John A. Long, "Eleven Years of Practice," 1855

John W. Maddin, "The Problem of Man's Proclivity to Live," 1856

William J. Miller, "Diagnosis," 1854

William A. Moody, "The Responsibility and Duty of the Physician," 1851

Richard Owen, "The Influence of Soil and Climate on Man," 1857

George W. Rives, "Death," 1857

M. A. Shackleford, "Gossipium," 1857

Thomas B. Springs, "Epidemic Dysentery as It Occurred in Warren County, Ten., during the Summer and Fall of 1851," 1851

Theo[dore] Westmoreland, "The Anatomical and Physiological Difference in the Ethiopian and White Man," 1855

Pinckney A. Williams, "Physical Diagnosis," 1854

Madison G. Woolridge, "The Medical Student," 1857

New Orleans, Louisiana

Tulane University

Howard-Tilton Memorial Library, Special Collections

Chaillé-Jamison Family Papers

George Colmer Papers

George Colmer Diary

Joseph Slemmons Copes Papers

Charles Colcock Jones Papers

Joseph Jones Collection

John Leonard Riddell Papers

Rudolph Matas Medical Library

Anonymous student notebook

Daniel Drake Diary and Commonplace Book (typescript)

Pendleton G. Huronymous Student Notebook

Charles E. Kennon Student Notebook

Samuel Logan, "Irregular Notes on the Principles and Practice of Medicine"

Benjamin Musser Student Notebook

R. W. Rea Student Notebook

Registre du Comité Medical de la N[ouv]elle Orleans

Baxter L. Thompson Student Notes

John Bernard Vandergriff, "Southern Practice of Medicine, Surgery, Obstetrics, Therapeutics, Toxicology, and Useful Notes on Various Methods of Treatment . . . ," n.d. [probably 1870s]

Thomas H. Wade Diary

Oxford, Mississippi

University of Mississippi, Special Collections

Stephen Duncan Ledgers

Hillary Moseley Diary and Memoirs (typescript)

Philadelphia, Pennsylvania

College of Physicians

William Gates Henderson Student Notes

Samuel H. Stout Student Notes

Richmond, Virginia
   Virginia Historical Society
      Elizabeth (Lumpkin) Motley Bagby Commonplace Book
      Philip Southall Blanton, "The Modus Operandi of Therapeutic Agents," M.D. thesis,
           Medical Department, Randolph-Macon College, n.d. [probably 1848]
      James Reed Branch Letter
      Joseph Decatur Campbell Papers
        Joseph Decatur Campbell Account Book and Diary (1836–84)
      Clark Family Papers
      Fayette Baker Spragins Letter
      Joseph Dupuy Commonplace Book
      Hundley Family Papers
      Joynes Family Papers
      John Peter Mettauer Papers
      Peyton Family Papers
      Philip Turner Southall Account Book (1817–46)
      George Hill Winfrey Genealogical Notes and Memoir
Rock Hill, South Carolina
   Dacus Library, Archives and Special Collections, Winthrop University
      Thomas and Mary Boulware Diary
      Emily Liles Harris Journals
      Knox-Wise Family Papers
      John Knox Medical Diaries and Account Book
Tallahassee, Florida
   Florida State Library
      [Thaddeus Hentz], "Diary of Dr. Hentz: Marianna and Quincy, Fla., May 3–31, 1863"
        (typescript)

Published Primary Sources

Affleck, Thomas. "On the Hygiene of Cotton Plantations and the Management of Negro
    Slaves." *Southern Medical Reports* 2 (1850): 429–36.
Alcott, William A. *The House I Live In; or, The Human Body, For the Use of Families and Schools*.
    2nd ed. Boston: Light and Stearns, 1837.
Alexander, John Brevard. *Reminiscences of the Past Sixty Years*. Charlotte, [N.C.]: Ray Printing
    Co., 1908.
American Gentleman's Medical Pocket-Book and Health Adviser. . . . Philadelphia: James Kay, Jun.
    and Brother, [ca. 1833].
"American Medical Association." *Virginia Medical Journal* 10 (May 1858): 425.
Anderson, John Q., ed. *Louisiana Swamp Doctor: the Writings of Henry Clay Lewis alias "Madison
    Tensas, M.D."* 1850. Baton Rouge: Louisiana State University Press, 1962.
Anderson, L. B. "Treatment of Cancer." *Virginia Medical Journal* 7 (July 1856): 48–51.
Anderson, William. "On the Uses of Cold Water in Scarlatina Maligna." *New Orleans Medical
    and Surgical Journal* 6 (September 1849): 193–97.

"Annual Announcement of the Jefferson Medical College." *New Orleans Medical and Surgical Journal* 5 (November 1848): 342–47.

Archer, Cauthorn. "Memoranda of Cases in Country Practice." *Virginia Medical Journal* 12 (January 1859): 1–11.

Arnold, W. E. "Random Thoughts on Conservative Medicine, Medical Reform, Young Physic, etc." *Nashville Journal of Medicine and Surgery* 17 (December 1859): 486–91.

Bailey, R[obert] S. "Essay on Medical Faith." In *Transactions of the South Carolina Medical Association*, 17–21. Charleston, S.C.: Walker and Evans, 1856.

Bailey, Robert S. "Three Cases of Puerperal Convulsions." In *Proceedings of the South Carolina Medical Association*, 144–50. Charleston, S.C.: Steam Power Press of Walker and James, 1852.

Baird, W. David, ed. *Years of Discontent: Doctor Frank L. James in Arkansas, 1877–1878.* Memphis, Tenn.: Memphis State University Press, 1977.

Bartlett, Elisha. *An Essay on the Philosophy of Medical Science.* Philadelphia: Lea and Blanchard, 1844.

Baruch, Simon. "Lessons of Half a Century in Medicine." Richmond, [Va.]: Old Dominion Publishing Corporation, 1910.

Bassett, John Y. "On the Climate and Diseases of Huntsville, Ala., and its Vicinity, for the Year 1850." *Southern Medical Reports* 2 (1850): 315–23.

——. "Report on the Topography, Climate, and Diseases of Madison County, Ala." *Southern Medical Reports* 1 (1849): 256–81.

Bates, F. A. "On the Prevailing Diseases of a Portion of Dallas County, [Alabama]. . . ." *Southern Medical Reports* 1 (1849): 303–15.

Becton, Frederick E. "An Essay on the Topography and Diseases of Rutherford County, Tennessee." *Transylvania Journal of Medicine and the Associate Sciences* 5 (April–June 1832): 157–80.

[Bell, John]. "Dr. Cartwright's Address—State-Rights Medicine." *Bulletin of Medical Science*, 3rd ser., 4 (1846): 207–13.

Bell, John, Charles Bell, and John D. Godman. *The Anatomy and Physiology of the Human Body.* 2 vols. Sixth American ed. New York: Collins and Co., 1827.

Bemiss, S[amuel] M. "Four Cases of Albuminaria Complicating Pregnancy." *New Orleans Medical and Surgical Journal*, n.s., 1 (September 1873): 207–19.

Bigelow, Jacob. "On Self-Limited Diseases." *Medical Communications of the Massachusetts Medical Society*, 2nd ser., 1(1836): 319–58.

Billingslea, James C. "An Appeal on Behalf of Southern Medical Colleges and Southern Medical Literature." *New Orleans Medical and Surgical Journal* 13 (September 1856): 214–17.

Blackburn, J. C. C. "A Case of Ruptured Uterus." *Southern Medical and Surgical Journal*, n.s., 5 (February 1849): 72–73.

Blackwell, Elizabeth, *Pioneer Work in Opening the Medical Profession to Women.* 1895. New York: Schocken Books, 1977.

Boardman, H. A. *The Claims of Religion upon Medical Men.* Philadelphia: Book and Job Printing Office, Ledger Building, 1844.

[Bowling, W. K.] "Female Doctors." *Nashville Journal of Medicine and Surgery* 2 (1852): 123–24.

Bowling, W. K. "Historical Address to the Graduating Class of 1868, in the Medical

Department of the University of Nashville." *Nashville Journal of Medicine and Surgery*, n.s., 3 (March 1868): 393–414.

Boykin, E. M. "Observations on the Medical Topography of the Middle or Sand-hill Region of South Carolina." *Charleston Medical Journal and Review* 6 (1851): 498–505.

Breckenridge, R. J. "Address [to the Medical Society of the University of Nashville]." *Nashville Journal of Medicine and Surgery* 2 (1852): 7–30.

Brickell, D. Warren. "Epidemic Typhoid Pneumonia amongst Negroes." *Monthly Stethoscope and Medical Reporter* 1 (April 1856): 244–60.

Briggs, William T. "A Case of Traumatic Tetanus—Treated by Inhalation of Chloroform—Result Unsuccessful." *Nashville Journal of Medicine and Surgery* 1 (February 1851): 30–38.

Brown, William A. "A Curious Case of Malingering." *Medical Journal of North Carolina* 3 (May 1860): 375–78.

Buchanan, A. H. "Remarks on Negro Consumption." *Western Medical and Surgical Journal*, 2nd ser., 2 (December 1840): 405–18.

Burr, Virginia Ingraham, ed. *The Secret Eye: The Journal of Ella Gertrude Clanton Thomas, 1848–1889*. Chapel Hill: University of North Carolina Press, 1990.

Burt, W. J. "Report on the Anatomical and Physiological Differences between the White and Negro Races; the Modification of their Respective Diseases and the Difference in the Treatment Resulting Therefrom." *Transactions of the Texas Medical Association* 8 (1876): 115–23.

Caldwell, Charles. *Autobiography of Charles Caldwell, M.D., with a Preface, Notes, and Appendix by Harriot W. Warner*. Philadelphia: Lippincott, Grambo, 1855.

——. "An Introductory Address, Intended as a Defence of the Medical Profession against the Charge of Irreligion and Infidelity, with Thoughts on the Truth and Importance of Natural Religion." Lexington, Ky.: At the Office of the Kentucky Whig, 1826.

——. "A Valedictory Address on Some of the Duties and Qualifications of a Physician, Delivered to the Graduates of the Medical Department of Transylvania University, on the 17th Day of March, 1830." *Transylvania Journal of Medicine and the Associate Sciences* 3 (August 1830): 309–30.

Calhoun, D. P. "Trismus Nascentium." *New Orleans Medical and Surgical Journal* 7 (1850): 124–26.

Camden, T. P. " 'Missed Labor.' " *New Orleans Journal of Medicine* 21 (January 1868): 150–54.

Campbell, George W. "On the Utility of Blood-letting in the Advanced Stages of Fever." *Transylvania Journal of Medicine and the Associate Sciences* 2 (August 1829): 332–43.

Carpenter, W. M. "Observations on Cachexia Africana, or the Habit and Effects of Dirt-eating in the Negro Race." *New Orleans Medical and Surgical Journal* 1 (October 1844): 146–68.

Cartwright, Samuel A. "Alcohol and the Ethiopian." *New Orleans Medical and Surgical Journal* 10 (September 1853): 150–65.

——. "Apoplexy of the South—its Pathology and Treatments." *Southern Medical and Surgical Journal*, n.s., 6 (March 1850): 158–67.

——. "Canaan Identified with the Ethiopian." *Southern Quarterly Review* 2 (October 1842): 321–83.

——. "The Diseases and Physical Peculiarities of the Negro Race." *Southern Medical Reports* 2 (1850): 421–29.

——. "The Diseases and Physical Peculiarities of the Negro Race." *Charleston Medical Journal and Review* 6 (1851): 643–52.

——. "Diseases and Physical Peculiarities of the Negro Race," *New Orleans Medical and Surgical Journal* 7 (May 1851): 691–715.

——. "The Diseases and Physical Peculiarities of the Negro Race." *New Orleans Medical and Surgical Journal* 8 (September 1851): 187–94.

——. "Hygienics of Temperance." *Boston Medical and Surgical Journal* 48 (1853): 373–77.

——. "Philosophy of the Negro Constitution." *New Orleans Medical and Surgical Journal* 9 (September 1852): 195–208.

——. "Remarks on Dysentery among Negroes." *New Orleans Medical and Surgical Journal* 11 (September 1854): 145–63.

——. "Report on the Diseases and Physical Peculiarities of the Negro Race." *New Orleans Medical and Surgical Journal* 7 (May 1851): 691–715.

——. "Report on the Diseases and Physical Peculiarities of the Negro Race." *New Orleans Medical and Surgical Journal* 8 (November 1851): 369–73.

——. "Report on the Diseases and Physical Peculiarities of the Negro Race." *DeBow's Review* 11 (1851): 64–69, 209–13, 331–36, 504–8.

——. "Report on the Locality of Plants." *New Orleans Medical and Surgical Journal* 10 (July 1853): 1–12.

——. "Synopsis of Medical Etiquette, Presented to the Natchez Medical Society." *New Orleans Medical and Surgical Journal* 1 (July 1844): 102–4.

"Cartwright on the Diseases and Physical Peculiarities of the Negro Race." *Charleston Medical Journal and Review* 7 (January 1852): 89–98.

Cauthorn, Richard S. "A New Anti-Periodic and a Substitute for Quinia." *Monthly Telescope* 2 (January 1857): 7–14.

Chaillé, Stanford E. "Address on the State Medicine and Medical Organization. . . ." New Orleans: Democrat Publishing Co., 1879.

——. "Anniversary Oration of the Physico-Medical Society." In Stanford E. Chaillé, *Collected Reprints*, vol. 1, [1855], 1–16.

——. *Collected Reprints, 1855–1908.* New Orleans: Tulane University of Louisiana Medical School. 2 vols. [1948–58].

——. "Historical Sketch of the Medical Department of the University of Louisiana: Its Professors and Alumni, from 1835 to 1862." New Orleans: Bulletin Book and Job Office, 1861.

——. "The Medical Colleges, the Medical Profession, and the Public." *New Orleans Medical and Surgical Journal*, n.s., 1 (May 1874): 818–41.

"Charleston Preparatory Medical School." *New Orleans Medical and Surgical Journal* 8 (March 1852): 684.

Chester, Charles. "Four Cases of Cerebro-Spinal Meningitis." *New Orleans Medical and Surgical Journal* 4 (November 1847): 314–17.

Churchill, Fleetwood. *On the Theory and Practice of Midwifery. . . .* Philadelphia: Blanchard and Lea, 1858.

Clark, C[ourtney] J. "Remarks on the Existence of Typhoid Fever in Alabama (Communicated to Dr. J. C. Harris, of Wetumpka)." *New Orleans Medical and Surgical Journal* 6 (January 1850): 461–71.

"Clinical Instruction." *Transylvania Medical Journal* 1 (April 1850): 457–62.

"Clinical Teaching in Virginia." *Virginia Medical Journal* 9 (September 1857): 248–54.

Cochran, Jerome. "Address of Dr. Jerome Cochran." In *Transactions of the Medical Association of the State of Alabama*, 57–66. Mobile: Printed at the Daily Register Office, 1871.

Cochran, W. A. "Topography and Diseases of Orrville [Alabama] and Vicinity." In *Transactions of the Medical Association of the State of Alabama*, 151–61. Mobile: Printed at the Daily Register Office, 1871.

Cooke, John Esten. "Essay on Autumnal Diseases." *Transylvania Journal of Medicine and the Associate Sciences* 1 (August 1828): 339–406.

Cooper, Thomas. *Lectures on the Elements of Political Economy*. Columbia, S.C.: D. E. Sweeny, 1826.

——. "A View of the Metaphysical and Physiological Arguments in Favour of Materialism, by a Physician." Philadelphia: [n.p.], 1824.

"Correspondence." *Nashville Journal of Medicine and Surgery*, n.s., 3 (October 1867): 182.

Cowling, Richard O. *The Relations of Medicine to Modern UnBelief. . . .* Louisville, Ky.: John P. Morton and Co., 1876.

Cox, A. B. *Footprints on the Sands of Time: A History of South-western Virginia and North-western North Carolina*. Sparta, N.C.: Star Publishing Co., 1900.

Cuttino, George Peddy. *Saddle Bag and Spinning Wheel: Being the Civil War Letters of George W. Peddy, M.D., Surgeon, 56th Georgia Volunteer Regiment, C.S.A., and His Wife, Kate Featherston Peddy*. Macon, Ga.: Mercer University Press, 1981.

"D." Review of *Indigenous Races of the Earth; or, A Few Chapters of Ethnological Inquiry*, by J. C. Nott and George R. Gliddon. *Southern Medical and Surgical Journal*, n.s., 15 (January 1858): 18–25.

Darby, John Thomson. "The Progress of Medicine and Surgery. An Address Before the South Carolina Medical Association. . . ." Columbia, S.C.: Printed at the Presbyterian Publishing House, 1873.

Davis, John. "Thoughts on the Medical Convention." *Southern Medical and Surgical Journal*, n.s., 4 (January 1848): 17–27.

Day, Richard H. "Obstetrical Cases." *New Orleans Medical and Surgical Journal* 4 (September 1847): 223–27.

DeGraffenreid, W. G. "On Brotherly Love in the Medical Profession." *New Orleans Medical and Surgical Journal* 12 (May 1856): 743–47.

Delony, Edward. "A Letter to the Editors." *Southern Medical and Surgical Journal* 1 (October 1836): 257–61.

Denman, Thomas. *Introduction to the Practice of Midwifery*. Brattleborough, Vt.: Published by William Fessenden, 1807.

Dewees, William P. *A Compendious System of Midwifery: Chiefly Designed to Facilitate the Inquiries of Those Who May Be Pursuing this Branch of Study*. Philadelphia: Lea and Blanchard, 1843.

Dickson, Samuel H. "Essay on Mania a Potu. . . ." Charleston, S.C.: A. E. Miller, 1836.

——. *Essays on Life, Sleep, Pain, etc.* Philadelphia: Blanchard and Lea, 1852.

——. "A Few Thoughts on Some Vexed Questions in Medical Ethics." *Charleston Medical Journal and Review* 13 (1858): 35–41.

——. "Introductory Lecture Delivered at the Commencement of the Second Session of the Medical College of South-Carolina." Charleston, S.C.: W. Riley, 1826.

——. "Introductory Lecture Read at the Commencement of the Course." Charleston, S.C.: Walker and Burke, 1846.

——. "Medical Ethics and the American Medical Gazette." *Charleston Medical Journal and Review* 13 (1858): 273–76.

——. "Statements in Reply to Certain Publications: From the Medical Society of South Carolina." Charleston, S.C.: Printed by J. S. Burges, 1834.

Dowler, Bennet. "Experimental Researches into Animal Heat, in the Living and in the Dead Body." *New Orleans Medical and Surgical Journal* 12 (November 1855): 289–308.

——. "Historical Retrospection of the Fundamental Principles and Polity of the American Medical Association." *New Orleans Medical and Surgical Journal* 11 (January 1855): 479–93.

——. "Progress of Medicine." *New Orleans Medical and Surgical Journal* 12 (September 1855): 220–21.

——. "Researches into the Natural History of the Mosquito." *New Orleans Medical and Surgical Journal* 12 (July 1855): 63–77; 12 (September 1855): 176–96.

——. "Researches on Meteorology." *New Orleans Medical and Surgical Journal* 4 (January 1848): 411–34.

——. Review of *Types of Mankind, or Ethnological Researches. . . .*, by Louis Agassiz. *New Orleans Medical and Surgical Journal* 11 (July 1854): 108–13.

——. "Transcendental Medicine." *New Orleans Medical and Surgical Journal* 13 (November 1856): 312–25.

——. "The Vital Statistics of Negroes in the United States." *New Orleans Medical and Surgical Journal* 13 (September 1856): 164–75.

——. "Worms in the Urinary Bladder." *New Orleans Medical and Surgical Journal* 11 (November 1854): 357–58.

Drake, Charles D., ed. *Pioneer Life in Kentucky. A Series of Reminiscential Letters from Daniel Drake, M.D., of Cincinnati, to His Children.* Cincinnati: Robert Clarke and Co., 1870.

[Drake, Daniel]. [Editorial]. *Western Journal of Medicine and Physical Science* 8 (1834–35): 323.

Drake, Daniel. "An Inaugural Discourse on Medical Education." Cincinnati: Printed by Looker, Palmer, and Reynolds, 1820.

——. "An Introductory Lecture, on the Means of Promoting the Intellectual Improvement of Students and Physicians, of the Valley of the Mississippi. . . ." Louisville, Ky.: Prentice and Weissinger, 1844.

——. "Strictures on Some of the Defects and Infirmities of Intellectual and Moral Character in Students of Medicine. . . ." Louisville, Ky.: Prentice and Weissinger, 1847.

——. *A Systematic Treatise, Historical, Etiological, and Practical, on the Principal Diseases of the Interior Valley of North America, as they Appear in the Caucasian, African, Indian, and Esquimaux Varieties of Its Population.* Cincinnati: Winthrop B. Smith and Co., 1850.

——. "To the Physicians and Meteorological Observers of the Valley of the Mississippi and the Lakes." *Western Journal of Medicine and Surgery*, n.s., 4 (December 1845): 541–42.

Dugas, L[ouis] A. "A Clinical Lecture Upon Some of the Effects of Intemperance; Delivered at the Augusta City Hospital. . . ." *Southern Medical and Surgical Journal* 15 (January 1858): 1–11.

——. "Purulent Ophthalmia of Infants." *Southern Medical and Surgical Journal* 1 (July 1836): 81–83.

Dungan, James B. "Report on the Topography, Climate, and Diseases of the Parish of St. Mary, La." *Southern Medical Reports* 1 (1849): 190–95.

Dunglison, Robley. *Dictionary of Medical Science*. 6th ed. Philadelphia: Lea and Blanchard, 1846.

———. *The Medical Student; or, Aids to the Study of Medicine. A Revised and Modified Edition*. Philadelphia: Lea and Blanchard, 1844.

Dyer, J. S. "Twins, with Enormous Quantity of Liquor Amnii." *Nashville Journal of Medicine and Surgery* 2 (1852): 46–47.

Eberle, John. *A Treatise of the Materia Medica and Therapeutics*. 2 vols. 4th ed. Philadelphia: Grigg and Elliot, 1834.

———. *A Treatise on the Practice of Medicine*. 2 vols. Philadelphia: John Grigg; William Brown, printer, 1830.

———. *A Treatise on the Practice of Medicine*. 2 vols. Philadelphia: John Grigg; Lydia R. Bailey, printer, 1831.

[Editorial on anesthesia]. *New Orleans Medical and Surgical Journal* 5 (July 1848): 130.

"Editorial" [on the "negro race"]. *Monthly Stethoscope and Medical Reporter* 1 (February 1856): 128–30.

"Editorial" [on race]. *Monthly Stethoscope and Medical Reporter* 1 (March 1856): 161–64.

"Editorial: Southern Medical and Surgical Journal." *Southern Medical and Surgical Journal* 21 (July 1866): 164–65.

"Editor's Table. The Sacredness of the Human Body." *Harper's New Monthly Magazine* 8 (April 1854): 690–93.

Elliott, Stephen. "An Address Delivered at the Opening of the Medical College in Charleston. . . ." Charleston, S.C.: Printed by A. E. Miller, 1826.

Ellzey, M. G. "Life-Work of the Modern Physician as a Member of Modern Society." *Transactions of the Medical Society of Virginia* 2 (1879): 344–50.

Eve, Joseph A. "Essay on Expectation. . . ." *Southern Medical and Surgical Journal* 2 (January 1838): 323–31.

———. "Medical Education." *Southern Medical and Surgical Journal* 1 (September 1836): 216–23.

Farrar, S. C. "General Report on the Topography, Meteorology, and Diseases of Jackson, the Capital of Mississippi." *Southern Medical Reports* 1 (1849): 345–59.

Faulkner, L. "Case of Homicide, by Severing the Atlas from the Head." *Virginia Medical Journal* 7 (December 1856): 485–90.

———. "Cases from My Note Book and Memory." *Virginia Medical Journal* 6 (June 1856): 461–65.

Fenner, E[rasmus] D. "Acclimation; and the Liability of Negroes to the Endemic Fevers of the South." *Southern Medical and Surgical Journal*, n.s., 15 (July 1858): 452–60.

———. "Brief Notes on a Medical Tour of the United States." *New Orleans Medical and Surgical Journal* 3 (September 1846): 195–212.

———. "On the Use of Quinine in Continued Fever." *New Orleans Medical and Surgical Journal* 9 (November 1852): 318–40.

[Fenner, Erasmus D.]. "Report on the New-Orleans Charity Hospital." *Southern Medical Reports* 2 (1850): 280–90.

———. "State Medical Society of Louisiana." *Southern Medical Reports* 2 (1850): 294–98.

Fessenden, Benjamin F. "A Case of Puerperal Apoplectic Convulsions, with Spontaneous

Expulsion of the Foetus after Death." *Medical Journal of North Carolina* 1 (August 1858): 16–17.

Fields, Annie, ed. *Life and Letters of Harriet Beecher Stowe*. Boston: Houghton, Mifflin and Co., 1897.

"First Annual Session of the American Medical Association." *Southern Medical and Surgical Journal*, n.s., 4 (June 1848): 376–83.

Flint, Austin. "Address at the Opening of the Session for 1854–55 in the Medical Department of the University of Louisville." *Western Journal of Medicine and Surgery*, 4th ser., 2 (December 1854): 410–28.

Folger, Alfred M. *The Family Physician, Being a Domestic Work, Written in Plain Style.* . . . Spartanburg C.H., S.C.: Z. D. Cottrell, 1845.

Forbes, S. S. "Diseases of Conecuh County [Alabama]." In *Transactions of the Medical Association of the State of Alabama*, 135–37. Mobile: Printed at the Daily Register Office, 1871.

Ford, Lewis D. "Remarks on the Pathology and Treatment of Intermittent and Remittent Fevers, with Cases." *Southern Medical and Surgical Journal* 1 (November 1836): 335–60.

"Franklin." "On the Preservation of Health of Negroes." *Southern Agriculturalist* 12 (September 1839): 492–93.

Freese, J. R. "Healing Art vs. the Knife." *New Orleans Medical and Surgical Journal* 13 (July 1856): 12–14.

Gage, R. J. "Plantation Hygiene." *Farmer and Planter* 8 (February 1857): 25–31.

Gaillard, E. S. "Medical Topography of Florida." *Charleston Medical Journal and Review* 10 (July 1855): 457–63; 10 (September 1855): 649–68; 10 (November 1855): 797–813; 11 (January 1856 [first page misdated 1855]): 23–47; 11 (March 1856): 198–213; 11 (July 1856): 568–80.

Gammage, W. L. "Topography, Settlement, Climate, Population, Botany, and Diseases of Cherokee County, Texas." *New Orleans Medical and Surgical Journal* 12 (January 1856): 626–45.

Geddings, Eli. "Report of the Committee of the Medical Association of South Carolina on the Medical Topography of the State of South Carolina." Charleston, S.C.: Walker, Richards and Co., 1852.

Gibbs, R. T. "On the Medical Topography and Diseases of the Parish of DeSoto, La., . . ." *Southern Medical Reports* 2 (1850): 185–204.

Goodlett, A. G. *The Family Physician; or, Everyman's Companion, Being a Compilation from the Most Approved Medical Authors, Adapted to the Southern and Western Climates.* . . . Nashville, Tenn.: Printed at Smith and Nesbit's Steam Press, 1838.

Grant, Geo[rge] R. "A Case in Which the Placenta was Retained Thirteen Days after Delivery at Full Term." *Southern Medical and Surgical Journal* 1 (September 1836): 193–97.

Grier, S. L. "The Negro and His Diseases." *New Orleans Medical and Surgical Journal* 9 (January 1853): 752–63.

Gross, Samuel D. *Elements of Pathological Anatomy*. 2 vols. Boston: Marsh, Capen, Lyon, and Webb, and James B. Dow, 1839.

——. *A System of Surgery: Pathological, Diagnostic, Therapeutic, and Operative*. Philadelphia: Blanchard and Lea, 1859.

"Gun-shot Wound of Heart." *Southern Medical and Surgical Journal* 21 (March 1867): 520–21.

Hamilton, J. M. "How Long Shall We Wait?" *Nashville Journal of Medicine and Surgery* 10 (January 1856): 33–34.

Harden, John M. B. "Observations on the Soil, Climate, and Diseases of Liberty County, Georgia." *Southern Medical and Surgical Journal*, n.s., 1 (October 1845): 481–569.

Harris, T. M. "A Contribution to the Curiosities of Medical Experience." *Western Journal of Medicine and Surgery*, 3rd ser., 2 (October 1848): 281–83.

Harvey, W. B. "Bilious Remittent Fever." *New Orleans Journal of Medicine* 21 (January 1868): 44–46.

"The Health of Augusta." *Southern Medical and Surgical Journal*, n.s., 15 (September 1858): 718–19.

Heard, T. S. "On the Topography, Climate, and Diseases of Washington, Texas." *New Orleans Medical and Surgical Journal* 13 (July 1856): 1–7.

"Herod Out-Heroded." *Nashville Journal of Medicine and Surgery* 5 (October 1857): 249–53.

Holcombe, William H. *How I Became a Homoeopath*. 1866. Philadelphia: Boericke and Tafel, 1892.

Holmes, Oliver Wendell. *Currents and Counter-Currents in Medical Science*. Boston: Ticknor and Fields, 1861.

Holmes, William Fletcher. "Two Cases of Pneumonia, Illustrating the Comparative Efficacy of Mercury and Tartar Emetic, in the Treatment of that Disease." *Charleston Medical Journal and Review* 4 (March 1849): 176–79.

Hope, Matthew Boyd. "A Discourse Designed to Show that Physiological Inquiries Are Not Unfriendly to Religious Sentiment. . . ." Philadelphia: Barrett and Jones, printers, 1845.

Hopkins, T. S. "A Remarkable Case of Feigned Disease." *Charleston Medical Journal and Review* 8 (March 1853): 173–76.

Hort, William P. "An Enquiry Whether There Is in the Southern States, a Specific Disease That Can Properly Be Called Congestive Fever; with Cases and Remarks." *New Orleans Medical and Surgical Journal* 4 (July 1847): 56–68.

———. "Medical Education &c." *New Orleans Medical and Surgical Journal* 8 (November 1851): 314–27.

Jarrot, Richard. "Amputation for Gangrene of the Foot, Successfully Performed on a Negro, at the Advanced Age of One Hundred and Two Years." *Charleston Medical Journal and Review* 4 (May 1849): 301–5.

Jennings, Samuel K. *A Compendium of Medical Science, or Fifty Years' Experience in the Art of Healing*. Tuscaloosa, Ala.: M. J. Slade, 1847.

Johnson, Joseph. "Advice to Persons Spending the Summer and Fall in the Low Countries." *Southern Agriculturalist* 3 (September 1830): 476–78.

———. "Some Account of the Origin and Prevention of Yellow Fever in Charleston, S.C." *Charleston Medical Journal and Review* 4 (March 1849): 154–69.

Johnson, N. B. "Passage of a Half-Dollar Through the Alimentary Canal." *Southern Medical and Surgical Journal*, n.s., 4 (June 1848): 342–43.

Jones, Joseph. "Suggestions on Medical Education: Introductory Lecture to the Course of 1859–60, in the Medical College of Georgia. . . ." Augusta, Ga.: Printed at the Constitutionalist Book and Job Office, 1860.

Jordan, C. H. "Thoughts on Cachexia Africana or Negro Consumption." *Transylvania Journal of Medicine and the Associate Sciences* 5 (January–March 1832): 18–30.

Kerr, W. J. W. "Letter from Mississippi," *Nashville Journal of Medicine and Surgery*, n.s., 5 (August 1869): 70.

Ketchum, George A. "Notes on the Topography, Sanitary Condition, and Vital Statistics of Mobile, Ala." *Southern Medical Reports* 2 (1850): 301–7.

Kilpatrick, Andrew R. "Report on the Medical Topography, Meteorology, and Diseases of Trinity, La., and its Vicinity, during the Year 1850." *Southern Medical Reports* 2 (1850): 157–85.

King, R[oswell], Jr. "On the Management of the Butler Estate, and the Cultivation of the Sugar Cane." *Southern Agriculturalist* 1 (December 1828): 523–29.

King, William R. "Diseases of Franklin County [N.C.]." *Medical Journal of North Carolina* 1 (August 1858): 1–11.

Kinloch, R. A. "Annual Address: a Plea for Education as the Means for Unifying the Profession and Strengthening the Association." In *Transactions of the South Carolina Medical Association*, 23–48. Charleston, S.C.: Edward Perry, 1884.

Koonce, Donald B., ed. *Doctor to the Front: the Recollections of Confederate Surgeon Thomas Fanning Wood, 1861–1865*. Knoxville: University of Tennessee Press, 2000.

Lavender, C. E. "Anthropo-toxicologia. Cases; with Remarks." *New Orleans Medical and Surgical Journal* 5 (July 1848): 33–37.

——. "On the Topography, Climate, and Diseases of Selma, Alabama." *New Orleans Medical and Surgical Journal* 6 (November 1849): 342–48.

Lawton, James S. "Case of Rupture of the Womb," *Charleston Medical Journal and Review* 9 (March 1854): 183–84.

Lebby, Robert. "Tetanus Occurring Ten Days After a Natural Labor." *Charleston Medical Journal and Review* 3 (May 1848): 283–86.

LeConte, John. "Observations on Geophagy." *Southern Medical and Surgical Journal*, n.s., 1 (August 1845): 417–44.

——. "The Philosophy of Medicine." *Southern Medical and Surgical Journal*, n.s., 5 (May 1849): 257–77.

LeConte, Joseph. "On the Science of Medicine and the Causes Which Have Retarded Its Progress." *Southern Medical and Surgical Journal*, n.s., 6 (August 1850): 456–74.

Lewis, Ernest Sydney. "Reminiscences." *New Orleans Medical and Surgical Journal* 74 (1922): 744–77.

Lewis, John Terrill. "Remarkable Case of Hemorrhage." *Transylvania Journal of Medicine and the Associate Sciences* 3 (May 1830): 260–62.

Macon, E. H. "On the Diuretic Virtues of the Azalea, or Honeysuckle." *Southern Medical and Surgical Journal* 2 (August 1837): 20–25.

Manson, O[tis] F. "On Malarial Pneumonia." *Medical Journal of North Carolina* 3 (August 1860): 465–94.

Massie, J. C. *A Treatise on the Eclectic Southern Practice of Medicine*. Philadelphia: Thomas, Cowperthwait & Co., 1854.

Matthews, Thomas M. "A Case of Gangrene Consequent upon Miasmatic, or Epidemic Bilious Fever." *New Orleans Journal of Medicine* 21 (January 1868): 30–35.

McCrady, Edward. "An Historical Address Delivered in Charleston, S.C. . . . Before the Graduating Class of the Medical College of the State of South Carolina." N.p., 1885 [revised . . . 1896].

McCullough, Joseph A. "The Effect of Religious Conceptions upon Science and Practice of Medicine. . . ." Columbia, S.C.: State Co., 1906.

"Medical Attendance on Families by the Year." *New Orleans Medical and Surgical Journal* 8 (January 1852): 543.

Medical College of Georgia. "Annual Announcement. . . ." Augusta, Ga.: Printed by Jas. McCafferty, 1848.

——. "Annual Announcement. . . ." [Augusta, Ga.: N.p., 1852].

——. "Annual Announcement. . . ." [Augusta, Ga.: N.p., 1855].

——. "Annual Announcement. . . ." [Augusta, Ga., N.p.], 1858.

——. "Annual Announcement. . . ." Augusta, Ga.: J. Morris, Book and Job Printers, 1859.

——. "Annual Announcement. . . ." Augusta, Ga.: James L. Gow Book and Job Printer, 1874.

——. "Annual Announcement. . . ." Augusta, Ga.: Chronicle and Const. Job Print., [1881].

"Medical College of Georgia, Augusta." *Southern Medical and Surgical Journal* 21 (July 1866): 181.

Medical College of the State of South Carolina. "Annual Announcement. . . ." Charleston, S.C.: Printed at Burges and James, 1840.

——. "Catalogue. . . ." Charleston, S.C.: J. B. Nixon, Printer, 1845.

——. "Catalogue. . . ." Charleston, S.C.: J. B. Nixon, Printer, 1848.

——. "Catalogue. . . ." Charleston, S.C.: Steam Power-Press of Walker and James, 1851.

——. "Catalogue. . . ." Charleston, S.C.: Steam Power-Press of Walker and James, 1852.

——. "Catalogue. . . ." Charleston, S.C.: Steam Power Press of Walker and James, 1853.

——. "Catalogue. . . ." Charleston, S.C.: Steam Power-Press Printers Office, 1854.

——. "Annual Circular. . . ." Charleston, S.C.: James and Williams, 1858.

——. "Annual Circular. . . ." Charleston, S.C.: James and Williams, 1860.

——. "Annual Circular. . . ." Charleston, S.C.: Joseph Walker, Printer, 1866.

——. "Annual Announcement. . . ." Charleston, S.C.: Walker, Evans, and Cogswell, Printers, 1873.

"Medical Convention of the State of South Carolina." *Charleston Medical Journal and Review* 3 (March 1848): 236–43.

"Medical Department of Louisville University." *Western Journal of Medicine and Surgery*, 3rd ser., 4 (December 1849): 545.

"Medical Ethics." *Medical Journal of North Carolina* 2 (February 1859): 389–99.

"Medical Ethics in Virginia." *Virginia Medical Journal* 7 (September 1856): 250–59.

"Medical Ethics in Virginia." *Virginia Medical Journal* 9 (September 1857): 263.

"Medical Intelligence," *Southern Medical and Surgical Journal* 2 (August 1837): 63–64.

"A Medical Pirate." *The Monthly Stethoscope and Medical Reporter* 1 (March 1856): 159–60.

Medical Society of Columbia [S.C.]. "Constitution, Code of Ethics, and Fee Bill of the Medical Society of Columbia, S.C. . . ." Columbia, S.C.: Steam-Power Press of R. W. Gibbes and Co., 1854.

"Medical Theses." *Charleston Medical Journal and Review*, n.s., 3 (1876): 327–29.

Merrill, A. P. "Distinctive Peculiarities of the Negro Race." *Monthly Stethoscope and Medical Reporter* 1 (January 1856): 23–34; 1 (February 1856): 89–98.

——. "Plantation Hygiene." *Southern Agriculturalist* 1 (September 1853): 267–71.

Minor, P. B. "Diseases of the Fork of Greene [County, Alabama]." In *Transactions of the Medical Association of the State of Alabama*, 199–202. Mobile: Printed at the Daily Register Office, 1871.

"Miscellaneous Intelligence." *Western Journal of the Medical and Physical Sciences* 11 (October 1837): 181–82.

A Mississippi Planter. "Management of Negroes upon Southern Estates." *DeBow's Review* 10 (June 1851): 621–25.

Monette, John W. "An Essay on the Summer and Autumnal Remittent Fevers of Mississippi." *Western Journal of Medicine and Surgery* 1 (February 1840): 87–130.

Moore, T. V. "Religion and Medicine." *Maryland and Virginia Medical Journal* 14 (1860): 89–99.

Morton, W. S. "Causes of Mortality amongst Negroes." *Monthly Stethoscope and Medical Reporter* 1 (May 1856): 289–92.

Moultrie, James, Jr. "Introductory Address Delivered at the Opening of the Medical College of the State of South-Carolina. . . ." Charleston, S.C.: Printed by J. S. Burges, 1834.

Musgrove, W. C. "Poisoning by Phytolaccoe Radix (Poke Root)—Four Cases." *Southern Medical and Surgical Journal*, n.s., 15 (April 1858): 230–31.

"The New Orleans Charity Hospital." *Harper's Weekly* 3 (September 3, 1859): 569–70.

Nott, J[osiah] C. "Instincts of Races." *New Orleans Medical and Surgical Journal* 19 (July 1866): 1–16; 19 (September 1866): 145–56.

Nott, Josiah C., and George R. Gliddon, eds. *Indigenous Races of the Earth; or, New Chapters of Ethnological Enquiry*. Philadelphia: J. B. Lippincott and Co., 1857.

——. *Types of Mankind; or, Ethnological Researches, Based upon the Ancient Monuments, Paintings, Sculptures, and Crania of Races. . . .* Philadelphia: Lippincott, Grambo, 1854.

O'Keeffe, D. C. "Experimental Researches on the Febrifuge Properties of the Extract of Dogwood Bark; Cornine Obtained—with Cases." *Southern Medical and Surgical Journal*, n.s., 5 (January 1849): 1–28.

"On the Treatment of Cholera on Plantations. By Dr. C. B. New." *New Orleans Medical and Surgical Journal* 7 (September 1850): 211–12.

Osler, William. "An Alabama Student." In *An Alabama Student and Other Biographical Essays*, 1–18. London: Oxford University Press, 1908.

——. "An Alabama Student." *Johns Hopkins Hospital Bulletin* 7, no. 58 (January 1896): 6–11.

Parvin, Theophilus. "The Physician Is a Good Man, Skilled in Healing." *Louisville Medical News* 15 (1883): 145–52.

P[atteson], A. A. "Patterson's Cases." *Transylvania Medical Journal* 1 (February 1850): 323–36.

Payne, Alban S. "Hydrography, Topography, Geology, and Climate of Paris [Virginia] and that Piedmont Region of the Country. . . ." *Virginia Medical Journal* 9 (July 1857): 33–43.

——. "On the Epidemics of Piedmont." *Virginia Medical Journal* 12 (April 1859): 273–82.

Pendleton, E. M. "General Report on the Topography, Climate, and Diseases of Middle Georgia." *Southern Medical Reports* 1 (1849): 315–42.

———. "On the Comparative Fecundity of the Caucasian and African Races." *Charleston Medical Journal and Review* 6 (May 1851): 351–56.

"People's Medical Gazette." *Charleston Medical Journal and Review* 9 (March 1854): 125.

Peter, Robert. *The History of the Medical Department of Transylvania University.* . . . Louisville, Ky.: John P. Morgan and Co., 1905.

Phillips, James. "A Plate of Artificial Teeth, Swallowed, and Subsequently Discharged Per Anum." *New Orleans Medical and Surgical Journal* 12 (January 1856): 543–44.

Physiological Temperance Society of the Medical Institute of Louisville. "Proceedings of the Physiological Temperance Society. . . ." Louisville, Ky.: Printed by N. H. White, Market Street, near the bank, 1842.

"Physiological Temperance Society of the University of Louisville." *Western Journal of Medicine and Surgery*, 3 ser., 1 (March 1848): 273.

"A Planter." "Notions on the Management of Negroes." *Southern Agriculturalist* 9 (November 1836): 580–84.

Pollack, Simon, "My Autobiography and Reminiscences." *St. Louis Medical Review*, February 20–July 30, 1904, passim.

Porcher, Francis Peyre. *Resources of the Southern Fields and Forests, Medical, Economical, and Agricultural.* . . . Richmond, Va.: Charles Evans and Cogswell, 1863.

———. "Suggestions Made to the Medical Department. Modifications of Treatment Required in the Management of the Confederate Soldier, Dependent upon His Peculiar Moral and Physical Condition; with Reference to Certain Points in Practice." *Southern Medical and Surgical Journal* 21 (September 1866): 248–86.

Posey, John F. "Report upon the Topography and Epidemic Diseases of the State of Georgia." *Southern Medical and Surgical Journal*, n.s., 15 (February 1858): 106–14.

Powell, Thomas S. "A Colloquy on the Duties and Elements of a Physician." Atlanta, Ga.: Franklin Printing House, 1860.

———. "The True Physician." In *Transactions of the Medical Association of Georgia*, 157–70. Atlanta, Ga.: 1878.

"Practical Anatomy." *Nashville Journal of Medicine and Surgery* 2 (1852): 187–88.

Pusey, William Allen. *A Doctor of the 1870's and 80's.* Springfield, Ill., and Baltimore, Md.: Charles C. Thomas, 1932.

Quintard, Charles T. "An Address Delivered before the Graduating Class of the Medical College of Georgia." Augusta, Ga.: Printed by Jas. McCafferty, 1851.

Ramsay, Henry A. "Inflammation of the Bladder, Gangrene, Death, Autopsy." *Charleston Medical Journal and Review* 5 (January 1850): 45–47.

———. *The Necrological Appearances of Southern Typhoid Fever in the Negro.* Columbia Co., Georgia: 1852.

Ramsay, W. G. "The Physiological Differences between the European (or White Man) and the Negro." *Southern Agriculturalist* 12 (June 1839): 286–94; 12 (August 1839): 411–19.

Rawick, George P., ed. *The American Slave: A Composite Autobiography.* Westport, Conn.: Greenwood, 1978.

Reese, W. P. "Proceedings of the Medical Association of the State of Alabama." *Southern Medical Reports* 2 (1850): 324–30.

Reynolds, Mark. "Concerning Southern Medicine: Its Duties and Responsibilities." *Charleston Medical Journal and Review*, n.s., 1 (1873): 133–37.

Riddell, A. A. J. "Epidemic Bloody Flux." *New Orleans Medical and Surgical Journal* 7 (July 1850): 99.

Robinson, John Havey. *Marietta; or, The Two Students, a Tale of the Dissecting Room and Body Snatching.* Boston: Jordan and Wiley, 1846.

Robinson, Victor. *Victory over Pain, a History of Anesthesia.* . . . New York: Schuman, 1946.

Roper, John Herbert, ed. *Repairing the "March of Mars": The Civil War Diaries of John Samuel Apperson, Hospital Steward in the Stonewall Brigade, 1861–1865.* Macon, Ga.: Mercer University Press, 2001.

Rouanet, M. "Popular Errors Exposed—Mothers Killing Their Children." *New Orleans Medical and Surgical Journal* 8 (September 1851): 199–200.

Rumph, J. D. "Thoughts on Malaria, and the Causes Generally of Fever." *Charleston Medical Journal and Review* 9 (July 1854): 438–50.

Savage, G. C. "Medical Education in the South." *Bulletin of the American Academy of Medicine* 4 (1899): 358–75.

Schenck, Ralph. *The Family Physician: Treating of the Diseases Which Assail the Human System at Different Periods of Life.* . . . Fincastle, Va.: O. Callaghan and W. E. M. Word, 1842.

Schmidt, H. D. "Observations on Diphtheria." *New Orleans Journal of Medicine* 21 (April 1868): 266–81.

Scruggs, R. L. "Clinical Notes from Private Practice." *New Orleans Medical and Surgical Journal* 9 (July 1852): 26–35.

"Sectional Medicine." *Western Journal of Medicine and Surgery,* 3rd ser., 3 (January 1849): 89.

Semmes, A. J. "Surgical Notes of the Late War." *New Orleans Medical and Surgical Journal* 19 (July 1866): 65–71.

Sevier, Jno. W. "Report of Cases Treated at the 'City Dispensary,' Medical Department, University of Nashville." *Nashville Journal of Medicine and Surgery* 10 (February 1856): 130–34.

Sharpe, W. R. "Report on the Diseases of Davie County [N.C.]" *Medical Journal of North Carolina* 3 ([February] 1860): 278–86.

Short, Charles Wilkins. *Duties of Medical Students during Attendance on Lectures.* Louisville, Ky.: Morton and Griswold, 1845.

Simons, John Hume. *Planter's Guide, and Family Book of Medicine: For the Instruction and Use of Planters, Families, Country People.* . . . Charleston, S.C.: M'Carter and Allen, 1848.

Simons, Manning. "Report on the Climatology and Epidemics of South Carolina. . . ." Philadelphia: Collins, 1872.

Simons, Thomas Y. "Observations on the Fever Which Is Developed in the City of Charleston after Exposure to Country Air, during the Summer and Autumn, and Which Is Hence Called Country Fever." *Southern Medical Reports* 1 (1849): 398–407.

Sims, J. Marion. *The Story of My Life.* New York: D. Appleton and Co., 1884.

Smedes, Susan Dabney. *Memorials of a Southern Planter.* Edited by Fletcher M. Green. Jackson, Miss.: University Press of Mississippi, 1981.

Smith, Bat. "Miasm; its Probable Origin and Action." *New Orleans Medical and Surgical Journal,* n.s., 1 (January 1874): 516–36.

Smith, D. D. Huger. *A Charlestonian's Recollections, 1846–1913.* Charleston, S.C.: Carolina Art Association, 1950.

Smith, James E. "Cases Illustrating the Practice of Medicine in the Counties of Rusk and

Panola [Texas]." *New Orleans Medical and Surgical Journal* 13 (January 1857): 443–48; 14 (September 1857): 166–70.

Smith, James T. "Review of Dr. Cartwright's Report on the Diseases and Physical Peculiarities of the Negro Race." *New Orleans Medical and Surgical Journal* 8 (September 1851): 228–37.

"A Southerner." "Dieting, &c. of Negroes." *Southern Agriculturalist* 9 (October 1836): 518–20.

"Southern Medical Students." *Medical Examiner*, n.s., 6 (November 1850): 662–64.

"Statistics of the Charity Hospital." *New Orleans Journal of Medicine* 21 (January 1868): 201.

Still, James. *Early Recollections and Life of Dr. James Still*. Philadelphia: J. B. Lippincott and Co., 1877.

Stowe, Steven M., ed. *A Southern Practice: The Diary and Autobiography of Charles A. Hentz, M.D.* Charlottesville: University Press of Virginia, 2000.

Suddarth, J. B. "Physical and Medical Topography, etc., of Simpson County [Kentucky]." *Nashville Journal of Medicine and Surgery* 11 (December 1856): 473–88.

"Summer Institute." *Nashville Journal of Medicine and Surgery* 11 (October 1856): 367–68.

Sutton, W. L. "A Case of Doubtful Paternity." *Southern Medical and Surgical Journal*, n.s., 8 (December 1852): 760–63.

———. "Medical Reform." *Western Journal of Medicine and Surgery* 8 (November 1847): 403–18.

Thompson, Hugh M. "Address on the Curative Value of High Character in the Physician." *Proceedings of the Louisiana Medical Association* 3 (1880): 12–22.

Trautman, Richard L., ed. *The Heavens Are Weeping: The Diaries of George Richard Browder, 1852–1886*. Grand Rapids, Mich.: Zondervan Publishing House, 1987.

"Tribute of Respect to a Member of the Present Medical Class." *Southern Medical and Surgical Journal*, n.s., 5 (February 1849): 127–28.

Troy, M. "Report on the Diseases of Cahaba [Alabama] and Its Vicinity." *New Orleans Medical and Surgical Journal* 12 (September 1855): 237–44.

Turner, William Mason. "A Record of Two Singular Cases, in Which the Positive Diagnosis Is Still in Doubt." *New Orleans Journal of Medicine* 21 (October 1868): 679–84.

"Types of Mankind." *Western Journal of Medicine and Surgery*, 4th ser., 2 (September 1854): 186–211.

Underwood, T. G. "Case of Extraordinary Hysteria." *Nashville Journal of Medicine and Surgery* 17 (July 1859): 9–14.

University of Louisiana. "Annual Circular. . . ." New Orleans, n.p., 1838.

———. "Catalogue from 1834 to 1872 of the Professors, Other Instructors, and Alumni." New Orleans: Printed at the Bronze Pen Book and Job Office, 1871.

[University of Louisville]. "Louisville Medical Institute [Circular]." Louisville, Ky.: Prentice and Weissinger, 1838.

University of Louisville. "Circular. . . ." Louisville, Ky.: Prentice and Weissinger, 1839.

———. "Annual Catalogue. . . ." Louisville, Ky.: Prentice and Weissinger, 1842.

———. "Annual Catalogue. . . ." Louisville, Ky.: Prentice and Weissinger, 1849.

———. "Annual Catalogue. . . ." Louisville, Ky.: Hanna and Company Printers, Corner Main and Third Streets, July 1862.

———. "Announcement. . . ." Louisville, Ky.: Escott, Stackhouse and Co., Printers, 231 Main Street, July 1864.

——. "Annual Announcement. . . ." Louisville, Ky.: John P. Morton and Company, 1872.

University of Nashville. "Second Annual Announcement. . . ." Nashville, Tenn.: A Nelson and Co., Printers, Cherry Street, 1852.

——. "Annual Announcement. . . ." Nashville, Tenn.: Cameron and Fall, 1855.

——. "Catalogue of the Medical Department. . . ." Nashville, Tenn.: John T. S. Fall, Book and Job Printer, Corner of College and Union Streets, 1860.

——. "Catalogue of the Medical Department. . . ." Nashville, Tenn.: John T. S. Fall, Book and Job Printer, Corner of College and Union Streets, 1861.

——. "Catalogue for the Session 1865–6. . . ." Nashville, Tenn.: J. T. S. Fall and Sons, Printers, Corner College and Union Streets, 1866.

"Vaccination from the Negro." *Nashville Journal of Medicine and Surgery* 6 (March 1854): 182.

Van Bibber, W. Chew. "A Case of Fatal Poisoning by Alcohol." *Virginia Medical Journal* 7 (August 1856): 101–3.

"W." "Contributions of a Country Doctor." *Virginia Medical Journal* 8 (January 1857): 1–8.

Walke, J. Wistar. "Continued Fever, of an Adynamic Form, Popularly Called 'Typhoid Fever,' as Met with in Chesterfield County [Virginia] during the Present Year—with Remarks, &c, &c." *Virginia Medical Journal* 12 (January 1859): 19–34.

Ward, B. F. "Medicine in the Cotton States." [Jackson, Miss.]: Mississippi State Medical Association, 1880.

Waring, Joseph Ioor, ed. *Excerpts from the Minute Book of the Medical Society of South Carolina.* 2 vols. Charleston, S.C.: Nelson's Southern Printing Co., 1956.

Watkins, M. S. "Case of Mrs. Watkins' Cure of Recto-Vaginal Laceration, by Dr. J. Marion Sims, of New-York; Reported by M. S. Watkins, M.D., of Jackson, Miss., the Husband of the Patient." *New Orleans Medical and Surgical Journal* 11 (March 1855): 645–47.

[Weatherly, Job Sobiesky]. "Address of Dr. Weatherly on Medical Education." In *Transactions of the Medical Association of the State of Alabama*, 32–44. Mobile, Ala.: Printed at the Daily Register Office, 1871.

"Western Medical Schools." *Western Journal of the Medical and Physical Sciences* 9 (1835–36): 607–18.

Wharton, R. G. "An Account of the Epidemic Erysipelas: With Cases." *New Orleans Medical and Surgical Journal* 2 (November 1845): 277–86.

Wilson, Jno. Stainback. "Female Medical Education." *Southern Medical and Surgical Journal*, n.s., 10 (January 1854): 5–17.

Wilson, John S. "Peculiarities and Diseases of Negroes." *DeBow's Review* 28 (May 1860): 597–99.

——. *Woman's Home Book of Health: A Work for Mothers and for Families.* . . . Philadelphia: J. B. Lippincott and Co., 1860.

Wooten, H. V. "Dysentery among Negroes." *New Orleans Medical and Surgical Journal* 11 (January 1855): 448–56.

——. "On the Topography and Diseases of Lowndesboro' [Alabama] and Its Vicinity, during the Year 1850." *Southern Medical Reports* 2 (1850): 330–45.

"A Word about Catalogues." *Nashville Journal of Medicine and Surgery* 9 (August 1855): 149–50.

Wragg, W. T. "Report on Closing the Roper Hospital after the Yellow Fever Epidemic of 1854." *Charleston Medical Journal and Review* 10 (January 1855): 67–85.

Wright, Isaac. *Wright's Family Medicine, or System of Domestic Practice.* . . . Madisonville, Tenn.: Printed at the Office of Henderson, Johnson and Co., 1833.

Yandell, David Wendel. *Notes on Medical Matters and Medical Men in London and Paris.* Louisville, Ky.: Prentice and Weissinger, 1848.

——. "The Progress of Medicine: an Introductory Lecture. . . ." Louisville, Ky.: Bradley and Gilbert, Printers, 1869.

Yandell, Lunsford P. "An Address on the Improvement of the Medical Profession. . . ." Louisville, Ky.: Prentice and Weissinger, 1841.

——. "Cases of Dysentery, with Remarks." *Transylvania Journal of Medicine and the Associate Sciences* 9 (April–June 1836): 240–50.

——. "An Introductory Lecture on the Advantages and Pleasures of the Study of Chemistry. . . ." Lexington, Ky.: Printed by N. L. Finnell and J. F. Herndon, 1831.

——. "An Introductory Lecture to the Medical Class of the University of Louisville." Louisville, Ky.: Prentice and Weissinger, 1848.

——. "A Narrative of the Dissolution of the Medical Faculty of Transylvania University." Nashville, Tenn.: W. Hasell Hunt, 1837.

——. "Remarks on Struma Africana, or the Disease Usually Called Negro Poison, or Negro Consumption." *Transylvania Journal of Medicine and the Associate Sciences* 4 (February 1831): 83–103.

SECONDARY SOURCES

Abel, Emily K. *Hearts of Wisdom: American Women Caring for Kin, 1850–1940.* Cambridge, Mass.: Harvard University Press, 2000.

——. "A Terrible and Exhausting Struggle: Family Caregiving during the Transformation of Medicine." *Journal of the History of Medicine and Allied Sciences* 50 (October 1995): 478–506.

Ackerknecht, Erwin H. *A Short History of Medicine.* Rev. ed. Baltimore: Johns Hopkins University Press, 1982.

Albanese, Catherine L. "Body Politic and Body Perfect: Religion, Politics, and Thomsonian Medicine in Nineteenth-Century America." In *New Dimensions in American Religious History: Essays in Honor of Martin E. Marty.* Edited by Jay P. Dolan and James P. Wind, 131–51. Grand Rapids, Mich.: W. B. Eerdmans, 1993.

——. *Nature Religion in America: From the Algonkion Indians to the New Age.* Chicago: University of Chicago Press, 1990.

Atlee, John Light. "The Education of a Physician in the Early Nineteenth Century." *Journal of the Lancaster County Historical Society* 91 (Easter 1987): 78–88.

Atwater, Edward C. "The Protracted Labor and Brief Life of a Country Medical School: The Auburn Medical Institution, 1825." *Journal of the History of Medicine and Allied Sciences* 34 (July 1979): 334–52.

Bakan, David. *Disease, Pain, and Sacrifice: Toward a Psychology of Suffering.* Chicago: University of Chicago Press, 1968.

Baker, Robert, Arthur L. Caplan, Linda L. Emanuel, and Stephen K. Latham, eds. *The American Medical Ethics Revolution: How the AMA's Code of Ethics has Transformed Physicians'*

Relationships to Patients, Professionals, and Society. Baltimore: Johns Hopkins University Press, 1999.

Barber, Bernard, and Walter Hirsch, eds. *The Sociology of Science*. New York: Free Press, 1962.

Barker-Benfield, G. J. *The Horrors of a Half-Known Life: Male Attitudes toward Women and Sexuality in Nineteenth-Century America*. New York: Harper and Row, 1976.

Barlow, William, and David O. Powell. "A Dedicated Medical Student: Solomon Mordecai, 1819–1822." *Journal of the Early Republic* (Winter 1987): 377–97.

———. "Malthus A. Ward, Frontier Physician, 1815–1823." *Journal of the History of Medicine and Allied Sciences* 32 (July 1977): 280–91.

Bassett, Victor H. "A Georgia Medical Student in the Year 1801." *Georgia Historical Quarterly* 22 (December 1938): 331–68.

Beaver, Donald deB. *The American Scientific Community, 1800–1860: A Statistical-Historical Study*. New York: Arno Press, 1980.

Beeson, Paul B., and Russell C. Maulitz. "The Inner History of Internal Medicine." In Maulitz and Long, eds., *Grand Rounds*, 15–54.

Beier, Lucinda McCray. *Sufferers and Healers: The Experience of Illness in Seventeenth-Century England*. London: Routledge and Kegan Paul, 1987.

Ben-David, Joseph. "Scientific Productivity and Academic Organization in Nineteenth-Century Medicine." In Barber and Hirsch, eds., *Sociology of Science*, 305–28.

Blake, John B. "Anatomy." In Numbers, ed., *Education of American Physicians*, 29–47.

———. "The Development of American Anatomy Acts." *Journal of Medical Education* 30 (August 1955): 431–39.

Blanton, Wyndham. *Medicine in Virginia in the Eighteenth Century*. Richmond, Va.: Garrett and Massie, 1931.

———. *Medicine in Virginia in the Nineteenth Century*. Richmond, Va.: Garrett and Massie, 1933.

Bliss, Michael. *William Osler: A Life in Medicine*. New York: Oxford University Press, 1999.

Breeden, James O., ed. *Advice among Masters: The Ideal of Slave Management in the Old South*. Westport, Conn.: Greenwood, 1980.

———. "Body Snatchers and Anatomy Professors: Medical Education in Nineteenth-Century Virginia." *Virginia Magazine of History and Biography* 83 (July 1975): 321–45.

———. "States-Rights Medicine in the Old South." *Bulletin of the New York Academy of Medicine* 52 (1968–69): 29–45.

Bridgforth, Lucie R. "Medicine in Antebellum Mississippi." *Journal of Mississippi History* 46 (May 1984): 82–107.

Brieger, Gert H. "The History of Medicine and the History of Science." *Isis* 72 (December 1981): 537–40.

———. "Therapeutic Conflicts and the American Medical Profession in the 1860s." *Bulletin of the History of Medicine* 41 (May–June 1967): 215–22.

Brody, Howard. *Stories of Sickness*. New Haven, Conn.: Yale University Press, 1987.

Brody, Janet Farrell. *Contraception and Abortion in Nineteenth-Century America*. Ithaca, N.Y.: Cornell University Press, 1994.

Burkett, Roberta O., W. A. Sawyer, and W. C. Worthington Jr., comps. "A Bibliography of Inaugural Theses of Graduating Students of the Medical College of (the State of) South Carolina." Charleston: Waring Historical Library of the Medical University of South Carolina, n.d.

Butler, Judith, and Joan W. Scott, eds. *Feminists Theorize the Political*. New York: Routledge, 1992.

Bynum, W. F. *Science and the Practice of Medicine in the Nineteenth Century*. Cambridge: Cambridge University Press, 1994.

Bynum, W. F., Stephen Lock, and Roy Porter, eds. *Medical Journals and Medical Knowledge: Historical Essays*. New York: Routledge, 1992.

Bynum, W. F., and Vivian Nutton, eds. *Essays in the History of Therapeutics*. Clio Medica 22. Atlanta, Ga.: Rodopi, 1991.

Bynum, W. F., and Roy Porter, eds. *William Hunter and the Eighteenth-Century Medical World*. Cambridge: Cambridge University Press, 1985.

Cadwallader, D. E., and F. J. Wilson. "Folklore Medicine among Georgia's Piedmont Negroes after the Civil War." *Georgia Historical Quarterly* 49 (June 1965): 217–27.

Calhoun, Daniel J. *Professional Lives in America*. Cambridge, Mass.: Harvard University Press, 1965.

Camino, Linda A. "The Cultural Epidemiology of Spiritual Heart Trouble." In Kirkland et al., eds., *Herbal and Magical Medicine*, 118–36.

Cassedy, James H. *Medicine and American Growth, 1800–1860*. Madison, Wisc.: University of Wisconsin Press, 1986.

———. *Medicine in America: A Short History*. Baltimore: Johns Hopkins University Press, 1991.

Catalogue of the Transylvania University Medical Library. Lexington, Ky.: Transylvania University, 1987.

Chaplin, Joyce E. *Subject Matter: Technology, the Body, and Science on the Anglo-American Frontier, 1500–1676*. Cambridge, Mass.: Harvard University Press, 2001.

Charon, Rita. "To Build a Case: Medical Histories as Traditions in Conflict." *Literature and Medicine* 11 (Spring 1992): 115–32.

Chireau, Yvonne. "The Uses of the Supernatural: Toward a History of Black Women's Magical Practices." In Juster and MacFarlane, eds., *Mighty Baptism*, 171–88.

Clarke, Edwin, ed. *Modern Methods in the History of Medicine*. London: Athlone Press, 1971.

Cleaveland, Clif. *Sacred Space: Stories from a Life in Medicine*. Philadelphia: American College of Physicians, 1998.

Cohen, Emily Jane. "Anatomy and the Dirty Philosopher." *Configurations* 5 (Fall 1997): 369–424.

Conkin, Paul K. *Gone with the Ivy: A Biography of Vanderbilt University*. Knoxville: University of Tennessee Press, 1985.

Conser, Walter H., Jr. *God and the Natural World: Religion and Science in Antebellum America*. Columbia: University of South Carolina Press, 1993.

Coombs, Jan. "Rural Medical Practice in the 1880s: A View from Central Wisconsin." *Bulletin of the History of Medicine* 64 (Spring 1990): 35–62.

Cowdrey, Albert E. *This Land, This South: An Environmental History*. Lexington: University Press of Kentucky, 1983.

Cox, Dwayne D. "A History of the University of Louisville." Ph.D. dissertation, University of Kentucky, 1984.

———. "The Louisville Medical Institute: A Case History in American Medical Education." *Filson Club History Quarterly* 62 (April 1988): 197–219.

Cox, Dwayne D., and William J. Morison. *The University of Louisville*. Lexington: University Press of Kentucky, 2000.

Croom, Edward M. "Herbal Medicine among the Lumbee Indians." In *Herbal and Magical Medicine: Traditional Healing Today*, edited by James Kirkland, Holly F. Matthews, C. W. Sullivan III and Karen Baldwin, 137–69. Durham, N.C.: Duke University Press, 1992.

Cunningham, H. H. *Doctors in Gray: The Confederate Medical Service*. Baton Rouge: Louisiana State University Press, 1958.

Davis, Curtis Carroll, ed. "Chronicler of the Cavaliers: Some Letters from and to William Alexander Caruthers, M.D. (1802–1846)." *Virginia Magazine of History and Biography* 55 (July 1947): 213–32.

Dear, Peter, ed. *The Literary Structure of Scientific Argument: Historical Studies*. Philadelphia: University of Pennsylvania Press, 1991.

Donnelly, William J. "Righting the Medical Record: Transforming Chronicle into Story." *Soundings* 72 (Spring 1989): 127–36.

Drachman, Virginia G. *Hospital with a Heart: Women Doctors and the Paradox of Separation at the New England Hospital, 1862–1969*. Ithaca, N.Y.: Cornell University Press, 1984.

Duden, Barbara. *The Woman Beneath the Skin: A Doctor's Patients in Eighteenth-Century Germany*. Translated by Howard Dunlap. Cambridge, Mass.: Harvard University Press, 1991.

Duffin, Jacalyn. "'In View of the Body of Job Broom': A Glimpse of the Medical Knowledge and Practice of John Rolf." *Canadian Bulletin of Medical History / Bulletin Canadien D'Historie de la Médecine* 7 (1990): 9–30.

——. *Langstaff: A Nineteenth-Century Medical Life*. Toronto: University of Toronto Press, 1993.

Duffin, Jacalyn, and Pierre René. "'Anti-moine; Anti-biotique': The Public Fortunes of the Secret Properties of Antimony Potassium Tartrate (Tartar Emetic)." *Journal of the History of Medicine and Allied Sciences* 46 (October 1991): 440–56.

Duffy, John. "American Perceptions of the Medical, Legal, and Theological Professions." *Bulletin of the History of Medicine* 58 (Spring 1984): 1–15.

——. *From Humors to Medical Science: A History of American Medicine*. 2nd ed. Urbana: University of Illinois Press, 1993.

——. "A Note on Ante-bellum Southern Nationalism and Medical Practice." *Journal of Southern History* 34 (May 1968): 274–76.

——, ed. *The Rudolph Matas History of Medicine in Louisiana*. 2 vols. Baton Rouge: Louisiana State University Press, 1958, 1962.

——. *The Tulane University Medical Center: One Hundred and Fifty Years of Medical Education*. Baton Rouge: Louisiana State University Press, 1984.

Dwyer, Ellen. "Stories of Epilepsy, 1880–1930." In *Framing Disease: Studies in Cultural History*, edited by Charles E. Rosenberg and Janet S. Golden, 248–72. New Brunswick, N.J.: Rutgers University Press, 1997.

Eamon, William. *Science and the Secrets of Nature: Books of Secrets in Medieval and Early Modern Culture*. Princeton, N.J.: Princeton University Press, 1994.

Elkin, Daniel C., ed. *The Medical Reports of John Y. Bassett, M.D., the Alabama Student*. Springfield, Ill.: C. C. Thomas, 1941.

Ellis, John H. *Medicine in Kentucky*. Lexington: University Press of Kentucky, 1977.

Estes, J. Worth. *Dictionary of Protopharmacology: Therapeutic Practices, 1700–1850*. Canton, Mass.: Science History Publications, 1990.

Fett, Sharla. " 'It's a Spirit in Me': Spiritual Power and the Healing Work of African American Women in Slavery." In Juster and MacFarlane, eds., *Mighty Baptism*, 189–209.

——. *Working Cures: Healing, Health, and Power on Southern Slave Plantations*. Chapel Hill: University of North Carolina Press, 2002.

Fisher, J. Walter. "Physicians and Slavery in the Antebellum Southern Medical Journal." *Journal of the History of Medicine and Allied Sciences* 23 (January 1968): 36–49.

Fissell, Mary. "Readers, Texts, and Contexts: Vernacular Medical Works in Early Modern 1England." In Porter, ed., *Popularization of Medicine*, 72–96.

Fleming, Donald. *William H. Welch and the Rise of Modern Medicine*. Boston: Little, Brown, 1954.

Flesher, Dale L., and Michael G. Schumacher. "A Natchez Doctor's Ledgers as a Source of History, 1804–1809." *Journal of Mississippi History* 58 (Summer 1996): 177–92.

Flexner, James Thomas. *Doctors on Horseback: Pioneers of American Medicine*. New York: Viking Press, 1937.

Fontenot, Wonda L. *Secret Doctors: Ethnomedicine of African Americans*. Westport, Conn.: Bergin and Garvey, 1994.

Fraser, Gertrude Jacinta. *African American Midwifery in the South: Dialogues of Birth, Race, and Memory*. Cambridge, Mass.: Harvard University Press, 1998.

Fulmer, Henry Griffin. "The Civil War Diary of Samuel Wells Leland, M.D., 1861–1865." Masters thesis, University of South Carolina, 1985.

Gamble, Vanessa. *Making a Place for Ourselves: The Black Hospital Movement, 1920–1945*. New York: Oxford University Press, 1995.

Gay, Evelyn Ward. *The Medical Profession in Georgia, 1733–1983*. Atlanta, Ga.: Auxiliary to the Medical Association of Georgia, 1986.

Geison, Gerald L. *Michael Foster and the Cambridge School of Physiology: The Scientific Enterprise in Late Victorian Society*. Princeton, N.J.: Princeton University Press, 1978.

——., ed. *Physiology in the American Context, 1850–1940*. Bethesda, Md.: American Physiological Society, 1987.

Genovese, Eugene D. *Roll, Jordan, Roll: The World the Slaves Made*. New York: Pantheon Books, 1974.

Gevitz, Norman, ed. *Other Healers: Unorthodox Medicine in America*. Baltimore: Johns Hopkins University Press, 1988.

Goler, Robert I., and Pascal James Imperato, eds. *Early American Medicine: A Symposium*. New York: Fraunces Tavern Museum, 1987.

Grob, Gerald N. *Edward Jarvis and the Medical World of Nineteenth-Century America*. Knoxville: University of Tennessee Press, 1978.

Gross, Ariela J. *Double Character: Slavery and Mastery in the Antebellum Southern Courtroom*. Princeton, N.J.: Princeton University Press, 2000.

Haber, Samuel. *The Quest for Authority and Honor in the American Professions, 1750–1900*. Chicago: University of Chicago Press, 1991.

Haller, John S., Jr. *Kindly Medicine: Physio-Medicalism in America, 1836–1911*. Kent, Ohio: Kent State University Press, 1997.

——. *Medical Protestants: The Eclectics in American Medicine, 1825–1939*. Carbondale: University of Southern Illinois Press, 1994.

Haygood, Tamara Miner. *Henry William Ravenel, 1814–1887: South Carolina Scientist in the Civil War Era*. Tuscaloosa: University of Alabama Press, 1987.

Holifield, E. Brooks. "The Wealth of Nineteenth-Century American Physicians." *Bulletin of the History of Medicine* 64 (Spring 1990): 79–85.

Holley, Howard L. *The History of Medicine in Alabama*. Birmingham: University of Alabama School of Medicine, 1982.

Holloway, Joseph E., ed. *Africanisms in American Culture*. Bloomington: Indiana University Press, 1991.

Horine, Emmet Field. "A History of the Louisville Medical Institute and of the Establishment of the University of Louisville and Its School of Medicine, 1833–1846." *Filson Club History Quarterly* 7 (July 1933): 133–47.

Horowitz, Helen Lefkowitz. *Rereading Sex: Battles over Sexual Knowledge and Suppression in Nineteenth-Century America*. New York: Knopf, 2002.

Horsman, Reginald. *Josiah Nott of Mobile: Southerner, Physician, and Racial Theorist*. Baton Rouge: Louisiana State University Press, 1987.

Humphreys, Margaret. *Malaria: Poverty, Race, and Public Health in the United States*. Baltimore: Johns Hopkins University Press, 2001.

——. *Yellow Fever in the South*. New Brunswick, N.J.: Rutgers University Press, 1992.

Hunt, Lynn, ed. *The New Cultural History*. Berkeley: University of California Press, 1989.

Hunter, Kathryn Montgomery. *Doctors' Stories: The Narrative Structure of Medical Knowledge*. Princeton, N.J.: Princeton University Press, 1991.

Index-Catalogue of the Library of the Surgeon-General's Office. Series I. Washington, D.C.: U.S. Government Printing Office, 1889.

Inkster, Ian. "Marginal Men: Aspects of the Social Role of the Medical Community in Sheffield, 1790–1850." In Woodward and Richard, eds., *Health Care and Popular Medicine*, 128–63.

Johnson, Thomas Cary, Jr. *Scientific Interests in the Old South*. New York: D. Appleton-Century, Inc., for the Institute for Research in the Social Sciences, University of Virginia, 1936.

Johnson, Walter. *Soul by Soul: Life Inside the Antebellum Slave Market*. Cambridge, Mass.: Harvard University Press, 1999.

Jones, Anne Goodwyn, and Susan V. Donaldson, eds. *Haunted Bodies: Gender and Southern Texts*. Charlottesville: University Press of Virginia, 1997.

Jones, James H. *Bad Blood: The Tuskegee Syphilis Experiment—A Tragedy of Race and Medicine*. New York: Free Press, 1981.

Jones, Norrece T. *Born a Child of Freedom, Yet a Slave: Mechanisms of Control and Strategies of Resistance in Antebellum South Carolina*. Hanover, N.H., and London, Eng.: Wesleyan University Press and University Press of New England, 1990.

Jones-Jackson, Patricia. *When Roots Die*. Athens: University of Georgia Press, 1987.

Jordan, Weymouth T. *Herbs, Hoecakes, and Husbandry: The Daybook of a Planter of the Old South*. Tallahassee: Florida State University Press, 1960.

——. "Herb Medicine." *Alabama Historical Quarterly* 2 (Winter 1940): 443–59.

———. "Homemade Medicine." *Alabama Historical Quarterly* 2 (Spring 1941): 117–29.

———. "Household Hints." *Alabama Historical Quarterly* 2 (Fall 1940): 318–30.

———. "Martin Marshall's Book: Introduction." *Alabama Historical Quarterly* 2 (Summer 1940): 158–68.

Jordanova, Ludmilla. *Sexual Visions: Images of Science and Medicine between the Eighteenth and Twentieth Centuries*. Madison: University of Wisconsin Press, 1989.

Juster, Susan, and Lisa MacFarlane, eds. *A Mighty Baptism: Race, Gender, and the Creation of American Protestantism*. Ithaca, N.Y.: Cornell University Press, 1996.

Kaufman, Martin. *American Medical Education: The Formative Years, 1765–1910*. Westport, Conn.: Greenwood, 1976.

Keeney, Elizabeth B. *The Botanizers: Amateur Scientists in Nineteenth-Century America*. Chapel Hill: University of North Carolina Press, 1992.

Kett, Joseph F. *The Formation of the American Medical Profession: The Role of Institutions*. New Haven, Conn.: Yale University Press, 1968.

Kevles, Daniel. *In the Name of Eugenics: Genetics and the Uses of Heredity*. New York: Knopf, 1985.

Kilbride, Daniel. "Southern Medical Students in Philadelphia, 1800–1861: Science and Sociability in the 'Republic of Medicine.'" *Journal of Southern History* 65 (November 1999): 697–732.

King, Nancy M. P., and Ann Folwell Stanford. "Patient Stories, Doctor Stories, and True Stories: A Cautionary Reading." *Literature and Medicine* 11 (Fall 1992): 185–99.

Kiple, Kenneth F., and Virginia Himmelsteib King. *Another Dimension of the Black Diaspora: Diet, Disease, and Racism*. Cambridge: Cambridge University Press, 1981.

Kirkland, James, Holly F. Mathews, C. W. Sullivan III, and Karen Baldwin, eds. *Herbal and Magical Medicine: Traditional Healing Today*. Durham, N.C.: Duke University Press, 1992.

Kleinman, Arthur. *The Illness Narratives: Suffering, Healing, and the Human Condition*. New York: Basic Books, 1988.

Kohlstedt, Sally. *The Formation of the American Scientific Community: The American Association for the Advancement of Science, 1848–60*. Urbana: University of Illinois Press, 1976.

Kunitz, Stephen J. "Classifications in Medicine." In Maulitz and Long, eds., *Grand Rounds*, 279–96.

Laderman, Gary. *The Sacred Remains: American Attitudes toward Death, 1799–1883*. New Haven, Conn.: Yale University Press, 1996.

Lane, Joan. "The Role of Apprenticeship in Eighteenth-Century Medical Education in England." In Bynum and Porter, eds., *William Hunter and the Eighteenth-Century Medical World*, 59–103.

Laqueur, Thomas W. "Bodies, Details, and the Humanitarian Narrative." In *The New Cultural History*, edited by Lynn Hunt, 176–204. Berkeley: University of California Press, 1989.

Lawrence, Christopher. "Ornate Physicians and Learned Medical Men, 1726–1776." In Bynum and Porter, eds., *William Hunter and the Eighteenth-Century Medical World*, 153–76.

Lawrence, Susan. *Charitable Knowledge: Hospital Pupils and Practitioners in Eighteenth-Century London*. Cambridge: Cambridge University Press, 1996.

Lawson, Hampden. "The Early Medical Schools of Kentucky." *Bulletin of the History of Medicine* 24 (March–April 1950): 168–75.

Leake, Chauncy D., ed. *Percival's Medical Ethics*. Baltimore: Williams and Wilkins Co., 1927.

Leavitt, Judith Walzer. *Brought to Bed: Childbearing in America, 1750 to 1950*. New York: Oxford University Press, 1986.

——. "Medicine in Context: A Review Essay of the History of Medicine." *American Historical Review* 95 (December 1990): 1471–84.

——. "Public Health and Preventive Medicine." In Numbers, ed., *Education of American Physicians*, 250–72.

——. " 'A Worrying Profession': The Domestic Environment of Medical Practice in Mid-Nineteenth-Century America." *Bulletin of the History of Medicine* 69 (Spring 1995): 1–29.

Leavitt, Judith Walzer, and Ronald L. Numbers, eds. *Sickness and Health in America: Readings in the History of Medicine and Public Health*. 3rd ed. Madison: University of Wisconsin Press, 1997.

Leder, Drew. *The Absent Body*. Chicago: University of Chicago Press, 1990.

Lederer, Susan E. *Subjected to Science: Human Experimentation in America before the Second World War*. Baltimore: Johns Hopkins University Press, 1995.

Loudon, Irvin. "A Doctor's Cash Book: The Economy of General Practice in the 1830s." *Medical History* 27 (July 1983): 249–68.

Ludmerer, Kenneth M. *Learning to Heal: The Development of American Medical Education*. New York: Basic Books, 1985.

Marshall, Tim. *Murdering to Dissect: Grave-Robbing, Frankenstein, and the Anatomy Literature*. Manchester, Eng.: Manchester University Press, 1995.

Mathews, Holly F. "Doctors and Root Doctors: Patients Who Use Both." In Kirkland et al., eds., *Herbal and Magical Medicine*, 68–98.

Maulitz, Russell C., and Diana E. Long, eds. *Grand Rounds: One Hundred Years of Internal Medicine*. Philadelphia: University of Pennsylvania Press, 1988.

McCandless, Peter. *Moonlight, Magnolias, and Madness: Insanity in South Carolina from the Colonial Period to the Progressive Era*. Chapel Hill: University of North Carolina Press, 1996.

McCullough, Laurence B. "Particularism in Medicine." *Criticism* 32 (Summer 1990): 361–70.

McGregor, Deborah Kuhn. *Sexual Surgery and the Origins of Gynecology: J. Marion Sims, His Hospital, and His Patients*. New York: Garland, 1989.

McLauren, Angus. "The Pleasures of Procreation: Traditional and Biomedical Theories of Conception." In Bynum and Porter, eds., *William Hunter and the Eighteenth-Century Medical World*, 323–41.

McMillen, Sally G. *Motherhood in the Old South: Pregnancy, Childbirth, and Infant Rearing*. Baton Rouge: Louisiana State University Press, 1990.

Meckel, Richard A. *Save the Babies: American Public Health Reform and the Prevention of Infant Mortality*. Baltimore: Johns Hopkins University Press, 1990.

Medicine and Its Development in Kentucky. Compiled and Written by the Medical Historical Research Project of the Works Projects Administration for the Commonwealth of Kentucky. Louisville: Standard Printing Co., 1940.

Melish, Joanne Pope. *Disowning Slavery: Gradual Emancipation and "Race" in New England, 1780–1860*. Ithaca, N.Y.: Cornell University Press, 1998.

Miller, Randall M., ed. *"Dear Master": Letters of a Slave Family*. Ithaca, N.Y.: Cornell University Press, 1978.

Mohr, James C. *Doctors and the Law: Medical Jurisprudence in Nineteenth-Century America*. New York: Oxford University Press, 1993.

Morais, Herbert. *The History of the Afro-American in Medicine*. Rev. ed. Cornwell Heights, Pa.: Publisher's Agency, 1978.

Morantz-Sanchez, Regina Markell. *Sympathy and Science: Women Physicians in American Medicine*. New York: Oxford University Press, 1985.

More, Ellen S. *Restoring the Balance: Women Physicians and the Profession of Medicine, 1850–1995*. Cambridge, Mass.: Harvard University Press, 1999.

Morgan, Philip D. *Slave Counterpoint: Black Culture in the Eighteenth-Century Chesapeake and Lowcountry*. Chapel Hill: University of North Carolina Press, 1998.

Moss, Kay K. *Southern Folk Medicine, 1750–1820*. Columbia: University of South Carolina Press, 1999.

Murphy, Lamar Riley. *Enter the Physician: The Transformation of Domestic Medicine, 1760–1860*. Tuscaloosa: University of Alabama Press, 1991.

Norwood, William Frederick. *Medical Education in the United States before the Civil War*. Philadelphia: University of Pennsylvania Press, 1944.

Numbers, Ronald L., ed. *The Education of American Physicians: Historical Essays*. Berkeley: University of California Press, 1980.

———. "The History of American Medicine: A Field in Ferment." *Reviews in American History* 10 (December 1982): 245–63.

Numbers, Ronald L., and Todd L. Savitt, eds. *Science and Medicine in the Old South*. Baton Rouge: Louisiana State University Press, 1989.

Numbers, Ronald L., and John Harley Warner. "The Maturation of American Medical Science." In Leavitt and Numbers, eds., *Sickness and Health in America*, 130–42.

O'Brien, Michael, and David Moltke-Hansen, eds. *Intellectual Life in Antebellum Charleston*. Knoxville: University of Tennessee Press, 1986.

Ott, Katherine. *Fevered Lives: Tuberculosis in American Culture Since 1870*. Cambridge, Mass.: Harvard University Press, 1996.

Parascandola, John. *The Development of American Pharmacology: John J. Abel and the Shaping of a Discipline*. Baltimore: Johns Hopkins University Press, 1992.

Pease, Jane H., and William H. Pease. "Intellectual Life in the 1830s: The Institutional Framework and the Charleston Style." In O'Brien and Moltke-Hansen, eds., *Intellectual Life in Antebellum Charleston*, 233–54.

Pernick, Martin S. *A Calculus of Suffering: Pain, Professionalism, and Anesthesia in Nineteenth-Century America*. New York: Columbia University Press, 1985.

Pickard, E. Madge, and R. Carlyle Buley. *The Midwest Pioneer: His Ills, Cures, and Doctors*. Crawfordsville, Ind., 1945.

Porter, Roy. *Health for Sale: Quackery in England, 1660–1850*. Manchester, Eng.: Manchester University Press, 1989.

———, ed. *The Popularization of Medicine, 1650–1850*. London: Routledge, 1992.

Reiser, Stanley Joel. *Medicine and the Reign of Technology*. Cambridge: Cambridge University Press, 1978.

Richardson, Ruth. *Death, Dissection, and the Destitute*. London: Penguin, 1988.

Risse, Guenter B., Ronald L. Numbers, and Judith Walzer Leavitt, eds. *Medicine without Doctors: Home Health Care in American History*. New York: Science History Publications/USA, 1977.

Risse, Guenter B., and John Harley Warner. "Reconstructing Clinical Activities: Patient Records in Medical History." *Social History of Medicine* 5 (August 1992): 183–205.

Roland, Charles G. "Diary of a Canadian Country Physician: Jonathan Woolverton (1811–1883)." *Medical History* 15 (April 1971): 168–80.

Rosen, George. *Fees and Fee Bills: Some Economic Aspects of Medical Practice in Nineteenth-Century America*. Baltimore: Johns Hopkins University Press, 1946.

Rosenberg, Charles E. *The Care of Strangers: The Rise of America's Hospital System*. New York: Basic Books, 1987.

———. *Explaining Epidemics and Other Studies in the History of Medicine*. Cambridge: Cambridge University Press, 1992.

———. Introduction to *Explaining Epidemics*, 1–6.

———. "Making It in Urban Medicine: A Career in the Age of Scientific Medicine." *Bulletin of the History of Medicine* 64 (Summer 1990): 163–86.

———. "The Medical Profession, Medical Practice, and the History of Medicine." In Clarke, ed., *Modern Methods in the History of Medicine*, 22–35.

———. "The Therapeutic Revolution: Medicine, Meaning, and Social Change in Nineteenth-Century America." In Vogel and Rosenberg, eds., *Therapeutic Revolution*, 3–25.

———, ed. *Right Living: An Anglo-American Tradition of Self-Help Medicine and Hygiene*. Baltimore: Johns Hopkins University Press, 2003.

Rosenberg, Charles E., and Janet Golden, eds. *Framing Disease: Studies in Cultural History*. New Brunswick, N.J.: Rutgers University Press, 1997.

Rosengarten, Theodore. *Tombee: Portrait of a Cotton Planter*. New York: William Morrow and Company, 1986.

Rosner, David. "Tempest in a Test Tube: Medical History and the Historian." *Radical History Review* 26 (1982): 166–71.

Rosner, Lisa. "Eighteenth-Century Medical Education and the Didactic Model of Experiment." In *The Literary Structure of Scientific Argument: Historical Studies*, edited by Peter Dear, 182–94. Philadelphia: University of Pennsylvania Press, 1991.

Rothman, Sheila M. *Living in the Shadow of Death: Tuberculosis and the Social Experience of Illness in American History*. Baltimore: Johns Hopkins University Press, 1994.

Rothstein, William G. *American Medical Schools and the Practice of Medicine: A History*. New York: Oxford University Press, 1987.

———. *American Physicians in the Nineteenth Century: From Sects to Science*. Baltimore: Johns Hopkins University Press, 1972.

Salvaggio, John. *The New Orleans Charity Hospital: A Story of Physicians, Politics, and Poverty*. Baton Rouge: Louisiana State University Press, 1992.

Sappol, Michael. *A Traffic of Dead Bodies: Anatomy and Embodied Social Identity in Nineteenth-Century America*. Princeton, N.J.: Princeton University Press, 2002.

Savitt, Todd L. "Four African-American Proprietary Medical Colleges: 1888–1923." *Journal of the History of Medicine and Allied Sciences* 55 (July 2000): 203–55.

———. " 'A Journal of Our Own': The *Medical and Surgical Observer* at the Beginnings of an African-American Medical Profession in Late 19th-Century America." *Journal of the National Medical Association* 88 (January 1996): 52–60.

———. *Medicine and Slavery: The Diseases and Health Care of Blacks in Antebellum Virginia*. Urbana: University of Illinois Press, 1978.

——. "Straight University Medical Department: The Short Life of a Black Medical School in Reconstruction New Orleans." *Louisiana History* 41 (Spring 2000): 175–201.

——. "The Use of Blacks for Medical Experimentation and Demonstration in the Old South." *Journal of Southern History* 45 (August 1982): 331–48.

Savitt, Todd L., and James Harvey Young, eds. *Disease and Distinctiveness in the American South*. Knoxville: University of Tennessee Press, 1988.

Scarry, Elaine. *The Body in Pain: The Making and Unmaking of the World*. New York: Oxford University Press, 1985.

Schweninger, Loren. "Doctor Jack: A Slave Physician on the Tennessee Frontier." *Tennessee Historical Quarterly* 57 (Spring/Summer 1998): 36–41.

Scott, Joan W. "Experience." In Butler and Scott, eds., *Feminists Theorize the Political*, 22–40.

Sewell, Jane Eliot. *Medicine in Maryland: The Practice and the Profession*. Baltimore: Johns Hopkins University Press, 1999.

Shorter, Edward. *Bedside Manners: The Troubled History of Doctors and Patients*. New York: Simon and Schuster, 1985.

Shryock, Richard H. "Empiricism and Rationalism in American Medicine, 1650–1950." Pt. 1. *Proceedings of the American Antiquarian Society*, n.s., 79 (April 15, 1969): 99–150.

——. "A Medical Perspective on the Civil War." In Shryock, *Medicine in America*, 90–110.

——. "Medical Practice in the Old South." In Shryock, *Medicine in America*, 49–70.

——. *Medicine in America: Historical Essays*. Baltimore: Johns Hopkins University Press, 1966.

Shultz, Suzanne M. *Body Snatching: The Robbing of Graves for the Education of Physicians*. Jefferson, N.C.: McFarland and Co., 1992.

Sigerist, Henry E. *Civilization and Disease*. Ithaca, N.Y.: Cornell University Press, 1943.

Snow, Loudell F. *Walkin' over Medicine: Traditional Health Practices in African-American Life*. Boulder, Colo.: Westview Press, 1993.

Spalding, Phinizy. *The History of the Medical College of Georgia*. Athens: University of Georgia Press, 1987.

Stafford, Barbara Maria. *Body Criticism: Imagining the Unseen in Enlightenment Art and Medicine*. Cambridge, Mass.: MIT Press, 1991.

Starr, Paul. *The Social Transformation of American Medicine: The Rise of a Sovereign Profession and the Making of a Vast Industry*. New York: Basic Books, 1982.

Stepan, Nancy Leys. "Race, Gender, Science, and Citizenship." *Gender and History* 10 (April 1998): 26–52.

Stephens Lester D. *Science, Race, and Religion in the American South: John Bachman and the Charleston Circle of Naturalists, 1815–1895*. Chapel Hill: University of North Carolina Press, 2000.

Stevens, Rosemary. *American Medicine and the Public Interest*. New Haven, Conn.: Yale University Press, 1971.

Stovall, Mary E. " 'To Be, To Do, and To Suffer': Responses to Illness and Death in the Nineteenth-Century Central South." *Journal of Mississippi History* 52 (May 1990): 95–109.

Stowe, Steven M. "Conflict and Self-Sufficiency: Domestic Medicine in the American South." In *Right Living: An Anglo-American Tradition of Self-Help Medicine and Hygiene*, edited by Charles E. Rosenberg, 147–69. Baltimore: Johns Hopkins University Press, 2003.

——. "Writing Sickness: A Southern Woman's Diary of Cares." In Jones and Donaldson, eds., *Haunted Bodies*, 257–84.

Street, John Phillips. *The Composition of Certain Patent and Proprietary Medicines*. Chicago: American Medical Association, 1917.

Tomes, Nancy. *The Gospel of Germs: Men, Women, and the Microbe in American Life*. Cambridge, Mass.: Harvard University Press, 1998.

Tyrrell, Ian R. "Drink and Temperance in the Antebellum South: An Overview and Interpretation." *Journal of Southern History* 48 (November 1982): 485–510.

U.S. Bureau of the Census. *Historical Statistics of the United States, Colonial Times to 1970. Bicentennial Edition*. Part 2. Washington, D.C.: U.S. Government Printing Office, 1975.

Valencius, Conevery Bolton. *The Health of the Country: How American Settlers Understood Themselves and Their Land*. New York: Basic Books, 2002.

Verbrugge, Martha. *Able-Bodied Womanhood: Personal Health and Social Change in Nineteenth-Century Boston*. New York: Oxford University Press, 1988.

Vogel, Morris J., and Charles E. Rosenberg, eds. *The Therapeutic Revolution: Essays in the Social History of American Medicine*. Philadelphia: University of Pennsylvania Press, 1979.

Walker, Helen Edith. *The Negro in the Medical Profession*. Charlottesville: University Press of Virginia, 1949.

Waring, Joseph Ioor. "Charleston Medicine, 1800–1860." *Journal of the History of Medicine and Allied Sciences* 31 (July 1976): 320–42.

———. *A History of Medicine in South Carolina, 1825–1900*. Columbia, S.C.: R. L. Bryan, 1967.

Warner, John Harley. *Against the Spirit of System: The French Impulse in Nineteenth-Century American Medicine*. Princeton, N.J.: Princeton University Press, 1998.

———. "The 1880s Rebellion against the AMA Code of Ethics: 'Scientific Democracy' and the Dissolution of Orthodoxy." In Baker et al., eds., *American Medical Ethics Revolution*, 52–69.

———. Foreword to *Bibliography of Inaugural Theses*, compiled by Burkett, Sawyer, and Worthington, i–vi.

———. "From Specificity to Universalism in Medical Therapeutics: Transformation in the Nineteenth Century United States." In Leavitt and Numbers, eds., *Sickness and Health in America*, 87–101.

———. "The Idea of Southern Medical Distinctiveness: Medical Knowledge and Practice in the Old South." In *Sickness and Health in America: Readings in the History of Medicine and Public Health*. 2nd ed., edited by Judith Walzer Leavitt and Ronald L. Numbers, 53–70. Madison: University of Wisconsin Press, 1985.

———. " 'The Nature-Trusting Heresy': American Physicians and the Concept of the Healing Power of Nature in the 1850's and 1860's." *Perspectives in American History* 11 (1977–78): 291–324.

———. "Science, Healing, and the Physician's Identity: A Problem of Professional Character in Nineteenth-Century America." In Bynum and Nutton, eds., *Essays in the History of Therapeutics*, 65–88.

———. "A Southern Medical Reform: The Meaning of the Antebellum Argument for Southern Medical Education." *Bulletin of the History of Medicine* 47 (Fall 1983): 364–81.

———. *The Therapeutic Perspective: Medical Practice, Knowledge, and Identity in America, 1820–1885*. Cambridge, Mass.: Harvard University Press, 1986.

Watson, Wilbur H., ed. *Black Folk Medicine*. New Brunswick, N.J.: Transaction Books, 1984.

Welch, Margaret. *The Book of Nature: Natural History in the United States, 1825–1875*. Boston: Northeastern University Press, 1998.

Wells, Susan. *Out of the Dead House: Nineteenth-Century Women Physicians and the Writing of Medicine*. Madison: University of Wisconsin Press, 2001.

Whorton, James C. *Inner Hygiene: Constipation and the Pursuit of Health in Modern Society*. New York: Oxford University Press, 2000.

Woodward, John, and David Richard, eds. *Health Care and Popular Medicine in Nineteenth-Century England*. New York: Holmes and Meier, 1977.

Wright, John D. *Transylvania: Tutor to the West*. Lexington: University Press of Kentucky, 1980.

~ Index ~

Affleck, Thomas, 211, 212
African Americans, 5, 9, 49–51, 54; and African healthways, 118–19, 134–35, 170, 173; and diagnosis, 144–45; and feigning ("possuming"), 51, 172–74, 216, 232; free, 107, 171–72, 260, 265–67; and risk of disease, 208–18. *See also* Patients; Race; Slaves (and slavery)
Agassiz, Louis, 240
Akens, T. M., 111
Allan, Algernon, 93
Allen, Joseph Eve, 35, 48
Alternative healers, 7, 22, 88, 122–23, 252–53. *See also* Country orthodoxy; Orthodox medicine: and vernacular medicine
American Medical Association, 23, 239
Anatomy. *See* Medical education: anatomy
Anderson, L. B., 158
Anderson, William, 129
Anesthesia. *See* Medical procedures: anesthesia
Ansley, Mary, 113
Anthony (slave), 31
Antisepsis. *See* Medical procedures: antisepsis
Antony, Milton, 36
Apprenticeship, 16, 20, 26, 27–31, 82. *See also* Medical education; Medical schools
Armstrong, A., 104
Army of Northern Virginia, 270
Arnold, Richard, 125–26, 129
Augusta, Ga. *See* Medical education; Medical schools; Southern places

Bachelor, Albert, 57, 97, 157
Bacon, Francis, 72
Baglivi, Georgio, 72

Bailey, R. S., 170
Bailey, Thomas P., 265–66
Bairel, Sudie, 125
Ball, Charles, 126
Barr, Jane, 114
Barton, Edward, 82
Baruch, Simon, 171, 270
Bassett, Isaphoena, 256
Bassett, John Young, 110, 203, 207, 249–57
Bates, F. A., 231
Battey, Martha, 129
Battey, Robert, 80, 264
Bayless, George, 65
Becton, Frederick, 206
Bedside notes, 102, 167–68, 175–99, 232. *See also* Case narratives; Daybooks
Bell, Elizabeth, 114
Ben (slave), 230
Berly, Joel, 139, 266
Bessie (slave), 135
Bets (slave), 180
Bibb, Dandridge, 64, 78–79
Blair, I. H., 36
Blistering. *See* Medical procedures: blistering
Bloodletting. *See* Medical procedures: venesection (bloodletting)
Bodies: and anatomy, 59–61, 64, 67–68, 216–17; in case narratives, 232–34; and diagnosis, 141–49, 183–85; and health talk, 114–15; physicians', 143–45; in physicians' notes, 179, 186–87, 191, 192; as signifiers, 96, 133, 142–44, 219, 223, 225; and violence, 159–62. *See also* Medical education: anatomy
Bonner, William, 54
Bowman, Ralph, 265

Boyd, Alfred, 144
Brandon, Zillah, 134
Briggs, James A., 205
Broyles, William, 62
Butler, Robert, 106

Caldwell, Charles, 36–37, 38, 221–22
Caldwell, W. Hugh, 111
Calomel. *See* Medicines: calomel
Campbell, Alexander, 111
Campbell, David, 114
Cantrell, Matilda, 244
Caregiving: in clinics, 53–54, 58; in homes, 6, 46–47, 73, 103, 131, 135, 151, 198–99, 247–48. *See also* Physicians: and bedside practice
Carrigan, A. V., 34
Cartwright, Samuel A., 209, 215–18
Case narratives, 3, 12, 102, 124, 167, 228–58, 269–70. *See also* Bedside notes; Daybooks
Castor oil. *See* Medicines: castor oil
Chaillé, Stanford, 129, 269
Chapman, James, 138
Charity Hospital (New Orleans, La.), 36, 53, 54, 287 (n. 20)
Charles (slave), 234–35
Charleston, S.C. *See* Medical education; Medical schools; Southern places
Chester, Charles, 147
Chicken soup, 80
Children, 5, 25, 46, 115–16, 171. *See also* Women
Childress, Pleasant, 123
Chisolm, Julian J., 268
Christmas, [Winfield?], 101, 103
City Hospital (Charleston, S.C.), 267
Civil War, 4, 9, 15, 81, 152, 201, 205, 251; aftermath of, 259–71
Clark, Courtney, 37, 43, 123, 176, 192–99, 234–35
Clark, J. E., 88
Class. *See* Social class
Climate (and weather), 117, 120, 133, 153, 202, 210, 285 (n. 11)
Cochran, W. A., 267
Cocke, John H., 117

Colmer, George, 101–3, 106, 110, 111, 112, 265–66
Communities: as ideal for practice, 3, 11, 24, 65, 78–79, 130, 205, 218, 221, 227, 239, 250; as influencing medicine, 7, 66, 69, 84–90, 92, 114, 127, 128, 148, 149, 199, 252, 253–55; and medical knowledge, 45, 47, 51–52, 58, 72–74, 95, 204, 242, 246. *See also* South; Southern places
Cooke, John Esten, 43, 150
Cooper, Thomas, 78, 219
Copes, James, 83
Copes, Joseph S., 28, 33, 81, 83–84, 137
Copes, Thomas, 83–84
Country orthodoxy: and local communities, 7, 69, 77, 102, 127–29, 259, 270; and medical knowledge, 2–3, 12, 114, 144, 146, 148, 176, 178, 198, 200, 214, 219, 235, 243, 250, 259; and practice, 42, 57, 59, 74–75, 97, 120, 131, 195, 196, 224. *See also* Communities; Orthodox medicine
Cousins, Frederick, 122
Cox, A. B., 269
Cox, Thomas, 107
Cozart, William, 57
Cullen, William, 72
Cunningham, Russell M., 17

Daniel (slave), 174
Darby, John T., 269
Davidson, Richard, 82
Davies, Maria, 135, 137
Davis, J. H., 112
Davis, Thomas, 104
Daybooks, 101–9 passim, 167, 265–66. *See also* Bedside notes; Case narratives
Death, 64, 92, 147, 219, 225–26, 239, 244, 256–57
Dewees, William Potts, 29
Dickson, Samuel H., 21, 27, 80, 82, 160, 223
Diet, 50, 51, 202, 210, 212–13, 231, 285 (n. 11)
Dillinger, Calvin, 125
Disease, 1–2, 4–5, 12, 58, 59–60, 62, 92, 115, 116, 196–99; diagnosis of, 141–49, 179; and diet, 5; and drugs, 149–55; as enemy, 93–94, 147–48, 159–60; and environment,

202; prevention of, 6, 115, 133–34; and race, 49–51, 214–16. *See also* Diseases; Illness

Diseases: bowel complaint, 136; cachexia africana, 50, 215; cancer, 236, 238, 243; cholera, 84, 244, 248; congestion, 49; consumption, 35, 136, 215, 225, 256; death mould, 136; delirium tremens, 38, 160; diphtheria, 46, 148; dropsy, 49, 136, 158; dysentery, 143, 148, 182, 217, 243–44, 247–48; dyspepsia, 206; erysipelas, 135, 161, 174; fevers, 5, 136, 138, 143, 148, 149, 170, 177, 182, 196–99, 204, 210–11; hemorrhoids, 92; hepatitis, 148, 177; indigestion, 136; influenza, 116; lumbago, 148; malaria, 5, 8, 152; marasmus, 215; masturbation, 48; obstruction, 136; opthalmia, 56; phrenzy, 148; piles, 136; plethora, 44; pleurisy, 46, 136, 148; pneumonia, 148, 182, 183, 187, 188, 189, 191; rheumatism, 148; scarlet fever, 135, 136, 157; shingles, 135; smallpox, 248; sore nipples, 136; spasm, 136; syphilis, 143; tonsillitis, 170; trismus nascentium, 215; typhoid, 144, 148, 192, 196–98, 215; typhus, 144, 148; whooping cough, 136; worms, 136. *See also* Disease; Illness

Dissection. *See* Medical education: anatomy

Doctors. *See* Physicians

Dowler, Bennet, 239–42, 243

Drake, Daniel, 17, 18, 21, 36, 37, 38, 43

Drunkenness, 38–39, 86, 206, 207, 241–42

Dudley, Benjamin, 37, 38, 43, 236

Dugas, Louis, 38, 47

Dunlap, George, 109

Dunlap, Mary, 177, 178, 180, 181

Dupuy, Joseph, 157

Dyer, J. S., 233

Dysentery. *See* Diseases: dysentery

Eberle, John, 29, 158

Efferson, Wilson, 101, 103

Efferson, Mrs. Wilson, 101–3

Egan, Frederick, 81

Eldee, Nancy, 180

Eliza (slave), 106

Elliott, Stephen, 36

Ellis, Abner, 107

Ellison, William, 107

Ely, S. Carswell, 95

Evans, Adaline, 117

Eve, Joseph A., 110, 113, 150

Ewing, Fayette, 70

Expectant therapy. *See* Physicians: and "expectant" medicine

"Experience": and community practice, 41, 102, 114, 120, 123, 124, 127–28, 191, 224; and country orthodoxy, 74–75, 97, 144, 149, 196; and medical knowledge, 59, 113, 151, 156, 172, 214, 217, 227, 228, 243, 249–50, 262; as physician's personal achievement, 3, 11, 70, 77, 132, 137, 155, 167. *See also* Country orthodoxy; Orthodox medicine; Physicians

Farrar, S. C., 204, 205

Fenner, Erasmus Darwin, 211, 217, 256

Fever. *See* Diseases: fevers

Flagg, E. Belin, 107, 155

Floyd (slave), 107

Ford, Louis D., 36, 38, 146

Forrest, Nathan Bedford, 261

Frank (slave), 92

Frank (slave), 174–75

Fretwell, James, 139

Galen, 72, 142

Galileo, 72

Galt, William, 146

Geddings, Edward, 45, 48–49

Gender, 5, 9, 28, 44, 49, 51, 53, 105, 106, 112, 115, 154, 161, 170. *See also* Sex (and sexuality); Women

Gibbes, R. T., 207

Gibson, James, 123

Goodlett, A. G., 209

Goodson, Mrs. Jesse W., 182–87, 188, 189, 191

Grant, Daniel, 116

Grant, George, 161

Grant, Leonidas, 198

Green, Fanny, 198

Green, Traill, 53

Gross, Samuel D., 37, 45, 56

Hamilton, Alfred T., 81, 82
Hamilton, J. M., 231
Hannah (slave), 177, 178, 180
Hannah (slave), 233
Harden, John, 205
Harriet (slave), 135
Harrod, Charles, 18
Hawkins, Josiah, 109
Heard, J. J., 206
Heard, J. M., 137
Henderson, Mary, 116, 135, 140–41
Henning, Samuel, 112
Henry (slave), 177, 178, 181
Henry, James, 92
Hentz, Charles A., 17, 19, 29, 34, 37–38, 39,
    56, 65–66, 81, 86, 98, 113, 120, 121, 122,
    147, 170, 176, 182–92, 196, 198, 232
Hippocrates, 72, 142, 207
Hoey, John, 241
Holbrook, J. Edwards, 61
Holcombe, William, 18, 110, 113, 120, 123,
    159, 222
Holley, Horace, 36
Holloway, Thomas, 139
Horses. See Physicians: and horses
Hort, William P., 233
Hosack, Phillip, 72
Hospitals. See Medical education: and clinics
Hundley, James, 92
Hundley, John, 98
Hunt, Thomas, 43

Illness, 1, 4, 6, 12, 19, 30, 77, 91–94, 136–37,
    141, 144–45, 146, 148, 162, 172–74, 180,
    191, 193–95, 219, 233, 236, 245–47. See also
    Disease; Diseases
Isaac (slave), 134
Ivy, Henry, 34, 62

Jackson, Frank, 119
Jacob (slave), 226
James, Frank, 110, 111, 125, 160, 221, 266
Jeffress, Nancy, 140
Jennings, Samuel, 209
Jennings family, 196–97
Jim (slave), 187–91
Jobe, Abraham, 30, 81–82, 88–90

Johns Hopkins University, 250
Johnson, Charles, 34, 35
Johnston, A. B., 137
Jones, Beverley, 137
Jones, Charles Colcock, 64–65
Jones, Francis, 54
Jones, Joseph, 33, 37, 43, 62, 64–65, 81
Jones, Mary Sharpe, 65
Jones, Theresa, 86
Jordan, C. H., 213
Joynes, Levin Smith, 168–69

Kean, M. S., 110
Keitt, J. W., 79
Keller, Thomas, 44
Kentucky School of Medicine, 66
Kilpatrick, Andrew, 169
Kimbrough, Marmaduke, 33, 55
King, Anna, 117
King, Washington, 101, 103
Kinloch, R. A., 269
Knox, John, 38, 47, 107, 121, 124, 176, 177–
    82, 185, 192, 196, 198

Laudanum. See Medicines: laudanum
Laura (slave), 117, 138
Lavender, C. E., 202
Laws, T. L., 54
Lebby, Robert, 28, 71
LeConte, Joseph, 63, 78, 221
Leland, Samuel, 86, 91–92, 113, 120, 123,
    126, 221, 226, 232
Lenah (slave), 105–6
Lewis, Henry Clay, 29, 37, 56, 63, 79, 91
Lexington, Ky. See Medical education; Medi-
    cal schools; Southern places
L'Fayette (slave), 65
Lindsley, John, 222
Little, Robert, 202
Lizzy (slave), 135
Logan, George, 28
Louisiana State Medical Society, 269
Louisville, Ky. See Medical education; Medi-
    cal schools; Southern places
Louisville Medical Institute (University of
    Louisville), 21, 26, 34, 36, 38, 43, 60, 61,
    262, 263

Lucas, Benjamin, 63
Lucy (slave), 106

MacRae, Agnes, 134
Malaria. *See* Diseases: malaria
Manning, J. R., 85
Marine Hospital (Louisville, Ky.), 53, 287
 (n. 20)
Martin, William, 225
Mary Ann (slave), 234
McCaa, William L., 211–12
McCarty, Thomas, 105
McCorkle, Lucila, 117, 135, 138
McGehee, E. L., 57
McKinney, Jeptha, 35, 36, 70, 224
McLure, Lydie, 129
M.D. thesis, 26, 69–74
Means, Alexander, 38
Medical College of Georgia, 21, 23, 35, 36,
 45, 46, 47, 48, 66, 78, 179, 262
Medical College of Louisiana (University of
 Louisiana), 21, 43, 48, 54, 60, 66, 262, 263
Medical College of (the State of) South Car-
 olina, 21, 36, 48, 53, 55, 61, 64, 72, 77, 78,
 262
Medical education: anatomy, 59–68, 78; bot-
 any, 44; and charity, 58–59, 68, 87, 112,
 171; chemistry, 43; and Civil War, 263; and
 clinics, 52–59; and lectures, 42–52; materia medica, 42, 44, 45, 50; and M.D. thesis,
 69–75, 290 (n. 46); obstetrics, 47–48, 53,
 60; pathology, 43, 60, 150; physiology, 43,
 48, 50, 60, 150; and race, 49–52; and the
 South as region, 21–22, 72; surgery, 42, 43,
 53, 55, 56, 59; therapeutics, 60; and urban
 poor, 55–57. *See also* Apprenticeship; Medical schools
Medical procedures: anesthesia, 8, 53, 56,
 238, 255, 263; antisepsis, 8; blistering, 56,
 73, 158, 161, 171, 183, 184, 186, 187, 189,
 193, 194, 195; childbirth, 110, 170–71;
 cupping, 161, 187, 188, 226; enema, 44,
 160, 186, 194; mustard bath, 161; ovariotomy, 55; purging, 160; sinapism, 231;
 tooth pulling, 108; tracheotomy, 46; vaccination, 152, venesection (bloodletting),
 53, 56, 73, 112, 157, 161

Medical profession, 3, 7, 9, 11, 16, 80, 227,
 257; and case narratives, 229–30, 232,
 234, 246, 249; and city life, 32–39; and
 clergy, 219–20, 255; and M.D. thesis, 69–
 70; and medical schools, 18, 22–23, 27, 36,
 37, 76–77; and religious faith, 220–21,
 255; and rural practice, 82, 88, 90, 113,
 122
Medical schools: and apprenticeship, 16, 27–
 31; after Civil War, 262–63; course of
 study in, 23–24; curriculum of, 20, 24–25,
 39, 42, 47, 49, 51; and graduation, 77–78;
 and intellectual life, 18, 20, 21, 22; as male
 world, 16, 26, 32–39, 54, 57–58, 77–78,
 82, 96; as urban institutions, 15, 21, 22–23,
 32–39, 52–53, 80–81. *See also* Medical
 education
Medical students: and city life, 32–39; and
 compassion, 57–58; deciding to study
 medicine, 16–19; and disease, 35; and
 manhood, 73–74; and medical history, 71–
 72; and teachers, 36–39, 58. *See also*
 Apprenticeship; Medical education
Medicine. *See* Country orthodoxy; Medical
 education; Medical schools; Orthodox
 medicine; Physicians
Medicines, 104, 133–34, 149–55, 156–58,
 302 (n. 4); asclepias root, 185; ale, 151;
 alum, 46; ammonia, 161; asafetida, 133;
 bacon fat, 157; bark tea, 181; bay rum, 157;
 beef broth, 161; blue pill, 177, 181; boneset tea, 183; brandy, 177, 181, 184, 186,
 189, 190, 191; caffeine, 160; calomel, 133,
 138, 157, 161, 177, 181, 183, 184, 187, 188,
 189, 203, 231, 243, 259; camphor, 133, 134,
 156, 181, 193; castor oil, 156, 161, 181,
 203; charcoal, 177, 181; chicken tea, 184,
 186; chloride potassium, 191; cinchona
 bark, 133; cod liver oil, 157, 256; coffee,
 184; cohosh, 184, 185; cologne, 157, 177,
 181; Cook's pills, 34, 157, 193; copaiba,
 177; cream of tartar, 134; croton oil, 190;
 digitalis, 152, 156; Dover's powder, 177;
 elixer of vitriol, 184, 186; epsom salts, 157;
 ergot, 156; flaxseed tea, 189; glycerine,
 134; Grave's tartar emetic, 189; gum water,
 183, 193; hellebore, 156; "heroic," 152–54;

hive syrup, 189; hydrargyrus cum creta, 184, 189; ipecac, 158, 243; iron, 151; laudanum, 156, 181, 189; lime water, 155; liverwort, 256; magnesia, 137; morphine, 152, 157, 160, 169, 193; muriatic morphine, 184; mustard poultice, 194; nitro muriatic acid, 46; opium, 152, 158, 161, 193, 231, 255, 267; pancakes, 157; Pancoast's pills, 157; paragoric, 134; poke root, 156; porter, 151; potassium chloride, 191; quinine, 133, 152, 155, 156, 177, 181, 184, 186, 203; red oak bark, 181; rose water, 157; sarsaparilla, 168; sassafras, 156, 181; scillae confection syrup, 183–89; Seidlitz powder, 177; seneka, 184, 185; silver nitrate, 46; snakeroot, 181; sugar of lead, 134; Swain's panacea, 112; sweet oil, 155, 157; tan, 256; tannin, 46; tobacco, 158; Tulley's powder, 177; turpentine, 155, 156, 161, 190; veratrum viride, 156, 161, 177, 183, 184, 186, 187, 188; water (and/or ice), 157, 160, 189, 244–45, 247–48; whiskey, 101, 134, 241, 255; wine, 151; wine whey, 184, 185, 186, 190, 191; Wright's pills, 177

Mettauer, John P., 139–40
Middleton, Eweretta, 225
Miller, William, 62
Milligan, J. A. S., 85, 126
Milligan, James, 86, 128, 130, 226
Mobley, Mary, 107
Mobley, W. W., 261
Montgomery, Robert, 28
Moody, William, 89–90
Moore, Fannie, 134
Moore, H. W., 213
Morality: and local practice, 12, 59, 68, 69, 78, 87, 92, 96–97, 102, 111, 113, 127–28, 132, 149, 150, 195, 227, 228, 231–32, 234, 239; and orthodox principles, 38, 41, 42, 45, 54, 57–58, 89, 207, 218, 253, 257; and physicians' personal character, 11, 64–65, 72–73, 79, 83, 155, 162, 242, 263
Mordecai, Solomon, 57, 63
Morphine. See Medicines: morphine
Moses (slave), 105–6
Muller, Gerhard, 110

Muller, Louisa, 135
Musser, Benjamin, 147

Nabors, Nancy, 198
Nashville, Tenn. See Medical education; Medical schools; Southern places
Nature, 19, 35, 43–44, 69, 71, 118, 120, 150, 157, 221, 222, 223
Neal, James, 139
New Orleans, La. See Medical education; Medical schools; Southern places
Nott, Josiah, 129–30, 209, 240

Obstetrics. See Medical education: obstetrics
Opium. See Medicines: opium
Orthodox medicine: as ideology, 2, 9, 11, 41, 43, 54, 61, 70–71, 127–28, 176, 250; and knowledge, 20, 26, 37, 38, 39–40, 57, 69, 207, 243; and practice, 8, 36, 91, 155, 187, 192, 196, 228, 257; and southern communities, 84–85, 97, 103, 149; and vernacular medicine, 2, 49, 75, 76, 124–25, 238, 168. See also Country orthodoxy
Osler, Sir William, 250–55

Palmetto Sharp Shooters, 261
Paracelsus, 72
Parramore, John, 168–69
Patients, 12, 19, 27, 29, 30, 46, 52–53, 54, 56, 58, 72, 129–30, 268; in case narratives, 232–34; co-attendance and conflict with, 168–75, 180, 188–91, 192, 195, 233–34, 247–48; in daybooks, 105–7, 265–66; and debt, 110–12; as the "first patient," 91–92; and health talk, 114–19, 168; and religious faith, 224–25, 238; on rounds, 124–26; summoning the physician, 137–41. See also Caregiving: in homes; Orthodox medicine: and vernacular medicine
Patteson, A. A., 236–39, 243
Peggy (slave), 107
Peterson, Mary, 110
Phebe (slave), 177, 178
Philadelphia, Pa., 72, 278 (n. 11)
Physicians: and anecdotes, 47, 124; and bedside practice, 24, 47, 50, 52, 57, 73, 94, 132, 141–51, 156–59, 162–63, 175–99, 246–

47; and co-attendance and conflict with
patients, 163, 167–75, 180, 185, 187, 190,
192, 194, 233–34, 247–48; and diagnosis,
59, 131–32, 141–49, 181, 185, 198, 220,
231, 256, 304 (n. 19); and drugs, 149–55,
182–95 passim; and "expectant" medicine,
43–44, 87, 93, 118, 150–51, 191, 193, 197,
203, 236–37, 239, 253, 267; and horses,
120–21; income of, 10, 82–83, 85, 101–2,
108–13; and intellect, 18, 25, 34–35, 42,
70, 74, 79, 86, 95–96, 192, 196–98, 200–
201, 207, 214, 218–19, 230, 232, 235; and
licensing, 9–10; and modernity, 2–3, 7, 20,
26, 69, 76, 127, 130, 132, 145, 148, 156,
168, 176, 192, 200, 203, 230, 232, 250, 251,
257, 260; numbers of, 8–9; and other
healers, 88–89, 122–23, 252–53; and religion, 45, 60, 64–65, 78, 85, 201, 218–27,
236, 245–46, 254–56; and rounds, 30, 47,
102, 119–27, 196, 220, 240; and rural life,
81, 85–87, 95, 112, 128–29, 260–62, 268;
and science, 8, 11, 19, 32, 39, 51, 57, 59–
60, 62, 63, 71, 132, 141, 148, 162, 191, 196,
200–201, 219, 239–40, 249; and subjectivity, 2–3, 40, 41–42, 74–75, 93–94, 104,
127–28, 143–44, 155, 162, 173, 192, 195,
198, 202, 227, 232, 243, 270; and surgery, 8,
9, 42, 56, 253, 263; and written texts, 3,
69–75, 101–9, 167–76, 200–201, 228–29.
See also Country orthodoxy; "Experience";
Morality; Orthodox medicine
Physick, Phillip Syng, 72
Polly (slave), 140–41
Pope, F. Perry, 50
Porcher, Francis Peyre, 45, 92, 96, 151, 267
Porcher, Walter, 37, 77
Posey, John F., 204
Powell, Gaston, 89
Powell, Joe, 89
Powell, Thomas S., 223
Pressly, S. H., 265
Price, Sallie, 133
Pricy (slave), 139
Prioleau, J. Ford, 36
Pusey, Robert B., 112, 169

Quinine. *See* Medicines: quinine

Race, 5, 9, 42, 49–52, 53, 55, 240; and bed-
side therapy, 170, 172–73, 187–89; in
daybooks, 105–7, 265; and diagnosis, 144–
45; as factor in disease, 208–18, 266–67;
and health talk, 117–18. *See also* African
Americans; Slaves (and slavery)
Ramsay, Frank, 264
Ramsay, Henry A., 230
Randolph Macon Medical College, 44
Ravenel, Henry, 121
Reed, Rachel Santee, 118
Reedy, J. A., 121, 124, 159
Reedy, William, 85, 121, 125
Reese, W. P., 171
Reynolds, Mark, 264–65
Richardson, John M., 29, 30, 91, 226
Riddell, James, 66
Robinson, John, 33, 39, 85, 111, 221
Roper Hospital (Charleston, S.C.), 53, 54,
287 (n. 20)
Rosenberg, Charles E., 260
Rouanet, M., 171
Rush, Benjamin, 18, 72
Ryland, Robert, 110, 112

Sally (slave), 140
Sam (slave), 147
Scruggs, R. L., 148
Sectarians. *See* Alternative healers
Sex (and sexuality), 33, 42, 47–49, 51–52, 63,
125–26, 213. *See also* Gender; Women
Shackleford, M. A., 70
Shands, W. A., 233
Sharpe, W. R., 146
Shaw, Samuel, 111
Shelton, Virginia, 117
Shenk, Louis, 101
Short, Charles, 44
Sickness. *See* Disease
Siewers, Nathaniel, 56, 65
Simmons, Smith, 119
Sims, J. Marion, 16, 17, 86, 88, 92–93, 222
Skipwith, Lucy, 117–18
Slaves (and slavery), 5, 30, 49–51, 54–55, 81,
87, 138–39, 155, 172, 201, 240–41, 265;
and abuse, 126–27, 213; and anatomical
dissection, 60; in bedside notes, 178; in

case narratives, 234–35, 254; in daybooks, 105–7; and health talk, 117–18; in medical topographies, 208–18; and therapies, 134–35, 170, 173–74, 188–89. *See also* African Americans; Patients; Race

Smedes, Susan, 135

Smith, Albert, 70

Smith, Bat, 266

Smith, J. E., 144, 169

Smith, James Strudwick, 137

Smith, James T., 217

Social class, 52–53, 56, 58, 78, 85–86, 87, 170, 172, 215, 232

Sophy (slave), 117

South, 21, 200, 202; as locus of disease, 4–5, 47, 54, 133, 210, 264; as a place to practice, 72–73, 81, 84–86, 95, 122, 128, 240, 250–52; and social context for health, 203, 205–7; and supply of cadavers, 60. *See also* Southern places

Southall, Philip, 109

Southern places: Abbeville Dist., S.C., 111, 203; Accomack Co., Va., 168; Americus, Ga., 260; Atlanta, Ga., 32; Augusta, Ga., 21; Baltimore, Md., 9, 250; Cahaba, Ala., 205; Carroll Co., Miss., 82; Charleston, S.C., 9, 21, 33, 34, 36, 53, 263, 267; Chester Dist., S.C., 176, 261; Columbia, S.C., 64; DeSoto Parish, La., 207; Due West, S.C., 85; Elizabethton, Tenn., 89; Elizabethtown, Ky., 169; Franklin Co., N.C., 104; Hanover Co., Va., 158; Harmony Grove, Ga., 85; Huntsville, Ala., 207, 250, 252, 261; Jackson, Miss., 204; Jacksonville, Ala., 176, 192; Knoxville, Tenn., 264; Lancaster Dist., S.C., 109; Lexington, Ky., 21; Liberty Co., Ga., 205; Louisville, Ky., 21, 53, 65; Lowndesboro, Ala., 202; Madison Co., Ala., 203; Manning's Roads, S.C., 85; Memphis, Tenn., 264; Mill Creek, S.C., 86; Mt. Meigs, Ala., 86; Murfreesboro, Tenn., 174, 243, 246; Nashville, Tenn., 21, 34; Natchez, Miss., 215; New Orleans, La., 9, 21, 32, 215, 241, 263; Orrville, Ala., 267; Osyka, Miss., 85; Prince Edward Co., Va., 139; Quincy, Fla., 176; Raysville, Ga., 230; Rome, Ga., 264; St. Charles, Mo., 83–84;

St. Louis, Mo., 83; Selma, Ala., 202; Simpson Co., Ky., 203, 210; Springfield, La., 101, 111; Statesburg, S.C., 264; Warren Co., Ky., 205; Washington, Tex., 206

Spann, James, 109

Spragins, Fayette, 32

Starr, Paul, 2

Steifer, G. F., 111

Sterrett, James, 223

Still, James, 19

Stone, Henry, 170

Stone, Warren, 46–47

Stout, Oliver, 77

Strait, Lafayette, 16, 18, 68–70, 261

Suddarth, J. B., 203, 210

Surgery. *See* Medical education: surgery

Sydenham, Thomas, 72

Taft, Willard, 79

Taylor, Thomas, 168–69

Taylor, Zachary, 110

Tennent, Gilbert, 203

Tensas, Madison. *See* Lewis, Henry Clay

Therapy. *See* Medical procedures; Medicines; Orthodox medicine

Thomas, Gertrude, 174

Thomason, E. W., 128–29

Thompson, Victoria, 134

Timmerman, W. H., 61

Transylvania Medical College, 21, 36, 38, 53, 70, 77, 79, 236

Trezevant, James D., 110

Turner, William, 159

Twain, Mark, 48

Tynes, W. E., 85

University of Nashville Medical School, 21, 25, 26, 60, 62, 70, 79, 262

University of Pennsylvania, 64, 278 (n. 11)

Van Bibber, W. Chew, 160–61

Van Wyck, Samuel, 76, 82, 261–62

Vaughn, William, 123

Wade, John, 174

Wade, Thomas, 30–31, 32, 33, 35, 38, 63

Walthall, J. E., 36

Ward, B. F., 268
Warner, John Harley, 259
Washington Medical College, 250
Weeden, Frederick, 122
Weeks, David, 112
Weever, Richard, 198
Whetstone, William, 29, 30, 53, 64, 81, 85
White, Mrs., 192–95, 197
Williams, Lizzie, 118
Winn, David, 260–61
Winn, Frances, 260
Women: as domestic caregivers, 6, 46–47; as physicians, 9; poor, in clinics, 55–56; pregnancy and childbirth, 5, 55, 103, 170–71, 210–11, 232, 254–55; and sexuality, 48–

49. *See also* Caregiving: in homes; Gender; Patients; Sex (and sexuality)
Wood, George, 256–57
Woodruff, Milford, 39
Wooten, H. V., 202, 217, 234
Wright, William C., 70, 113
Wylie, William, 18

Yandell, David W., 263–64
Yandell, Lunsford P., 17, 18, 19, 35, 38, 52, 79, 220, 225, 243–49
Yandell, Susan, 244–49
Yandell, Willie, 244–49
Yandell, Wilson, 77, 79, 123, 125, 126, 171, 174

STUDIES IN SOCIAL MEDICINE

NANCY M. P. KING, GAIL E. HENDERSON, AND JANE STEIN, EDS.,
Beyond Regulations: Ethics in Human Subjects Research (1999).

LAURIE ZOLOTH, *Health Care and the Ethics of Encounter:
A Jewish Discussion of Social Justice* (1999).

SUSAN M. REVERBY, ED., *Tuskegee's Truths:
Rethinking the Tuskegee Syphilis Study* (2000).

BEATRIX HOFFMAN, *The Wages of Sickness:
The Politics of Health Insurance in Progressive America* (2000).

MARGARETE SANDELOWSKI, *Devices and Desires:
Gender, Technology, and American Nursing* (2000).

KEITH WAILOO, *Dying in the City of the Blues:
Sickle Cell Anemia and the Politics of Race and Health* (2001).

JUDITH ANDRE, *Bioethics as Practice* (2002).

CHRIS FEUDTNER, *Bittersweet: Diabetes, Insulin,
and the Transformation of Illness* (2003).

ANN FOLWELL STANFORD, *Bodies in a Broken World:
Women Novelists of Color and the Politics of Medicine* (2003).

LAWRENCE O. GOSTIN, *The AIDS Pandemic:
Complacency, Injustice, and Unfulfilled Expectations* (2004).

ARTHUR A. DAEMMRICH, *Pharmacopolitics:
Drug Regulation in the United States and Germany* (2004).

CARL ELLIOTT AND TOD CHAMBERS, EDS.,
Prozac as a Way of Life (2004).

STEVEN M. STOWE, *Doctoring the South: Southern Physicians and
Everyday Medicine in the Mid-Nineteenth Century* (2004).

ML   6/05